LECTURES ON MATERIA MEDICA

BY
CARROLL DUNHAM, M. D.
AUTHOR OF "HOMŒOPATHY THE SCIENCE OF THERAPEUTICS," ETC.

FIFTH EDITION

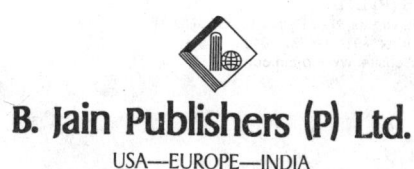

B. Jain Publishers (P) Ltd.
USA—EUROPE—INDIA

LECTURES ON MATERIA MEDICA
7th Impression: 2014

NOTE FROM THE PUBLISHERS
Any information given in this book is not intended to be taken as a replacement for medical advice. Any person with a condition requiring medical attention should consult a qualified practitioner or therapist.

All rights reserved. No part of this book may be reproduced, stored in a retrieval system or transmitted, in any form or by any means, mechanical, photocopying, recording or otherwise, without any prior written permission of the publisher.

© with the publisher

Published by Kuldeep Jain for
B. JAIN PUBLISHERS (P) LTD.
1921/10, Chuna Mandi, Paharganj, New Delhi 110 055 (INDIA)
Tel.: +91-11-4567 1000   Fax: +91-11-4567 1010
Email: info@bjain.com   Website: **www.bjain.com**

Printed in India by
JJ Imprints Pvt. Ltd.

ISBN: 978-81-319-0728-3

CONTENTS.
(VOL. I)

		PAGE.
PREFACE	. . . .	v
MEMOIR OF THE AUTHOR, BY E. M. KELLOGG, M. D.		vii
I.	MATERIA MEDICA AND THERAPEUTICS .	1
II.	STUDY OF MATERIA MEDICA . . .	19
III.	THE THERAPEUTIC LAW	39
IV.	PRELIMINARY OBSERVATIONS . . .	61
V.	ACONITUM NAPELLUS	66
VI.	BRYONIA ALBA	89
VII.	EUPATORIUM	115
VIII.	RHUS TOXICODENDRON	121
IX.	COLCHICUM	157
X.	LEDUM PALUSTRE	173
XI.	RHODODENDRON CHRYSANTHUM . .	182
XII.	KALMIA LATIFOLIA	187
XIII.	SPIGELIA ANTHELMIA	196
XIV.	ARTOPA BELLADONNA	213
XV.	HYOSCYAMUS NIGER	278
XVI.	DATURA STRAMONIUM	288
XVII.	OPIUM	301
XVIII.	HELLEBORUS NIGER	311
XIX.	SILICEA	316
XX.	STRYCHNOS NUX VOMICA	349
XXI.	ALOES	366
XXII.	SULPHUR	381
XXIII.	GRAPHITES	393
XXIV.	LACHESIS	401

CONTENTS.
(VOL. II)

		PAGE.
I.	PRINCIPLES OF HOMŒOPATHY—PRINCIPLES *vs.* PRACTICAL KNOWLEDGE	1
II.	SYMPTOMS, THEIR STUDY; OR "HOW TO TAKE THE CASE"	25
III.	THE ANAMNESIS	49
IV.	PULSATILLA	57
V.	CYCLAMEN EUROPÆUM	80
VI.	EUPHRASIA OFFICINALIS	98
VII.	ALLIUM CEPA	105
VIII.	MATRICARIA CHAMOMILLA	108
IX.	IGNATIA AMARA	122
X.	PLATINA	129
XI.	SEPIA	138
XII.	MUREX PURPUREA	158
XIII.	KREASOTUM	164
XIV.	SECALE CORNUTUM	169
XV.	JUNIPERUS SABINA	175
XVI.	ACHILLÆA MILLEFOLIUM	177
XVII.	ARSENICUM ALBUM	178
XVIII.	HYDRARGYRUM	208
XIX.	CUCUMIS COLOCYNTHIS	231
XX.	PODOPHYLLUM PELTATUM	239
XXI.	LACHESIS	243
XXII.	LYCOPODIUM CLAVATUM	256

CONTENTS.

		PAGE.
XXIII.	Natrum Muriaticum	266
XXIV.	Veratrum Alrum	272
XXV.	Hepar Sulphuris Calcareum	280
XXVI.	Dulcamara	287
XXVII.	Calcarea Carbonica	307
XXVIII.	Causticum	317
XXIX.	Nitric Acid	320
XXX.	Carbo Vegetabilis	325
XXXI.	Carbo Animalis	332
XXXII.	Apium Virus	333
XXXIII.	Phosphorus	338
XXXIV.	Cocculus Indicus	346
XXXV.	Conium Maculatum	362
XXXVI.	Cina	367
XXXVII.	The Art and Mode of Prescribing	386
XXXVIII.	Pathognomonic Symptoms and Characteristic Symptoms	392
XXXIX.	Valedictory Address	402

INTRODUCTORY.

"SEVERAL Editions" speak more conveniently in praise of a book than any words reviewer or publishers could utter. Dr. Caroll Dunham, after graduating himself from the Columbia College, New York, made the aquaintance of Dr. Constantine Hering, one of the greatest physicians ever born, who became too helpful to him as well as generous and genial friend. In the meantime he continued his study under Dr. Boenninghausen with a desire to know every thing within the enclosure of the school of Homœopathy. Subsequently he gratified himself with Doctorate from College of Physicians and Surgeons of New York.

But did he stop there? No. He wanted to drink the cup of knowledge upto its last drop. He began to study under many of the Great Physicians and Specialists of Europe for Years. And then when he was convinced that the knowledge of Homœopathy was already well known to him he returned to his homeland and began practicing Homœopathy.

The fruit of all these toil and effort, study and research came, Dr. Dunham rapidly rose and became one of the leaders of the Great school of Homœopathy.

Dr. Dunham delivered his knowledge in his book "Lectures on Materia Medica," an immortal part of Homœopathic literature, an indispensable library aid to the practicing Homœopathic practitioners. The personality of the author croped out every where. We beg to convey our sincere thanks to our friends for their kind co-operations and active help in bringing out this new edition. We believe, our efforts will meet with success.

PUBLISHERS.

PREFACE.

THE lectures contained in these volumes were delivered by Dr. Dunham while he occupied the chair of Materia Medica in the New-York Homœopathic Medical College.

They have been edited from his note-books, practically verbatim, and are the ripe fruit of his thought and experience,—in his own latest words, "too valuable to be lost."

His wife, now also deceased, made arrangements for their publication, hoping thereby to render his labors more available to the profession, and thus promote a chief object of his life,—the benefit of his fellow-men through the development and dissemination of a rational and scientific Therapeutics.

MEMOIR OF THE AUTHOR.

"His life was gentle; and the elements
So mixed in him, that Nature might stand up
And say to all the world—THIS WAS A MAN!"

THE memory of this great and good man is enshrined in the work he accomplished on earth, as well as in the hearts of all who came within the circle of his wise and helpful benevolence.

"Si monumentum quæris, circumspice!" Although no words can enrich such a record, they may serve, even in a fragmentary review, to present the leading traits of this noble life with sufficient distinctness for profitable study.

Carroll Dunham was the youngest of four sons of Edward Wood Dunham and Maria Smyth Parker, and was born in the city of New-York, October 29, 1828. The families of both parents were old and prominent residents of New Brunswick, in the State of New Jersey. Mr. Dunham was for many years a successful merchant, and was distinguished for his intelligence, energy, probity and methodical habits of business. About the year 1820 he removed with his family from New Brunswick to New York, and in 1853 he retired from business with an ample fortune, honorably acquired. He soon afterward became president of the Corn Exchange Bank, which position he retained until his death. His wife was a lady whose character happily combined gentleness with prudence and firmness; qualities which her son Carroll seems to have inherited along with the business aptitude, energy and uprightness of his father. Mrs. Dunham died during the cholera epidemic of 1832, when Carroll was but four years old.

Those who remember Carroll Dunham as a boy, speak of him as remarkably docile, bright and cheerful, and considerate of the feelings of others. His general health was good, but he usually avoided the rough sports of his companions. "He was always," says one of his elder brothers, "looking into things, with an eager desire to know all about their qualities and uses." As as youth he was affectionate, truthful and energetic, more fond of books than play; and even at that time, his demeanor, toward his fellows was marked by that same modest reserve—far removed from timidity—which was a prominent characteristic throughout his whole life.

He entered Columbia College in 1843, and graduated with honor in 1847. Immediately afterward, he commenced the study of medicine under Dr. Whittaker, an old-school practitioner, very capable, and at that time of high repute as a trainer of students. In 1850 he received his degree of M. D. from the College of Physicians and Surgeons of New-York, then located in Crosby street. His previous mental training, as well as his greater natural ability, enabled him, during his student life, to outstrip his fellows; and the cheerful readiness and patience with which he smoothed the difficulties of those who sought his aid soon drew around him a select number of followers, to whom he explained, in his own way, the lectures of the day.

About this period of his life, Carroll was cured of a dangerous illness by a homœopathic physician, after eminent practitioners of the "regular" school had failed. This circumstance made a deep impression upon both father and son, and led the latter to investigate the principles of homœopathy, and to institute comparisons between the old and new methods of treatment. In furtherance of this inquiry, after completing his college studies, he went to Philadelphia to seek the acquaintance of Dr. Constanitine Hering, as one of the most learned physicians of the new school; and not only profited largely by his teachings and advice, but (to use his own words) "I gained the most helpful, generous and genial friend I have ever made."

It was the wise desire of both his father and himself that his preparation for the arduous duties of his profession should be as complete as possible. After graduating, therefore, instead of beginning to practice, he sailed for Europe, to glean a further harvest of observation and study in foreign hospitals, and from the leaders of medical and surgical science abroad. In Dublin, he served as an "interne" in the Lying-in-Hospital; he also investigated the Stokes treatment of fevers in Meath Hospital. While in Dublin he received a dissecting-wound, which nearly ended his career; but, after the resident physicians had given him up to die, he called homœopathy to his aid, and cured himself with Lachesis.

From Dublin, Dr, Dunham went to Paris, where he studid specialties under such instructors as Bouillard, Velpeau, Trousseau, Ricord, Simon, Heurteloup, and others, while he also regularly visited the Homœopathic Hospital under the charge of Tessier. From Paris he went to Berlin, and thence, after a brief stay, to Vienna, where he remained several months, attending the hospital cliniques of Wurmb, and the lectures of Kaspar on Materia Medica. From Vienna he directed his course to Münster, to visit Bœnninghausen, who received the young physician with cordiality, and very soon learned to appreciate his tireless industry and active intelligence, and prophesied for him a brilliant future. Here the eager student remained long enough to watch numerous cases treated by Bœnninghausen, and to become thoroughly familiar with the methods of examining and prescribing for patients practised by that distinguished German.

Having thus liberally availed himself of the advantages of foreign culture, Dr. Dunham turned his steps homeward. During the whole period of his absence he was in close correspondence with his father, between whom and himself there existed a rare degree of affection and confidence. I had been his practice from his boyhood, when absent from home, to correspond almost daily with his father, and thus he acquired the habit of clear and terse expression, which is characteristic of all his writings., At a later period, his most elaborate articles were rarely re-written, so effectual was his early training in intellectual work. It is worthy of remark, that wherever the young physician tarried for a season in his travels, he was sure to make warm and constant friends, with many of whom, eminent in the homœopathic world, he kept up a life-long correspondence.

On his return to America, he began practice in Brooklyn; and at the very outset, so marked were his ability and success, that Dr. P. P. Wells, who had been an esteemed friend, as well as the physician, of the Dunham family for many years, says of Carroll: "He was always my friend, never my pupil." In February, 1854, Dr. Dunham married Miss Harriet E. Kellogg, daughter of Edward and Esther F. Kellogg,—a woman of rare personal beauty and highly endowed mind. From this union resulted many years of domestic happiness, a helpful companionship and co-operation in his arduous labors,. and the prolongation of his useful life through her tender watchfulness and devotion. So thoroughly were their two lives intertwined and identified, that they repeatedly told their children—as if to prepare them for the future— that should one parent die, they must expect the other soon to follow,—a prediction which was literally fulfilled, as in less than a year after Dr. Dnham's death, his wife was laid by his side in Greenwood. Her sad, brief widowhood was spent in an an attempt to continue his life-labors by collecting and publishing in book-form his numerous, but scattered, contributions to medical science.

In the year 1858, a severe attack of illness necessitated a removal from Brooklyn, and he took up his residence at Newburgh, N. Y. In this removal he sought rest of mind as well as of body, and it was not his intention to resume practice until fully restored; but the remarkable success which attended his prescriptions in one or two cases which were pressed upon him with an urgency not to be denied, brought other claimants to his door; and thus, in spite of the delicate state of his health, he soon became professionally busy. After residing in Newburgh about six years, his health again gave way under an attack of cardiac rheumatism, and he removed for a short time to New-York. While there he had the assurance of leading specialists of the old school, whose prognosis was invited, that he could not long survive. Upon this he sought the advice of Dr. Hering who, after a careful and exhaustive examination of the symptoms, prescribed a single remedy (Lithium carbonicum), which promptly conquered the disease. His own case thus, more than once, forcibly illustrated the soundness of the medical rule which he so often advocated, "a single remedy, and if possible, a single dose." Soon after, he moved his residence to Irvington-on-Hudson, which he made his home, for the most part, until his death, having, however, an office and consulting practice in New-York to which he attended upon certain days in the week.

During the whole of his active professional career, his health often gave way under the strain he put upon it, and he was several times compelled to seek to change of scene and climate. He visited Europe thrice in the pursuit of health; also, Nassau and other foreign resorts; but no suffering or sickness could prevent his active mind from utilizing his travels in the acquisition of knowledge, or blunt his zeal in the promotion of medical interests. During his last visit to Europe, though so weak and worn as to contemplate an unusually long absence, he exerted himself successfully to secure the good-will and co-operation of foreign physicians in his project of a "World's Homœopathic Convention."

The confidence in his ability to manage this scheme and carry it to a successful issue was so general among his colleagues, that our National Society conferred on him plenary power to arrange its details and to choose his associate workers. And in 1875, as has been truthfully said, "Our National Institute honored itself by electing him President for 1876, when the fruit of his special labor should be fully ripe." How efficiently he performed the duties of that office, and with what dignity, courtesy and fine tact he presided over that convention, few who were present will ever forget. A detailed history of that convention would show that in planning, arranging and executing his plans, he performed an amount of labor which few men could have borne. On April 27, 1876, he thus wrote to a professional friend: "The responses of our friends from abroad are very gratifying. Two years ago I had not much confidence; but when I found that the thing was to be, I determined that it should be a success." And this letter contained a list of foreign communications aggregating one thousand four hundred and fifty-six pages of large paper, and in half a dozen different languages. More came in May and the first week of June, from foreign and home contributors, presenting a mass of manuscript to be translated, abridged, corrected and put through the press, before which a literary Hercules might have stood appalled. This work was done by him or under his personal supervision; every article was carefully re-read by him, and the proofs were finally corrected by his pen; and all this material was collected by him through a voluminous correspondence. In addition, he assumed the care of the general arrangements for the sessions of the convention in Philadephia. "Of ocourse," he wrote at this time to a friend, "I have convention on the brain. I eat, sleep and live it; and have put some of my best blood into it;" adding words which now have a peculiar pathos, "but hope to have some left, when all is over."

During the sessions of the convention in the latter part of June, 1876, the heat was extreme, being often not less than 100° Fahr. in the shade; but he clung to his post, though in daily danger of utter prostration, performing all his duties to the end. He left Philadelphia, exhausted by his labors, and took a trip to the Upper Lakes from which he returned so much improved that he thought himself strong enough for the remaining work of the convention. But he was immediately stricken down by a severe attack of diphtheria, from which, in his enfeebled condition, he convalesced slowly. He resumed his labors too soon; but in the presence of duties unfulfilled, it was simply impossible for him to be idle. On June 19th he had written to a friend: "I am better, but not yet in working order. I hope to be in New-work on Wednesday, however, and to be fit for work next week". The central desire in his mind, the one thing to strive for, was "to be fit for work." On September 11, while confined to his bed at Irvington, he dictated to a friend at his bedside clear and definite instructions concerning the revisal of some manuscripts for the Centennial volume, and, nine days after, writes: "I am convalescent, but miserably feeble. It seems as if I never should feel strong again. I sit up part of the day." Again, on October 6th: "Strength comes slowly, but it comes."

He took to his bed, for the last time, on December 2d, 1876, where he lingered, under the devoted care of his family, and his physicians Drs. Wells and Joslin, until February 18th following, when he passed peacefully to his rest, in his 49th year. "Though his death," says Dr. Joslin, "was obviously caused by exhausted vitality, consequent on his labors in connection with the Worlds's Homœopathic Convention, and though the nervous system must be looked upon as the main seat of trouble, still the mind remained clear to the last, and was never clouded during any period of his illness. His old friend and physician, Dr. Wells, who attended Dr. Dunham with me, remarked to me that he died of no disease, but from exhaustion produced by excessive and protracted labor. He had a certain irritating cough, originating apparently in a small spot in the larger bronchi, and relieved after a time by the expectoration of a small quantity of tough mucus. This was an annoyance, but could not be said to have had much influence on his decline. An irregular fever was present, evidently varying with every slight strain on his nervous system. His kidneys showed evidence of acute disease for several weeks, but this difficulty seemed to be passing off before his death. His old enemy, rheumatism, appeared in slight degree several times during his last illness. He had for many years been a sufferer from valvular disease of the heart; but this was apparently rather improved than otherwise. He said he had kept watch over his heart with a flexible stethoscope, and was confident that no hypertrophy had taken place, which he attributed to the fact of his always being careful to keep well nourished, contrary, as he remarked, to some advice he had received."

In a private letter, written to correct some misapprehensions about his last illness, his wife writes thus: "A mind so acute as Dr. Dunham's could not have death approach his body and be unaware of it. Neither could a mind so exalted fail to submit tranquilly to an inevitable fate, from which the spirituality of his life took away all fear. He passed as from one phase of life to another of equal or greater activity; from one room in his Father's house to another. He said: 'I do not see my way through this illness;' and at the end of the seventh week, a month before he died, he said with perfect tranquillity; 'I shall go on in this way two weeks longer, and then I shall slip into my grave.' And again: 'I shall go on in this way through the ninth week, and then I shall go to Greenwood.' Any one who knew the correctness of his professional prophecy, must, after these remarks, have struggled against conviction, to have any hope of his recovery. * * * He complained of no pain; but from the beginning of his confinement, he constantly spoke of being 'perfectly wretched,' he could not tell how; but he never showed, as in former illnesses, any vigor underneath. * * * About five days before the last morning, I noticed a change in his complexion, and this deepened and became more permanent every day until the last moment. Up to that time he had wished the room cool; from that time he frequently asked if it was warm enough. Sunday morning, about eight o'clock, he asked the temperature. When told that it was between 69° and 70°, he said: 'There is an unfriendly feeling in the air; you had better light the fire.' He lay and looked into the flame, saying: 'That is very pleasant;' and he watched us feed the flame, and seemed to enjoy the cheery influence, speaking now and then. And so he passed away a little before nine o'clock, without any struggle. He peacefully ceased to breathe."

In some characters, opposing principles contend with varying fortune for mastery, and thus produce a complexity of contradictory phenomena, very difficulty of analysis. It is not easy, out of such conflicting elements, to form a just judgment of the man they constitute. But the character of Carroll Dunham was like a clear crystal, many-sided, indeed, but transparent throughout; and his whole life was so harmonious, his consecration of himself to a noble ideal of duty so evident, that the friend of a few weeks and the friend of a life-time would form, essentially, the same judgment of him; differing only in the degree in which they would comprehend and revere the rare nobility of his nature.

Dr. Dunham was a voluminous writer, though he never concentrated his energies on the production of a single large work. He began to contribute articles to the medical journals when in Europe in 1852, and continued to do steadily for twenty-five years, until death ended his labors. He devoted his efforts principally to the elaboration and perfection of the materia medica; though many of his writings are of a miscellaneous character, being reports, reviews, clinical cases, public addresses, lectures, monographs and translations; the most notable of the last being Bœnninghausen's work on whooping-cough. But these productions of his pen are not to be classed among the lighter or more ephemeral growths of medical literature. His faculty of giving his best powers to whatever he found to do, great or small, confers a permanent value on all that he wrote. He touched no subject without revealing something new and instructive, while the confidence he inspires in his statements, the judicial impartiality with which he treats matters in debate, and the lucid and manly language which he employs, give a rare zest to his compositions. There was no flaw in the fabric of his thought. He never said an unkind word or a silly one; and his opponents (he had no enemies) always admitted that his criticisms were just and manly. Every utterance of his was as perfect as the workings of that noble mind could make it. All his speeches, all his writings, all his labors were, in every part, symmetrical; for all were born of his earnest desire to "do good and communicate." Many of these contributions to our literature appeared in the "American Homœopathic Review," of which he was editor for some years; but all the prominent journals of our school, with scarcely an exception, were frequently enriched by articles from his pen. Besides his published writings, he maintained a more or less active correspondence with professional friends at home and abroad; in which way his great influence was the more widely and thoroughly felt, in the advancement of medical science and especially of homœopathic therapeutics.

Always subordinating his private interests to his elevated sense of duty, Dr. Dunham never sought titular honors or any public recognition of what he was or what he had done. But honors found him out; and he was, at various times, elected to high positions in many learned and scientific societies, both foreign and domestic; testimonials to his reputation as a physician and a scholar which were fully deserved.

When the death of Dr. Dunham was announced, so general and profound was the sense of an irreparable loss, that the whole homœopathic profession rose up as one man, both in this country and in Europe, to give utterance to their sorrow, to do honor to his memory, and to commemorate his character and services. Every one felt that we had "lost our best man." Special memorial meetings were called in many of our cities; all our societies paid their mournful tribute to his worth; obituary notices from the pens of our most distinguished men appeared in all our journals. Not even the death of Hahnemann stirred up such depths of grief; for Dunham, stricken down in the prime of his manhood, was nearly as widely known and admired, and was vastly more beloved. Perhaps we cannot give a better idea of the man, and of the impression which he made, than by quoting from some of the remarks and addresses which were then made as an offering to his memory.

A life-long friend remarked: "He was many-sided to such an extent as I have never seen in any other man. His learning was surprising, his literary culture great, and his modesty great as either. He spoke the languages of modern Europe as his own. His insight into the elements of disease, and into the nature of the agents by which they are cured, was wonderful. He has left an example which may God help us to follow!"

Another friend said of him: "Not long after the beginning of our acquaintance, we were associated in the

MEMOIR OF THE AUTHOR.   xix

investigation of some professional controversies. I confess I was hardly prepared for the display of clear, discriminating sagacity with which he took up the subject in dispute; and the earnestness with which he pursued the delicate and unpleasant task to a logical conclusion. * * * Most of the members of this society know something of the important part he took in the reorganization of our medical college. But few are aware of the amount of arduous labor which he gave to that business, or ˏof the peculiar difficulties he surmounted in its accomplishment. * * * His opinions always commanded respect, and usually controlled the course of action. And it may be said, without hesitation, that the existing laws of the State for regulating medical practice and for suppressing quackery owe much of their fair and liberal character to the influence he exerted. * * * Though the functions of arbitrator or inquisitor were not congenial to his modest and retiring disposition, yet he never hesitated to occupy any position or perform any duty legitimately imposed upon him. * * * In the social circle, amongst neighbors and friends, his genial nature shone conspicuous. With a vast fund of curious and interesting information, gathered from books and travel, he possessed a rare wit, and a fine appreciation of humor, which gave to his conversation a delightful charm and freshness."

The committee of the New-York County Homœopathic Medical Society, after bearing grateful testimony to his invaluable contributions to the materia medica, in the knowledge and practical application of which he was almost without a peer, speak thus of his qualities: "Possessing intellectual capacities of the highest order, he never exerted them for selfish ends, but always for the public good. Pure in his private life, exceptionally modest and retiring in his demeanor, ever gentle and kind, he knew not how to stoop to meanness and detraction; generous and larg-hearted, he was always ready to aid others, and all who were brought in contact with his noble and tender nature were compelled not only to admire and venerate the accomplished physician, but to trust and love the true-hearted Christian man."

From a Western physician we have this testimony: "At the meetings of our institute, he was the one who moved about the most quietly, who came and went with the least parade, and who, while he spoke very seldom in debate, always spoke to the purpose. He was the member whose committee never failed to report, and whose papers were always well digested, clear, concise, practical, and ready for the printer. He was the source of appeal for men on both sides of mooted questions. His influence was almost unbounded. He had the skill and tact of a great diplomatist, but these were never used for his own personal purposes. His pen was his sword,—the sword of Melancthon and not of Luther, bright, keen, trenchant,—but it can truly be said that it 'never carried a heart-stain away on its blade'."

Another friend said: "His life was one of truth and goodness. His name can never be mentioned without awakening feelings of love and reverence. His action in all matters, great or small, was prompted by purity of heart and love of right. By years of devotion to his profession, by his searching investigations, by his lucid writings, by his spotless integrity, and by his sincerity of purpose, he acquired unequaled influence among his colleagues; and I truly believe that Carroll Dunham has done more for the interests of homœopathy, not only in this city or country, but in the world at large, than any other man since the time of Hahnemann."

His life-long friend, Dr. P. P. Wells, said, after his death: "I would willingly have died for him."

One who had known him from his boyhood thus spoke of him: "When I pass in review the thirty-five years of our friendship, I can honestly and heartily say, that I do not remember a single word or act of his for which any of his friends need blush, or which he, now gone to his last account, would wish to be unsaid or undone. The only impatience I ever felt toward him during this long period, arose a few times because his calm, deliberative nature refused to plunge into the arena of medical polemics. But he was so magnanimous, or to use the more expressive Saxon word, so large-minded, that he could not be partisan; he could not but view both sides of every question at issue, and, as a consequence, he was liberal and generous even to his opponents, always ready to make allowance for the opinions and acts of those who differed with him. He was truly one of the 'blessed peace-markers.' The character of his mind was essentially judicial; approaching a subject impartially, he calmly weighed it in all its bearings; and had he been educated for the bar, his keen intellect and sound judgment would have graced the highest bench in the land. Actuated by an earnest love of truth and justice, he was thoroughly unselfish and always subordinated his private interests to the good of the cause with which he was identified. More than this: his whole lift was devoted, in a most self-sacrificing spirit, to the duties which the profession laid upon his willing shoulders; duties and responsibilities which he never refused and which came to him unsought, simply because all recognized his eminent fitness for their discharge. Thus he was often overburdened, and on several occasions his failing health compelled him to break off from all labor, and go abroad to rest and recuperate. But the moment he returned, those labors were resumed; and when, at last, exhausted nature succumbed, his death was merely the crowning act of a whole life of self-sacrifice. Though not physically strong, he was a steady worker and close student; and though independent of his income as a practitioner, and possessed of a competence by inheritance, which would, especially in view of his impaired health, have justified him in leading a life of elegant leisure, he accomplished an immense amount of literary labor; more, in fact, than most men, in full health and impelled by necessity, could have performed.

"His judgment was so sound, his convictions so sincere, his aims so unselfish, his life so pure, his sympathies so tender; he was so free from conceit or arrogance, so modest and unobtrusive, so devoid of petty ambitions, so intent on doing his whole duty, so liberal and tolerant toward those who differed with him, that he commanded the respect and won the affection of all who knew him. He wielded an immense power for good, not only by what he actually did, but by the mere force of his example, of a quiet, honest, thoughtful life.

"I have spoken of him as unselfish; I may add, from my private knowledge, that he was very generous and open-handed to all in need, imparting freely not only of his stores of knowledge, but of his purse. I could recount many acts of kindly charity and timely aid to poor struggling brethren; but I refrain, for he was one of those who never let their right hand know what their left hand gives.

"His unvarying cheerfulness was another marked characteristic. Notwithstanding his physical infirmities and his engrossing labors, he always seemed to dwell in a bright and serene atmosphere, full of hope and peace.

His very presence was refreshing and inspiriting; he went in and out among us, impressing all with the conviction that he was a true man, who had consecrated his life to a noble ideal of duty.

"Yes, friends and colleagues, we have lost our noblest and best man, one who was the heart and soul of the highest work done in our profession. In him we lose more than we now know; for, 'take him all in all, we ne'er shall look upon his like again.' But those who were so blessed as to call him friend, will always be thankful for his life and example; for such a man as he ennobles not only the age in which he lived, but humanity itself."

Much more might be quoted of the same purport; but these extracts will suffice to show how great and good a man was Carroll Dunham; as true a hero as ever fell in the front of battle, fighting for the right.

We cannot close this brief memorial more fitly than by quoting his parting words to his class, for they strike the key-note of his own life:

"May you have the pleasant consciousness, not only that you have made some permanent additions to the common stock of knowledge for the common good, but also that many men and women have been the happier for your lives."

E. M. KELLOGG, M. D.

MATERIA MEDICA AND THERAPEUTICS.

IN the exercise of any art which involves the use of tools or implements of any kind, the first condition essential to success is this:

That the scope and limits of the art be clearly defined and well understood, in order that no attempt may be made to exercise the art under circumstances which do not call for it, and which would necessarily preclude success.

A second condition no less essential is a thorough familiarity with the tools or implements of the art;, the origin, nature, powers and capabilities of each, and their relations to each other. This knowledge will teach us properly to select our tools according to the work we have to perform.

The problems before the artisan, then, are these:
1. When to use his tools.
2. What tools to select for each piece of work.
3. When selected, how to use them.

The practitioner of medicine, in the exercise of his profession, performs many functions. He may act simply as a diagnosticator of disease, detecting and explaining the seat and effects of disease, but without undertaking to treat it. Or, if he undertake to restore the sick to health, he may act simply as a surgeon, employing mechanical means alone, doing, as the etymology of the word surgeon or chirurgeon implies, handiwork. Or, he may act as the chemist, antidoting by chemical re-agents, noxious substances that are acting injuriously upon the body. Or, he may act as hygienist, bringing the laws of physiology to bear upon the regimen of his patient, and so ordering his mode of life as to eliminate the discoverable cause of disease. Or, finally, he may act as a therapeutist, by introducing into the organism of the patient certain substances from the external world which have the power of producing special modifications in the condition of the organism; and by means of these modifications he aims to cause the diseased action of the organism to cease and to be supplanted by the normal healthy action.

It is only with the practitioner of medicine in his last-named capacity, viz., as therapeutist, or curer of disease by means of drugs, that we have to do in the study of the sciences of materia medica and therapeutics.

The practitioner of medicine, in this capacity, employs certain tools or implements called drugs. These are the tools of his art. The problems before him are to determine:

1. When these tools are to be employed.
2. Their nature, history, and properties, collectively and individually.

3. How they are to be used.

The first of these problems, viz.: When and under what circumstances are drugs to be employed in taking care of the sick? has met with a variety of practical answer at different periods in medical history. At one time by a certain class of physicians, as is well known, drugs were universally and most lavishly employed in all cases of sickness. Another school in our own day goes to the opposite extreme of denying the power of drugs to control the course or result of disease, and altogether abstains from using them. Between these extremes there are all degrees of opinion and practice.

One might think that as this is a practical question, it might be settled by an appeal to experiment. But it is obvious that no experiments can be decisive, unless the experimenters agree upon the mode of making them. Two series of experiments cannot be compared unless their conditions are identical.

If one carpenter should use a plane to make smooth the surface of a plank, and another should use a gouge for the same purpose, these two artisans, on comparing results, would be found to have formed very different opinions respecting the efficiency of tools. Now, it is notorious that physicians have been altogether at variance in respect of the principles upon which drugs should be selected and the mode in which they should be used in treating disease. This will account for the unsettled state of the problem we are considering.

As has been said, there is an influential school of medicine—the expectant or physiological—which professes to abstain altogether from the use of drugs. Some advocates of this school argue, upon theoretical physiological grounds, that it is impossible for drugs to alter the course of action upon which the organism has entered in disease; that the organism must be allowed to carry out this course of action to its physiological conclusions,—indeed cannot be prevented from so doing. The fallacy of these arguments will be shown hereafter.

Others of this school point to the great successes of homœopathic and hydropathic physicians as proofs that drugs are a mischief and a mischief only. But this argument rests on the erroneous assumption that homœopathists use no drugs.

The legitimate conclusion from the successes of homœopathists and hydropathists is, that drugs unnecessarily and wrongly used are potent for evil; and the practical lesson to be drawn from this conclusion is, that it is a matter of the first importance to learn when it is necessary to use drugs and how to select and use the right drug for each case.

When called upon to take charge of a sick person, the first business of the practitioner is to make a diagnosis,—in homely words, to find out what ails the sufferer. The prognosis follows upon the diagnosis, and may be called a part of it. In doing this the practitioner observes the objective condition and surroundings of the patient, hears his subjective symptoms from the patient himself if he is able to state them, or from his friends; and listens to the previous history of the case. He inquires into the previous habits and occupations of the patient, ascertains whether he has been subjected to exposure or fatigue of mind or body, has been in the way of contagions or miasms of any kind, has been guilty of excesses or subjected to privations. Again, he looks for indications of any taint of constitution, any morbid diathesis inherited or acquired. In this way he endeavors to add to direct observations of the patient's present condition a knowledge of the pre-disposing and exciting causes of the disease under which he is laboring. Upon these data he forms his diagnosis. And up to a certain point his treatment is governed by his diagnosis. If, for instance, he finds the patient lying at the point of death from a mortal wound, or from cerebral apoplexy, or from whatever cause, he can do no more than communicate to the friends his diagnosis and prognosis, his view of the nature of the disease and his prediction of its course and termination, and leave the patient to their kind offices. Or if he find a wound, a fracture, a hernia, his diagnosis will be made accordingly; and, whatever his prognosis, he will employ the appropriate surgical means for closing the wound, adjusting the fractured parts, or reducing the hernia; and herewith, if there be no complication, his business will come to an end. Or if, again, he find as the exciting cause of the disease, some violation of the laws of health, his first business will be to cause this violation to cease. If it have been an error in diet, the diet must be regulated. If an unduly small or unduly great amount of exercise, this must be corrected; if an improper exposure to heat or cold, light or darkness, this must be adjusted; excesses must be curbed, deficiencies made up. In a great many cases, such an attention as this to the hygienic needs of the body will suffice to restore the patient's health. In every case it is to be the first concern of the physician; for, you may be well assured, without this care all administration of drugs will be in vain.

How to do in detail all that has been briefly alluded to as the duty of the practitioner in certain specified and in all similar cases, will be taught from the chairs of surgery, physiology, chemistry, and theory and practice. But from each of these chairs save that of chemistry, and, above all, from the chair of pathology, it will every day be taught that in a large number, I might say in a large majority, of cases of sickness, no amount of attention to the hygienic needs of the patient will be sufficient to put an end to his illness and restore him to health. Should his habits be regulated with the strictest observance of physiological laws, there will still be observed in him a diseased action of the organism, which, unless arrested or changed into a healthy action, will result in some kind of injury or deformity of one or more organs of the body, or may result in death.

Now, since in the case supposed the procedures of hygiene have failed to effect this necessary change of the morbid action into healthy action; since, although the conditions and surroundings and diet and habits of the patient are just what they should be, nevertheless the disease continues to progress and to injure or even destroy the organs of his body, we must either leave him to his fate, trust to nature to cure him,—a cruel step-mother, as I shall show, sometimes called kind and benignant, but only so because less cruel than a false and monstrous system of therapeutics, now happily declining,—I say we must leave him to his fate, or else we must find some particular means of bringing to bear on the diseased organism an influence capable of converting its morbid action into healthy action.

An influence of this kind is that which is exerted by drugs. Cases requiring the exercise of this influence,—cases in which hygiene has failed, or in which experience has shown that hygiene will fail, to arrest the morbid action of the organism,—these are the province of therapeutics, these are the cases in which drugs should be employed.

This may be made more clear by illustrations. Suppose a case of inflammation of the lungs. The patient is seen in the first stage, that of congestion. The physician ascertains the exciting cause, which has probably been undue exposure to cold winds or to a wet atmosphere, conjoined to a predisposing weakness of the lungs. All means are at once employed to adjust the temperature of the apartment, so as to supplement the deficiency of heat, by which in part the malady was induced. Experience has abundantly demonstrated that this care will not be sufficient to restore the lung to its normal state. Pathology teaches that in this stage the capillaries of the lungs are gorged to their utmost capacity; that the blood has almost if not altogether ceased to course through these capillaries; that the lining membrane of the air-cell in the part affected has ceased to perform its normal function; and that if this state of things continue, the membrane of capillaries and air-cells will assume a new function and will pour out an exudation which will fill up and obliterate the air-cell. If, in this state of things, we could bring to bear upon the patient some influence capable of acting just exactly upon the part affected by the disease, and of so acting as to resolve this stasis and set the blood in motion again; thus to relieve the gorged capillaries and to restore to the membrane of the air-cell the peculiar power which nature gave it, this influence would promptly effect a cure. It is an influence of this kind which we exert when we give a drug which is a specific for any diseased condition. And the object of the science of materia medica is to discover drugs which possess properties of this character, to ascertain the particular properties of each drug, and to learn how to give each drug in just those cases in which its peculiar properties will enable it to exercise such an influence as has been described.

If, in the case of inflammation of the lungs which has been supposed, we know of no such drug, but leave the case to nature, as the saying is, why then, either the inflammation and the consequent exudation are so extensive as to consolidate a larger part of the lung than the patient can spare, and death follows; or else after a long and tedious illness the exudation ceases to be poured out, and then becomes more or less completely absorbed again. This absorption, however, is rarely complete. The lung is left more or less consolidated and unfit for purposes of respiration, and more or less prone to the formation of secondary abscesses or of a nidus for the deposit of tubercle, while the patient goes forth again more or less a cripple in his respiratory organs.

Such is the benignity of nature, to whose curative power we are counseled to intrust our patients rather than endeavor to produce specific cures by means of drugs.

Let us meet, at once and for all, this question of nature as the great curer, superseding all the appliances of art.

How does nature amputate a limb? First she rots the skin, then she rots the muscles, then she rots the fasciæ and the vessels and the nerves, leaving them hanging out from the stump; last of all, after a long period, the bone, becoming dead and brittle, by some happy chance gets broken off. There is left a conical stump that will not bear to be touched, that will not tolerate an artificial limb, that is a torment to the patient, if indeed the months of suffering which the operation involves, or the drain of the constant discharges have not before this time carried him off. Compare this process and result with the expeditious amputations, the convenient stumps and the shapely and helpful artificial limbs of modern surgery! Dr. John Ware says that "the business of the medical practitioner is to stand between the patient and his friends and prevent the latter from interfering with the processes of nature!"

He would not think of applying this doctrine to the case of amputation! But he can be justified in applying it to cases of internal disease only on the assumption that he has as yet no knowledge of any better method than nature's. If this be so, then it should be stated as a fact affecting present time only, not laid down as a principle to hold good forever!

How does nature relieve a non-inflammatory congestion of the lung? By opening a blood-vessel into one of the air-tubes and causing an hæmoptysis. We very well known the ordinary sequelæ of pulmonary hæmorrhage, and how few are they who escape its termination in consumption! Is nature to be imitated in this?

How does nature cure a surplus of acid in the blood? By deposits in the joints, inflaming their synovial membranes and destroying the function of the joints, or by deposits in the kidneys or bladder causing nephritis or cystitis or calculi, or both. Shall we, from a superstitious devotion to nature, withhold ourselves from seeking out a better mode of cure?

It may be objected that this is not a fair statement of the doctrine which is, that we are to imitate nature, not in her mode of eliminating the proximate cause of the disease, but in the fact of its elimination. This reduces natures's teaching to the simple lesson that we are to "get rid of what annoys us," leaving us to find out the ways and means. So axiomatic a piece of advice as this would hardly seem to call for the admiration which has been expended on "nature, the great healer of diseases!"

The manner in which it has been proposed to imitate nature in the cases alluded to is this: Whereas in case of pulmonary congestion, she abstracts blood from the lungs, the doctors take it from the arm; whereas she gets rid of the excess of acid in the blood by pouring it into the joints and the kidneys, the doctors neutralize it by introducing an alkali into the blood.

But the result of this indirect imitation of nature does not differ much from that of a direct imitation. The cause of the pulmonary congestion being left unaffected, this congestion continues to be produced, notwithstanding that the doctor abstracts blood from the arm to relieve it. The continued congestion exhausts the patient by interfering with respiration. The doctor at the same time exhausts him, taking away his blood to cure the ever-reproduced congestion. Between disease and doctor the patient dies! And in this termination, there is still an imitation of nature! For does not nature put an end to the life of every living creature?

Let us take a higher view of these matters. Let us take a lesson from the Creator alike of ourselves and of that which we call nature!

Man comes into the world the most helpless of all living creatures, the feeblest, apparently the least provided for. If we look no higher than to the operations of external nature, we should say that his race must perish from off the earth, a victim of cold, of starvation, of maladies to which more than any other creature he is subject. The very opposite of all this happens. Every apparent law of nature is controverted. Man, the feeblest creature, dominates the earth. Every animal is subject to him. The three kingdoms of nature, throughout the globe, minister to his needs. How comes this contradiction? By the exercise of the intellectual faculties with which man has been endowed, man the feeble becomes mighty. Naked, he clothes himself with the spoils of animal and vegetable creation. Surrounded by crude food, yet unable to digest it in its natural state, his inventive faculties contrive for him the means of converting raw flesh and crude vegetables into delicate and savory nutriment, for which he gathers condiments from the ends of the earth. An easy victim of a host of miasms, he is endowed with intelligence to discover and with energy to procure, from distant climes if need be, specific remedies for the cure of every malady and the alleviation of every physical suffering. That he has to some extent succeeded in applying this intelligence to this beneficent end, is a guarantee of a success that may increase until we shall have a remedy for every ailment.

That we hitherto lack a great number of specifics,

this fact, instead of throwing us back into that stolid reliance upon nature, that stolid submission to the ills of our original state which is characteristic of the unenlightened savage, may well incite us to renewed exertions in this path of investigation and discovery so fruitful of blessings to our race!

To return now from this digression, we perceive that our first question may be answered as follows:

Drugs are to be used in cases in which disease persists after the employment of such mechanical, chemical or hygienic means, or all of them, as the laws of physiology may indicate, shall have proved ineffectual or insufficient to change the morbid action of the organism into a healthy action.

The employment of drugs must always be secondary and subordinate to a resort to hygienic measures.

Having thus determined when drugs are to be employed, viz.: when, after the exciting causes of disease have been removed, the disease still persists, and when some special influence from without the body is needed to bring it back into the way of healthy action, we come now to the second problem, viz.:

What is the nature of drugs in general, and how to ascertain the nature and properties of each particular drug.

The organism is made up of organs which perform their functions by virtue of a susceptibility which the tissues of which they are composed posses to certain stimuli which are necessary to life, and which are called general stimuli. These general stimuli are light, heat, electricity, air, moisture, aliment. The tissues of the lung are endowed with a susceptibility to the atmospheric air which acts as a stimulus to them, and under the influence of which they perform the function of respiration If this stimulus be withdrawn, the lungs cease to perform this function, and the animal perishes. If the quantity or quality of this stimulus be much altered, the function is performed in an unnatural or diseased manner, and sickness results. Heat is also a stimulus to the lungs as well as to other organs. Aliment is a stimulus to the digestive apparatus. Instances of this kind might be multiplied.

Now, it is well understood that when one of these stimuli has been in excess or in deficit, and consequently the function of the corresponding organ or apparatus comes to be abnormally performed, it will often be sufficient to re-adjust the proportion of the stimuli, for the organism to recur to its normal condition. To accomplish this re-adjustment is the task of the science of hygiene.

But, furthermore, it is also well known, as has been already stated, that hygiene, though it may with perfect nicety re-adjust the proportions of the general stimuli by virtue of which life goes on, is not always able by this re-adjustment to restore the organism to its former healthy condition. The organ or apparatus, which, through some deficiency or excess or perversion of some stimulus or other, became diseased, will often remain diseased after hygiene has corrected the disproportioned stimulus. Permanent disease exists, and hygiene has done all it can do.

In this state of things we are powerless unless we can bring to bear upon the diseased organ some influence which may have the power to directly convert its diseased action into the pristine healthy action. This, it will be conceded, is the desideratum and this must, in some way or other, be accomplished. The substances in which such influences reside are what we call drugs.

We now perceive the two requisite conditions for the successful employment of drugs in treating sickness.

1. We must possess substances which are capable of exerting such an influence upon the different organs of the body as to be able to produce definite changes in the mode of action of these organs: and

2. We must know how to apply this knowledge of the action of drugs to particular cases of sickness.

As a consequence of what has been said, then, a drug may, in general, be defined as being any substance which is capable of changing or definitely modifying the mode in which any organ or system of the body performs its functions, or of changing or modifying the tissues of the body.

The study of materia medica is the study of the nature and properties of drugs. How, then, are these to be ascertained? It may not be unprofitable to glance briefly at the history of the materia medica at this point.

There was a time when it was supposed that the properties of drugs were indicated by their physical properties, their color, odor, shape or taste. Thus, aloes, from the yellow color of its solution and from its bitter taste, was conceived to act pre-eminently upon the liver.

This was the famous doctrine of the Signature, most groundless and fanciful, and yet, like every other visionary notion, it was not without some semblance of support in analogy.

The chemical properties of substances furnished another supposed means of ascertaining their supposed properties as drugs. If they were to be employed as chemical re-agents in the cure of disease nothing could be more rational. But it must be remembered that we know but little about the chemistry of disease; indeed, that chemistry deals only with the results of organic action, while we aim, by the action of drugs, to modify organic action itself. Furthermore, experience shows us that substances possessing analogous chemical action produce very different effects as drugs. And, finally, when we come to the vegetable kingdom, we find the chemical composition and reactions of the different varieties to be nearly identical, while their action upon the vital organism is as various as could be imagined.

But leaving the history of materia medica, let us ask ourselves again what it is that we seek? To find out the properties of substances that we suppose to be drugs, to ascertain whether substances which we are investigating be really drugs or not, *i.e.,* whether they be capable of modifying the action of the organs of the body. What method so direct, so simple, so certain, as to test them on the living body; not on the lower animals, for these are often variously affected by drugs; but on the human beings for whose benefit they are to be employed as medicines.

But shall they be tested on the sick? This might be regarded as hardly justifiable, or if it were justifiable, it would be difficult to draw an inference from the action upon one case of sickness respecting its action upon another case of sickness; since each case of sickness is different from every other case. And then again, if we were to gain knowledge of drugs only by experimenting on the sick, and this knowledge were to serve us only in case we should meet a similar case of sickness again, our knowledge would be always too late to be of service. We should know well what had happened, but should have no store of general knowledge ready for any case that might occur.

It is a general rule in physics, that when we try an experiment we should have every element that enters into the experiment in as normal a condition as possible. This can only be done if we experiment on the body in health.

Accordingly, all trustworthy and useful knowledge of drugs has been obtained by experiments upon the healthy subject.

Such experiments are what we call provings of drugs. They are made by greater or less numbers of independent observers. The coincidences of effects observed by independent provers are cheering evidences of the correctness of this method. By the application of physiological knowledge to the results of these provings, a more or less complete appreciation of the action of a drug may be gathered.

It is in this way that we ascertain the nature and properties of drugs.

The special method and importance of drug-proving will form the subject of a future lecture.

STUDY OF MATERIA MEDICA.

IN our last lecture we discussed the nature of the sciences of materia medica and therapeutics, defining the one to comprise a knowledge of the properties of drugs, and the other a knowledge of the method of using drugs to cure sick people.

We then discussed two of the three general problems which present themselves to the medical practitioner in his capacity as a curer of disease by means of drugs. These were:

1. Under what circumstances of sickness he is called upon and required to resort to the use of drugs in treating disease.

2. The means of ascertaining the properties of drugs. To this second problem I wish to devote a few more words, for I greatly desire that you should very clearly understand the impossibility of acquiring a definite and complete knowledge of the absolute and positive properties of drugs in any other way than by provings upon the healthy subject.

Observations of the action of drugs upon the sick teach the properties of the drug in relation to the organism when in that particular abnormal condition, but give us no absolute knowledge of its constant action upon the organism. Yet we can have no science of therapeutics without some such knowledge of the constant and uniform properties of drugs.

If we give mercury to a patient laboring under Bright's disease, we find that an exceedingly small quantity produces a very powerful and remarkable effect, and such an effect as we see from mercury under no other circumstances.

Now, this knowledge would be of service to us if we should contemplate giving mercury in another case of Bright's disease; but it would not help us at all if the question were whether or not we should give mercury in some other disease, as for example, pericarditis. And yet you will perceive that one great essential of a science of therapeutics is, that it shall enable us to predict the effect of the application of a drug in a new case; to know before-hand what effect we shall be able to produce; and by this knowledge to select a drug capable of producing the effect we desire.

Now, on the other hand, if a dozen or a hundred healthy persons take mercury, the effects produced on them are, with the exception of slight differences depending on the idiosyncrasies of the provers, identical. This method then enables us to gain an absolute knowledge of the constant and uniform properties of drugs in their relation to the living organism.

If now, having gained this knowledge, we could advance a step farther, and find out what relation the effects which a drug produces on the healthy subject bear to those symptoms of disease which the drug is capable of removing, we should possess the elements of the much desired science. For, then, having the symptoms of the disease before us, and knowing the relationship which these symptoms bear to the effects of a drug capable of removing them, we could select our drug with *a priori* certainty of curing our patient.

Having thus considered the problem of the general nature and properties of drugs, and the method of ascertaining these properties, we come now to the third problem: How to use drugs.

Let us suppose that by the method already pointed out, viz.: experiment on the healthy human subject, we have gained a tolerably accurate knowledge of the properties and powers of certain drugs to modify the action of the organism.

Let us further suppose that a sick person is under our charge, in whose case the resources of hygiene have already been exhausted and to no purpose. His regimen and food have been regulated as well as could be desired. Still he does not recover. The interposition of some influence from without is needed to restore him to health. In short, drugs are required. We know the properties of a variety of drugs, their action on the healthy subject. The question now is how, on the basis of this knowledge, shall we select a suitable remedy for the sick man? How shall we apply our knowledge of the action of the drug on the healthy subject, so as to know what drug to select for this particular case of sickness? We demand, in other words, a principle or law for the selection of remedies. The selection and administration of remedies constitute the science of therapeutics, as the investigation of the properties of drugs constitutes the science of materia medica; and the principle or law of which we are in quest would be the great central principle of the science of therapeutics, just as the law of attraction is the central principle of the science of mechanics, and the law of the diffusion of light is the central principle of optics. It is impossible to conceive of a science (properly so called) without some such fundamental principle. A collection of facts bearing on therapeutics might be made which would be an interesting historical *résumé* of what had been done in the past, but which would be of but little or no service to the physician in the treatment of any new case,—which would not enable him to predict the result of treatment in a new case. And yet there are some medical men who deny the necessity for any therapeutic law and rely only on unmethodized experience. Of these we shall presently speak at greater length.

I wish now to speak of the physiological school, so called, as that which makes, just now, the loudest claims to exclusive possession of the truly scientific method of treating diseases. I shall speak of it at some length, because it is of the greatest importance that you learn as early in your studies as possible to analyze closely and fearlessly all claims and pretensions of this kind, and that you learn to distinguish clearly between assumptions and facts.

The physiological school scoffs at a therapeutic law, because a law of this kind is empirical, and does not rest on a rational understanding of the causes of disease. And this is true. It is likewise true of physics. The laws of the attraction of gravitation, and of the diffusion of light and of chemical affinity, in definite proportions, are empirical laws. They do not rest on a rational understanding of the causes of the phenomena with which they deal respectively, for, in truth, we know nothing about the causes of these phenomena, and have never been able to find out anything about them. These laws are simply inductions from a multitude of observed facts. But the physiological school undertakes to find out the causes of the phenomena of disease; to trace the symptoms of disease back to their ultimate origin, and then acting on the general principle, "remove the cause and the effect will cease," to remove the cause thus discovered and so cure the disease.

We have shown that in matters of hygiene this is possible and is the true method. It would be the true method in therapeutics if it were possible. But it is not possible, as we shall best show by an example.

Suppose a fully developed inflammation of the

lungs. The rational symptoms are: heat of the skin, accelerated and hardened pulse, difficult respiration, oppressing pain in the thorax, dry cough, tough, rusty expectoration. The physical signs are: dullness on percussion, bronchial respiration, and on the margins of the dullness, fine crepitation. The pathological condition is: locally, a deposit of fibrine in the air-cells and tubes, consolidating the lung; and generally, a marked excess of fibrine in the blood. Now, the physiological school assumes this general pathological condition to be the essential cause of the disease; to lie at the foundation of all its symptoms; and it therefore proposes, as the method of cure, to get rid of this pathological condition, viz., the excess of fibrine in the blood and the local deposit of fibrine in the lung. To accomplish this several means may be resorted to, which, though apparently different, are the same in principle. Blood may be abstracted from the arm. This will diminish the quantity of the circulating fluid, and thereby diminish the actual, although not the relative, quantity of fibrine. But as the quantity of the circulating fluid must always be the same, water is poured into the vessels from the surrounding tissues or from the intestines, and thus the blood is really diluted. All other antiphlogistic or derivative methods or medicines act in the same way. But does this method reach the real ultimate cause of the disease? By no means. In health the blood does not contain too much fibrine. How came it to do so in disease? This leads us to the question:

Where is the fibrine manufactured, and how came so much to be made, or by what means is fibrine generally removed from the blood, and how happens it that it is not more rapidly removed? To these questions the physiologists can return no certain responses as yet. But if they could do so, is it not obvious that in order that the blood should contain too much fibrine, there must have been either too much made or too little consumed. Now, if either of these be the case, how unwise to think of rectifying matters by merely conveying away the surplus. It is like endeavoring to pump out a leaking vessel while the leak is still open. The pumping out is only a palliation,—can never be a cure. The cause of the disease must lie in the secretion of the fibrine. But this process is conducted, as you learn from the chair of physiology, through the agency of a structureless cell-wall, and by a process of which we know, and can know, absolutely nothing. It is an ultimate fact, a part of the fact of life. Such are all the ultimate causes of disease. And as diseased organic action is merely a modification of healthy organic action, as disease is only modified life, we can never hope to attain a knowledge of the real causes of disease, and can never base a therapeutics on the rational method of removing the cause. We must fall back, as all investigators of natural science have done, on an empirical science and an empirical law.

The great majority, however, even of the old school of medicine, regard a therapeutic law as a great desideratum, as something essential to the constitution of medicine as a science.

But to return to our patient. How shall we determine what drug to give him? We have probably made a diagnosis, and given to the collective symptoms which he presents some name of a disease, although, if we have much experience at the bedside we shall undoubtedly have remarked that though the same name may be given to a large number of apparently similar cases of sickness, yet in reality no two of them are in all respects alike; indeed they often differ very widely. This is because the peculiarities of the individual patient are superadded to the general symptoms of the disease under which he is regarded as laboring.

But having formed our diagnosis and given a name to the case, we might recall from the annals of medicine a number of cases to which a similar name had been given, and which had been cured by such or such drugs. Now, there is a school of medicine, and it includes some very brilliant names, which teaches that such clinical experience as this is our only trustworthy source of therapeutic knowledge, that we must gather up reports of cases and analyze them, find out what mode of treatment cured the greatest number of cases, and adopt this as the right mode.

Louis, in Europe, and Bartlett and La Roche, in this country, are the representatives of this methodical or numerical school.

Now, it will be easily shown, I believe, that

while this method may be better than nothing, while it may answer as a make-shift until some better be discovered, it is very far from being in any true sense a science of therapeutics. One objection is this: Its aim is too low. It aims to cure only a majority of cases of any disease; for it avails itself of a method that succeeded only in a majority, not in all; it does not provide for the minority that were not cured by this favorite mode of treatment. It makes no provision for the investigation of the reason why it was that the mode in question failed in a certain number of cases, although it succeeded in a majority. And yet this failure could not have been accidental. There are no accidents in nature. There must have been some good reason for the failure, a reason to be ascertained by investigation and so turned to account as to diminish the minority, and finally altogether to eliminate the failures.

This point may be illustrated by example. If we gather the clinical records of intermittent fever, we shall find that a large majority of the cures recorded were effected by cinchona or its derivatives. The methodical school would therefore pronounce cinchona the cure for intermittent, still a minority of cases will be found which cinchona failed to cure. There must be a good reason for this failure, and a true science of therapeutics should make provision for the searching out and the finding of this reason. The science of the methodists makes no such provision. The highest ideal of the methodists, then, would be to cure a majority of the cases intrusted to them. This is too low an ideal to satisfy a reasoning creature.

To find out this reason why cinchona, which cures so many cases, yet fails to cure other cases bearing the same name, one must evidently examine curefully the cases cured, on the one hand, and the cases which failed to be cured, on the other hand, in the hope of finding some traits of difference among the many features of resemblance. It will be found that such points of difference exist; that while the symptoms of chill, fever and sweat may exist in all, thus entitling all to the generic name of intermittent fever, there are, neverthelesss, minor differences between the two classes of cases sufficient to make them quite distinct. Thus, for example, some cases have thirst, while others have none. Some have gastro-intestinal complications, while others have none. Or, complications of other organs or systems may exist. We thus see differences in cases grouped under the same nosological name. But as yet this does not help us to a reason why cinchona should cure some of these cases and not others. And yet this is the very "pith and marrow" of the question. This is the all-important question for solution. For it is obvious that if we could find out why cinchona cures certain cases presenting certain symptoms, we should know with certainty whether to give cinchona or not in a new case. We should have established a relation between cinchona or its properties and the

STUDY OF MATERIA MEDICA. 29

symptoms presented by cases of sickness. Such a relation is a law. We should then have discovered the great desideratum, the therapeutic law. What we seek to know then is this: What relation is there between the physiological action, the absolute properties of drugs, as ascertained by provings on the healthy subject, and the symptoms of disease? We have shown that the properties of drugs, in the sense in which we use the term, are accurately ascertained only by the symptoms they produce on the healthy subject. The question, then, may be expressed as follows: What relation subsists between the symptoms which a drug produces on the healthy subject and those which it will remove from a sick man? If we could answer this question, we should know what drug to select for our sick man, who has been waiting for a prescription while we have been discussing this subject.

Very long ago, an answer was given to this question in the words: *Contraria contrariis opponenda,* which means that the relation of contrariety or opposition should exist between the symptoms of the patient and the symptoms which the drug that we are to select to cure him is capable of producing. This was assumed to be the natural solution of the question. It was argued, and still is argued, that if a patient be heated, he seeks that which will cool him; if thirsty, that which will make him not thirsty; if constipated, a laxative; if loose in the bowels, an astringent, etc., etc.

The objection to this proposed law is twofold:

1. It rests upon a confusion of ideas. The procedures of hygiene are confounded with those of therapeutics. In hygienic treatment the problem is to find out which of the natural general stimuli necessary to maintain health has been deficient or in excess or perverted, and to restore or regulate it. By this method, if there be too much heat, from this stimulus having been in excess, the obvious remedy is a diminution of the supply. If thirst spring from a too sparing supply of water, it is obvious that this must be made up, etc. And the test of a successful judgment in such cases is the cessation of the symptom. So in the case of constipation, if the impacted fæces act merely as a mechanical irritant, as a foreign body in the intestine, their removal by direct mechanical means or indirectly through an irritation produced in the intestine by drugs, is purely a hygienic procedure, and may be effected in accordance with the law *Contraria contrariis.*

2. But when we come to symptoms which result not directly from abnormal supply of stimuli, but from a modification of the vital forces, and which consist in alterations of sensation, of function, of tissue, how can we find the contraries, the opposites of these symptoms? What symptom produced on the healthy subject by a drug can be the opposite or contrary of a sore throat, of a gastralgia, of a toothache, of a miliary rash, of a delirium, of a nausea, of a small-pox pustule, of a scarlatina eruption, of a varicose ulcer?

No more words are needed to show the absurdity of the maxim viewed in this light,—the impossibility of the proposed law. But it may be said that this interpretation does not do it justice. It may be urged that we are to seek not the contraries of the symptoms themselves, but the opposites of that physiological or pathological state which gave rise to the symptoms.

In considering the subject from this point we shall be able to pronounce an opinion at the same time upon another principle of therapeutics, that indeed which is at the present day regarded with almost universal favor,—the method, it may be called, of treating diseases upon general principles.

This method ignores any therapeutic law, its possibility or necessity. The reliance of this method is upon pathology, by means of which science it proposes to ascertain the interior changes in tissue and structure, which lie at the foundation of, and give rise to, the symptoms of the patient, and thus get a rational appreciation of the symptoms. It studies the symptoms produced by the drug in the same way. After having formed a theory of the conditions which produce these symptoms respectively, this mode of treatment proposes to select a drug capable of producing a pathological condition opposite or contrary to that which gave rise to the symptoms of the patient.

Except in words, this method does not differ from that which we have discussed. Instead of opposing symptoms to symptoms directly, a theory is formed respecting each series of symptoms, and these theories are opposed to each other.

Using the word symptom as we do, in its broadest sense, to include every fact that can be ascertained or observed by the medical practitioner, both objective and subjective, the symptoms of a patient comprise all that can be known respecting the patient's disease. To theorize upon the proximate or ultimate cause of these symptoms is not to add anything to our knowledge. It is indeed interposing an hypothesis, the probable result of which will be to lead us astray. In no possible event can it facilitate the cure.

Let us suppose a case: A patient presents a series of symptoms, among which paleness, palpitation, want of appetite, loss of strength, perhaps hæmorrhage from various surfaces, are prominent. These, with the other symptoms, furnish all that can be ascertained about this patient. Physiology and pathology enable us to comprehend how these symptoms are connected with each other, and with certain states of the solid and fluid tissues of the body; and thus these sciences enable us to form a diagnosis and a prognosis and to institute a hygienic treatment. But when we come to therapeutics, if we adopt the method of treating on "general principles," we shall say, the blood is deficient in red globules, hence the paleness and palpitation. The serum is in excess, hence the anasarca and the loss of strength. There are laxity and flaccidity of the surface membranes, and of the muscles and nerves, hence the hæmorrhages and the debility.

The indication is to give a remedy which will increase the red globules and will give tone to membranes, muscles and nerves.

This sounds wise and practical. But on analysis it proves to be mere verbiage. The pathological statement is a mere restatement of the symptoms, adding nothing to their force or significance.

The indication may be reduced to this simple general indication: Give a drug that will cure the patient,—a thing we all wish to do. We know of no drug that will, in the healthy subject, increase the red globules of the blood; nor can we ever know a drug that will give tone to the healthy membrane, muscle and nerve. For what do we mean by tone? Nothing more nor less than healthy normal condition. Can any drug ever produce this condition in a healthy subject? Can we reproduce what is already in active existence? It is manifest, then, that this method is, after all its parade of science, its pathological analysis, its indication, and its appeal to general principles, nothing else but the raw and crude resort to unmethodized, empirical experience. Iron, which in the case supposed, would of course be the drug selected, will in reality be chosen, not because its symptoms sustain, or their hypothetical, pathological cause bears, any relation of contrariety to the symptoms of the patient or their hypothetical, pathological cause; but solely because it was found out in some manner unknown that iron would cure such cases; and manifold experience has corroborated the discovery. Just as it was found out that cinchona would cure intermittent fever and mercury syphilis. The fact that iron cures the case, and that iron is a constituent of the red globule, is a mere curious coincidence. But unless a law should be induced from such experience, we have shown that the experience alone cannot serve as the basis of a science of therapeutics.

It is clear, then, that the relation between the symptoms of a disease and the symptoms of the drug that will remove them, cannot be that of contrariety or opposition.

How may we ascertain what it is if indeed there be any fixed relation?

If we had no knowledge of any drugs that almost uniformly cure certain diseases, it would be almost impossible to find an answer to this question. But, fortunately, we possess several drugs of which we know by long and often-repeated experience, indeed by common consent, that they do cause the disappearance of certain definite groups of symptoms. Now, is it not probable that if we avail ourselves of these facts, and if we prove some such drug upon the healthy organism, and compare the symptoms thus produced by it with the symptoms which we know it to be capable of curing, we shall thus at last, after a number of such trials, arrive at a knowledge of the relation which exists between the symptoms which a drug can produce on the healthy, and those which it can remove in the sick? This relation, if constantly observed, would serve as a therapeutic law. For, by provings upon the healthy we have it in our power to ascertain the symptoms which every drug is capable of producing. We can have thus an armament in reserve to meet any symptoms that may present themselves in a patient. And there is no limit to the extent to which this may be carried.

Now, this has actually been done with respect to all the well-known and conceded specific medicines, and indeed to nearly all known drugs. It has been observed that a constant relation exists between the symptoms which a drug will produce in the healthy subject and those which it will cure in the sick. This relation is that of similarity.

It is not necessary to adduce at this time instances in corroboration of this statement. They will occur during every lecture of this course when we come to the study of individual drugs.

From the fact of this constant relationship of similarity springs the therapeutic law which I believe to be the universal and only one,—*Similia similibus curantur*. Diseases are to be cured by drugs which are capable of producing in the healthy subject symptoms similar to those of the disease in question.

The homœopathic materia medica is made up, theoretically at least, of the objective and subjective symptoms produced upon healthy persons by drugs, taken with a view to ascertain their physiological or pathogenetic effects. I say theoretically, because our materia medica being as yet incomplete and imperfect, whereas the exigencies of practice are as wide and various as the distribution and the diseases of the human race, we are under the present necessity of supplementing our pure provings by observations of the action of remedies on the sick (called clinical symptoms), by toxicological records which are involuntary provings made in a rougher way than we could desire, and even by hypothetical conclusions from the scanty data of incomplete provings, as, for example, when from the action of a drug upon the mamma we infer its effect upon the ovary, etc., etc. The necessities for the temporary expedients will be less frequent in proportion as we are able to carry forward the development of the science of materia medica. This is a work which requires much time, labor and self-sacrifice of those who engage in it, and several generations must pass away before the science will have attained tolerable completeness. Were it never so complete, we are called upon to deal with bedside problems that would severely tax its resources. And we are compelled to base our prescriptions frequently upon clinical observations, upon analogies, upon some trivial symptoms in some region of the body quite remote from the pathological center of the disease; certainly such cases as these most brilliantly illustrate the value of our grand therapeutic law, which leads us to success through many dark places on which pathology would shed no light. Nevertheless, as students of science we cannot but desire that our materia medica should be as complete, and should present us pictures of drug diseases, as numerous and varied as the maladies for which we are called to prescribe; as workers in the domain of science, we cannot but determine to give ourselves to this task of developing the materia medica. It behooves us then to examine our present materia medica, and mark where it is weak and defective, that our earnest efforts may be given first to those points. Before specifying some of these points, let me speak for a moment of others on which I think the materia medica is strong, since by these we may exemplify the characteristics of a serviceable pathogenesis.

I consider that in its account of the action of drugs upon the alimentary canal as compared with other regions, the homœopathic materia medica is reasonably complete and definite. As regards the stomach, the symptoms of drugs are, in general, so clearly stated that we can distinguish, as Dr. Hirschel has shown in his prize essay on cardialgia, the neuroses from the various organic affections, and in each of these departments it is not often necessary to hesitate long in the selection of the remedy.

If this be true of the stomach, it may be still more emphatically stated of the lower portions of the alimentary canal. Among the points upon which the symptoms of the materia medica give data which enable us to distinguish the indications of one drug from those of another, may be named: the sensations and pains, both those felt by the patient irrespective of his actions, and such as are induced by motion, touch, etc.; second, performance of function; third, contents of the intestine, as evidenced by evacuations; fourth, symptoms attendant upon evacuation.

THE THERAPEUTIC LAW.

ANALYSIS.

History—Definition—Empirical, requiring evidence—Evidence furnished by physiological and the therapeutic effects of drugs, and to be given, in extenso, in the course of the lectures on special drugs—Practical application of the law—It involves a twofold study, each branch of which may be a distinct and independent study, viz.: 1. Study of the phenomena of natural disease, and 2. Study of the phenomena of the action of drugs on the healthy subject—These studies must be empirical and positive, recognizing only facts and disregarding hypotheses—Symptoms in the broad sense the only object of study—Similarity being the object of our search, cases are to be individualized, and nosologies to be disregarded—Each case studied in and for itself—Same with diseases and pathogeneses—What are symptoms?—How are physiology and pathology to be employed?—Varieties of symptoms—Generic, specific, characteristic—The same of diseases as of drugs—What is a proving?—How to study a drug.

THE last lecture concluded with a statement of what I regard as the universal therapeutic law; that commonly expressed by the words *"Similia similibus curantur,"* or, "Sick persons are to be cured by drugs which produce in the healthy symptoms similar to those of the sick persons."

Adherence to this law as the universal law of cure is distinctive of the homœopathic school of medicine. Nevertheless, the statement of the law did not by any means originate with Hahnemann, the founder of homœopathy; nor is the acceptance of the law as a law of cure confined to homœopathicians. Many most distinguished physicians of the old school, as Pereira, Watson, Trousseau, Bouchut, and many others, accept it as a law of cure, of wide application, although they deny its universality. I believe their denial springs from a confusion in their minds between the procedures of hygiene and therapeutics. The law was clearly expressed in a very remarkable passage of a work ascribed to Hippocrates. Paracelsus had a glimpse of this truth, and expressed it in his quaint and mystical fashion; and in so far as the imperfect state of the materia medica allowed, it is believed that he practiced in accordance with it. "Stoerck was struck with the idea that if stramonium disturbs the senses, and produces mental derangement in persons who are healthy, it might very easily be administered to maniacs for the purpose of restoring the senses by effecting a change of ideas." (Hahnemann's "Organon," 4th American Edition, p. 76.) This was a perception of a particular instance, but not of the general law.

Stahl expresses himself as follows: "The received method in medicine, of treating diseases by opposite remedies—that is to say, by medicines which are opposed to the effects they pro-

THE THERAPEUTIC LAW.   41

duce (*contraria contrariis*)—is completely false and absurd. I am convinced, on the contrary, that diseases are subdued by agents which produce a similar affection (*similia similibus*); burns by the heat of a fire to which the parts are exposed; the frost-bite by snow or icy-cold water; and inflammations and contusions by spirituous applications. It is by these means I have succeeded in curing a disposition to acidity of the stomach by using very small doses of sulphuric acid in cases where a multitude of absorbing powders had been administered to no purpose."

This was written in Denmark in 1738, nearly fifty years before Hahneman's first publication on the subject. It is a distinct statement of the law.

Hahnemann, who was a very learned man and a very highly educated physician, became, early in his practice, deeply and painfully convinced of the great uncertainty of medical science as it was then taught and practiced, and of the serious injuries that were often inflicted on the patients by the improper use of drugs. He fully indorsed the saying of his predecessor, Girtanner, that "the doctor with his drugs is like a blind man with a club. He aims to crush the disease, but is quite as likely to destroy the patient." Hahnemann was by no means singular in this view of actual medical science. Most of his contemporaries agreed with him. And from his day to the present, eminent physicians of the old school have expressed similar convictions. What fruits did this conviction bear?

It is related of Sir Isaac Newton that when asked to account for his transcendent genius and its wonderful achievements, he modestly replied that it consisted in nothing but this: that he had a little more patience and perseverance than some other men.

So Hahnemann, when convinced of the uncertainty and unsafeness of the medical science of his day, rested not in his search for something more safe and sure. "He that seeketh shall find." To the receptive, eager mind, a trivial incident may serve as the clue to a brilliant discovery, just as the falling apple did in Newton's case and the swinging chandelier in Galileo's.

Hahnemann, having taken a dose of tincture cinchonæ, observed the symptoms which resulted from it. He was struck with their similarity to the symptoms of an attack of intermittent fever, from which he had suffered years before. He knew that cinchona was the great specific for intermittent fever. The question at once occurred to him, Can it be that this similarity is a mere coincidence in the case of this particular drug and the disease which it cures, or is it an example of a general law of nature? If it be indeed a general law of nature, may it not be the great therapeutic law of which we are in so great need? Up to this point of perceiving or suspecting the law, *Similia similibus curantur*, Hahnemann had been preceded, as he very well knew and openly stated, by Hippocrates, Stoerck and Stahl, and others. They, however, contented themselves with throwing out the intimation or conjecture and abandoning it. Not so Hahnemann. He argued: if this be a general law, it is capable of demonstration in two ways:

1. *A posteriori,*—by searching and analyzing the records of medicine,—a task which he forthwith undertook with great success, and,

2. *A priori,*—by the direct experiment,—by ascertaining the effects of some drugs on the healthy subject, and then giving them to sick people whose symptoms happened to be similar to those which the drugs had produced.

By experiments and observations of these kinds, carried on for twenty years, Hahnemann satisfied himself of the truth of the law The points of evidence will be laid before you when we study the different drugs of the materia medica.

But now, please take notice that this law requires that the sick person shall receive a drug which is capable of producing in the healthy subject symptoms similar to those of the patient. This law can never be applied in practice unless we possess a materia medica which contains a record of the symptoms which drugs produce in the healthy. No such materia medica existed in Hahnemann's day. All that there was, was a mere record of the effects upon the sick, and of hypotheses and guesses. Now came into operation that infinite patience and that perseverance which mark transcendent genius. Hahnemann undertook the Titanic labor of creating this indispensable materia medica. Proving more than a hundred drugs upon himself and his friends, subjecting himself therby to toil and suffering indescribable, he compiled for us the "Materia Medica Pura," in six volumes, and the "Chronic Diseases," in five volumes,—an imperishable monument to his genius and self-devotion.

This materia medica, founded by Hahnemann, and enlarged and enriched by the labors of his successors and by the addition of all that is trustworthy in ancient or contemporary literary literature, is our treasury of knowledge of the action of drugs upon the human organism.

You will observe that the therapeutic law we have laid down speaks of two classes of symptoms:

1. Those of the patient; and,
2. Those produced in the healthy subject by a drug. If the latter be similar to the former, then the drug which produced the latter will remove the former.

This statement points to two subjects for our study,—the symptoms respectively of sick persons and of drug-provings.

The law, it will be noticed, is empirical. It is based on no theory of the action of drugs, and it involves no theory whatever. It merely states that a coincidence has been observed to exist between the symptoms which a drug will cause in the healthy and those which it will remove in the sick. In this respect it is analogous to the laws of gravitation and of chemical affinity, and in definite proportions indeed to the great central laws of all the natural sciences.

In like manner the studies of the two classes of symptoms to which the law points us, are to be made in a positive and empirical manner; and we are to take care that no hypothesis respecting the nature and ultimate cause of the symptoms which we observe in the sick, be allowed to come in and modify or pervert our pure observation.

In order to apply the therapeutic law in the treatment of disease, we have then to study.

1. The symptoms of patients; and,
2. The symptoms of healthy persons who have taken drugs for the purpose of ascertaining their effects.

These studies are similar in their character, but they are wholly independent of each other, and may be pursued separately; indeed, are only conjoined when the subject of the study is to be qualified to practice the art of curing. This being one object, we cannot do better than devote some time to an investigation of the modes of studying symptoms.

By a symptom of disease, whether it be a natural disease or a diseased state produced upon himself intentionally by a prover of drugs, we mean any deviation from a normal condition in any organ or function of the body, which deviation is capable of being observed by the physician or by the attendants, or by the patient himself. The senses of the observers may be assisted by any implements or processes, such as the stethoscope, the microscope, the ophthalmoscope, chemical analysis, etc., etc. If every function of the body be performed in a proper, healthy manner, there can of course be no symptoms of disease. If any function be not performed in a proper, healthy manner, the facts by which we perceive and which enable us to know that this is so, are the symptoms of the case. We sometimes hear of the existence of latent disease of which no symptom exists. This may be, but its existence is only hypothesis, and is afterward inferred from the subsequent occurrence of symptoms. To detect its existence when thus latent would be impossible, for if it gave in any way the least token of its existence, that token would be a symptom.

Symptoms may be objective or subjective. Objective symptoms are those which are observed and taken note of by the physician or by the attendants of the patient. They could be observed whether the patient were conscious or not. The aid of his intelligence is not invoked in gaining a knowledge of them. They are the color, texture, temperature of the skin and membranes, the expression of the eyes and features generally, position, motions and attitudes of the body, secretions and excretions of glands and surfaces; in short, objective symptoms comprise everything which the physician can take cognizance of in the sick man, by the aid of his five senses assisted or unassisted. Physical and chemical and microscopic analyses are included. Subjective symptoms are those of which we get a knowledge through the medium of the patient's own intelligence and testimony. They comprise the various sensations, pains and abnormal feelings, the infinite variety of unwonted thoughts, emotions, sentiments, dreams and visions which diversify the existence of the sick man. If the patient be ill of a disease which makes him stupid or unconscious, we cannot get any subjective symptoms,—as in typhoid fever sometimes. If he be delirious we have to receive his expressions with due caution.

To these varieties of symptoms must be added a third, which modifies the former, viz., the symptoms comprised in the previous history of the case. These will show us any constitutional taint or miasm in the patient; and by teaching us his habits and idiosyncrasies may often enable us to decide how much weight to attach to one or another subjective or objective symptom.

We have thus briefly described the classes of symptoms. The law requires us to compare the aggregate of symptoms presented by the patient with the symptoms produced by drugs that are known to us; and to select for the case the drug of which the symptoms are most similar to those of the patient. It is objected to this very empirical and almost mechanical method, that it takes no account of the causes of symptoms, does not undertake to trace them to their causes; that it entirely ignores physiology and pathology, sciences which have thrown so much light on the nature and causes of disease; that it exposes the prescriber to the hazard of making great errors, inasmuch as the same external symptoms may be due to very different internal causes; and finally, that it virtually makes out disease as consisting of an aggregate of external symptoms, whereas it is universally conceded that disease exists by virtue of an internal dynamic cause, no less a cause than a deranged condition of some of the vital forces or susceptibilities.

Now, I hold strictly to the therapeutic law. I maintain that, viewed from the stand-point of the prescriber, the aggregate of the symptoms does constitute the disease. That in no other way than by selecting his drugs in strict accordance with the similarity of the symptoms, can he so surely prescribe accurately, and cure his patient quickly. Nevertheless, I shall endeavor to show you that this adherence to the law is by no means equivalent to a declaration that the symptoms are really the disease; I shall show you that we are in no danger of confounding different diseases—misled by a similarity of their symptoms—if we strictly follow the law. And then, if I do not show you as we proceed in our course, that for the proper study of symptoms before we get ready to prescribe for our patient, we have need of and must employ our knowledge of physiology and pathology to the utmost extent of our resources, bringing every auxiliary medical science to bear on our study of symptoms, I shall submit to be offered a sacrifice to the offended divinities of these respectable

THE THERAPEUTIC LAW. 49

sciences—auxiliary merely and subsidiary as they are to the great practical end and aim of medicine, the application of drugs to the cure of the sick.

The symptoms which a patient presents do not constitute the essence of the disease; they are not the disease itself, they are only a result of the disease. This we freely admit. We have already stated that the essential nature of the disease is to be sought in a modification of that mysterious property of the organic cell-walls, by virtue of which the respective organs of the body perform their functions. In the healthy body we know nothing of the nature of this property or vital force. We should not know of its existence were it not for the functions which, by virtue of its exercise, the organs of the body perform. But in like manner, we should not know that the action of this mysterious force was perverted in disease, were it not that in consequence of its perversion the functions of the organs of the body are performed in an abnormal manner. But the abnormal performance of its function by any organ of the body constitutes a symptom of disease. It is, therefore, from the existence of symptoms of disease that we argue the existence of disease. *Per contra,* if no symptoms of disease present themselves to our scrutiny, we cannot know that disease exists. It is, therefore, strictly correct to say that we recognize the existence of disease only through the existence of its symptoms. It is manifest, then, that if we can cause the permanent cessation and disappearance of symptoms we shall have effected an annihilation of the disease, in so far as it is possible to judge of this matter. And it follows that the declaration that the aggregate of the symptoms is, from the practical stand-point, equivalent to the disease, is correct, because, the aggregate of the symptoms being permanently removed, we are justified in assuming that their cause has been removed.

It has been objected to the mode of prescribing which the law, *Similia similibus curantur,* enjoins, that it is a prescribing for the symptoms and not for the disease. This is not a fair criticism. The symptoms are our guide in selecting the remedy. It does not follow that they are the object of our prescription. This no more follows than it follows that because a traveler in a strange road goes from guide-post to guide-post, from mile-stone to mile-stone, therefore the guide-posts and mile-stones are the object of his journey, that his sole purpose is to find and come up with one after another of these useful indicators, these symptoms that he is on the right road.

The objection of which we are speaking, viz., to the treatment of symptoms, is well grounded only in cases where one or a very few symptoms are taken as the basis of the prescription, while the remaining symptoms are ignored. Where this is done, we often see deplorable mistakes committed. A remarkable instance of this is furnished by a celebrated surgical case. When Mr. Perceval was short, as he came out from the House of Commons, being mistaken for Sir Robert Peel, he came under the care of the celebrated surgeon, Mr. Guthrie. The wound was of the thoracic walls. The public interest in the case was very great. Daily bulletins were required, and were issued. Mr. Guthrie reported that his patient's wound was doing well and that his prospects of recovery were excellent. One day, after such a report, the patient died; and it was discovered at the autopsy that he died of empyema (or pus in the cavity of the pleura). How came Mr. Guthrie to blunder so terribly? Why, it was explained in this way. His specialty being surgery, he had confined his attention to the wound and had overlooked the symptoms of pleuritis which had no doubt been present for a number of days, obvious to whomsoever had eyes to see. To give this case as an instance of the impropriety of judging and prescribing according to the symptoms of a case, is to lose sight of the fact that our law requires that the aggregrate or totality of the symptoms be made the basis of the prescription. This is the all-important point.

Not only will care in this respect prevent our overlooking and failing to meet the real nature of the case; but it will obviate another objection which is raised against a prescription based on the symptoms, to wit: that the same symptom may depend upon any one of several morbid states, and that therefore we may be led to adopt a mode of treatment very suitable for one form of disease that often presents the symptoms before us, while in reality a very different disease is at the foundation of the symptoms of the case in hand. We admit this to be true of isolated symptoms or groups of symptoms, but we deny that it is true of aggregates of symptoms. The same aggregate or totality of symptoms can be produced only by the same morbific cause, acting in the same manner and direction. Were it otherwise, it would be impossible to distinguish between the two causes, since these imponderable causes are recognized only by their effects, the disease only by the totality of its symptoms.

This position should be illustrated by examples. The disease known as acute hydrocephalus has well-marked symptoms, indicating first, inflammation of the meninges of the brain, and then effusion with its resultant symptoms of oppression.

Now there is an affection, which is pathologically of a precisely opposite character, and which is not unfrequently met with, the hydrocephaloid affection described by Marshall Hall. The signs of irritation in the first stage and of oppression in the second stage, are so very similar to those of hydrocephalus acutus, as to deceive all but the most wary practitioners. Yet the symptoms of hydrocephalus acutus result from a true inflammation of the meninges of the brain, while those of the hydrocephaloid affection depend altogether upon a depressed state of the vegetative system,

THE THERAPEUTIC LAW. 53

in fact upon a starved condition of the organism, caused by either a too severe antiphlogistic course of treatment, or a too abstemious regimen during some general disease (not cerebral). The pathological difference is world-wide. The difference in the symptoms, so far as the brain symptoms are concerned, is hardly perceptible. Yet it is of the utmost importance, so far as the treatment is concerned, that these affections should be clearly distinguished. How shall it be done? Why, if we confine our attention to the brain symptoms alone (and a careless writer calls these the important symptoms), to the symptoms of that organ which seems to be chiefly affected, I hazard nothing in saying that the distinction cannot be made and the treatment cannot be judiciously selected.

But we have repeatedly stated that the aggregate of the symptoms, the totality of the symptoms, is to be regarded. Now, in this aggregate or totality are included not merely the brain symptoms, but likewise all other symptoms, and not merely the present state but also the past history or anamnesis of the patient. If we turn from the cerebral symptoms to the history and to the other symptoms of the patient, we shall find that whereas in the case of true hydrocephalus there is a hard, full, and rather frequent pulse with evident inflammatory fever, and the disease has come out from a state of tolerable, sometimes of what is called "ruddy," health; in the other affection the pulse is small, or, if full, is very soft, infrequent and irregular, the skin is cool, and the history of the patient discloses that the affection is always a sequel of some acute and exhausting malady, quite frequently of some one of the exanthematous fevers. Thus, a study of the totality of the symptoms rescues us from the danger into which we might fall from a study of a few prominent symptoms only,—the danger, namely, of confounding one disease with another, and of thus forming and adopting an erroneous plan of treatment.

Now, while these remarks are fresh in your minds, let me ask you to notice these facts. The example just cited shows you that while observations of symptoms may be correct, yet the conclusions drawn from them when we reason upon them may be altogether erroneous; and a treatment based upon this reasoning would be course be injudicious. Now, if we can base our plan of treatment directly upon the aggregate of the symptoms, without the interposition of a course of reasoning which may or may not be erroneous, but which is always liable to be false, shall we not be much more sure of success?

Another instance of an error in treatment from the exclusive observation of a few symptoms and the neglect of the aggregate, is so common among old-school practitioners that I may do you a service in mentioning it.

Young girls who have just become young women, and have grown rapidly, and have been perhaps assiduous at school, often complain of dyspnœa, of stitch in the side, of a slight cough, of lassitude. Their complexion may be very fair and a high color may give brilliancy to their cheeks, particularly in the afternoon. The doctor is called. The chest is the part complained of, and so he addresses his power of observation to the chest. He observes dyspnœa; ah! that shows infiltration in the air-cells; cough, irritation of the mucous surface; stitch in the side, circumscribed pleurisy of course; heightened color in the afternoon, what can this be but hectic? No more is needed to be looked for or asked about. He diagnosticates at once tuberculous deposit, inflammation around it, and incipient phthisis. Now is the very time for antiphlogistic measures, that we may nip it in the bud. Accordingly, if the doctor be of the very old school, he bleeds; if not so very old, he depletes in some less obvious, less sanguinary manner. But the patient does not improve. She grows steadily worse. If I had not very frequently seen such cases, were not indeed in the habit of seeing them, I should not venture to give such grows instances of error from forming a judgment on the basis of a few symptoms only. In truth, there is no tuberculosis, no inflammation about these cases. If the doctor had studied the totality of the symptoms, he would have found in the history of the case a fine state of health, gradually impaired by too close application at school; menstruation free and frequent, gradually diminished in quantity and frequency, and deteriorated in quality; the stitch in the side not, like that of pleurisy, aggravated by motion and pressure, but actually relieved by exertion in the open air; the supposed hectic no such thing, the pulse being actually at that time small, and though frequent, yet very soft and compressible, and the lungs, on percussion and auscultation, normal, showing that there can be no deposit in them. In addition to all this there will be a change in temperament and disposition, a timid, despondent, sighing and longing disposition, which makes the patient melancholy, prone to tears and easily discouraged, the very reverse of that which characterizes incipient phthisis. These symptoms all taken together clearly indicate the remedies required, if indeed any be needed. I express this doubt, because often a mere change of diet, regimen and associations will work the desired cure; while the antiphlogistic treatment, by rendering still more serious the existing debility, may induce the very state of things which, under an erroneous diagnosis, it supposes to exist and seeks to remove.

Be never content, then, to prescribe without carefully collecting and study the totality of the symptoms.

We know nothing about life, except through its manifestations in the functions of the living organism. Disease has been defined as modified life. Whatever life may be, disease is the same thing modified so as to have become abnormal. As life is known only through its manifestations, so can

THE THERAPEUTIC LAW. 57

disease be known only through its manifestations, which are the perverted functions of organs or the modified and altered tissues of the body. But we cannot have any knowledge of, or ability to recognize, a perverted function unless we be familiar with the healthy or normal function. We cannot recognize a changed or diseased tissue unless we be familiar with the healthy tissue. But we derive a knowledge of healthy tissue through the science of anatomy, and of healthy and normal functions through the science of physiology. It is, therefore, I think, a logical necessity to admit that we cannot recognize and study symptoms which are the manifestations of disease unless we be familiar with anatomy and physiology.

It is clear, then, that no matter in what way we may propose to use our symptoms in making a prescription, whether we compare them directly with those of drugs in order to find a simile, or whether we use them as the basis of theory, in correspondence with which we are to prescribe "on general principles," —it is clear, I say, that we cannot recognize nor obtain our symptoms without the aid of physiology.

Furthermore, we are to get the totality of the symptoms. So numerous are the organs of the body, so complex their functions, so intimate their relations to each other, so various their mutual reactions, that unless we follow some guiding method in the examination of the patient, we shall be in great danger of letting some symptom, or group of symptoms, obscure perhaps but all important, elude our vigilance.

Now, the relations of different organs of the body are so intimate, that when the functions of certain organs are altered it invariably happens that certain other organs likewise are affected. A knowledge of such facts as these affords us incalculable aid in getting at the true state of our patient, and it is indispensable. Knowledge of this kind belongs to the science of pathology which treats of the perverted functions and relations of the diseased organism.

Again, the function of an organ may be so modified as that, under certain conditions and circumstances, this modification must be regarded as a symptom of disease, while under other conditions it should not be so regarded. An enormous appetite which, under ordinary circumstances, would be a symptom of disease, might, during convalescence from a typhoid fever, be looked upon as not abnormal in any degree. So, too, of the cough in hypostatic pneumonia. So, likewise, of many alterations of taste and appetite, *e. g.*, for fruit at the close of rheumatic fever. But with the significance of the functions of the organism under various circumstances it is the special province of pathology to deal.

We perceive, then, that without the aid of physiology and pathology, we are utterly unable to recognize and to discriminate and estimate symptoms.

Now, I think, with these points settled, we may pass with quiet confidence to the practical question: How shall we study and arrange this totality of the symptoms, so as to make a prescription in accordance with it?

The therapeutic law requires us to select a drug of which the symptoms produced on the healthy are most similar to those of the patient. It appears, then, that we are to make a comparison between the aggregate of the patient's symptoms and the symptoms of the drugs in the materia medica, in order that we may find among these drugs that one drug of which the symptoms are the most similar. It is probable—indeed we well know—that the symptoms of a large number of drugs may present some similarity to each other and to the case in hand. A few will be very similar, and it may be very difficult to select from these that one which is most similar. The spirit of the whole process is evidently one of individualization. We take groups of drugs and analyze the symptoms they present, and select the one or the few that seem similar, and if there are several we analyze again, and select from among these that one which is the most similar. The process is the reverse of generalizing.

It is evident that for the convenience of this process, through which the prescriber must go at each prescription, drugs will naturally divide themselves into groups, the members of which resemble each other pretty closely, but which, nevertheless, may be distinguished from each other, and from all others by a few symptoms. Now, the symptoms which the members of these groups have in common are generic symptoms. These symptoms could never enable us to select the remedy, but they would point out to us a group of drugs, all of which possess these symptoms, and all of which are therefore tolerably similar; but which of these is most similar, we can only ascertain by finding some symptom or collocation of symptoms possessed by that drug alone, and which serves to distinguish it from all other drugs. Such symptoms are what are called characteristic symptoms, and are of the greatest importance to the prescriber.

They are different from those symptoms which the diagnostician would call characteristic, and which are pathognomonic symptoms.

Our next lecture will be on *Aconitum napellus.*

PRELIMINARY OBSERVATIONS.

DR. HERING has very happily explained that Hahnemann called his materia medica "pure," not as claiming that it is "spotless" or faultless, but that it is "free from fiction," from preconceived theory, from hypothetical notions; but it embodies the result of the pure observation of phenomena produced by drugs upon the healthy organism.

Such is our materia medica,—a record of actual occurrences, of events that really took place, of results that were unquestionably produced upon the healthy subject. It can never grow obsolete. Theories may be originated, may flourish and grow antiquated, and at last fade into oblivion. The hypotheses that constitute the science of pathology, after passing current for a generation or two, are sure to be rejected in favor of some newer issue, and the very terms in which they are expressed may become unintelligible as time goes on. But the facts of our materia medica, expressed in the ever-comprehensible vernacular language, are always fresh. Being the results of pure observation, and therefore absolutely true, no modifications in philosophy, no changes of theory, can supersede them. Our materia medica is an ever-enduring work.

It is of the utmost importance that it should always retain this quality of "purity," this freedom from fiction and from hypothesis. Very justly, therefore, do the leaders of our school denounce and discourage all attempts to incorporate into the materia medica speculations upon the *modus operandi* of remedies, and inferences, concerning the diseases which they may be likely to cure.

But we, whose business it is to encounter disease, the foe we are to grapple and to overcome, receive in our hands this weapon—the pure materia medica. And before we sally forth to encounter the Philistine, we need to "prove" our weapon, to test its strength, to feel its sharpness and to form an estimate of the feats we may reasonably hope to be able to accomplish with it,—to what tasks it will probably be equal, and for what others we shall need to look elsewhere for an implement. Now, as regards the result of the use of a weapon, much depends upon its shape, texture and temper. But much, likewise, depends on the strength and dexterity of him who uses it. The same sword that would serve only to trip up an awkward wearer may execute wonders of prowess in the hand of a master.

And thus it is with the records that make up our materia medica. The facts are the same to the eye of every reader. But where one mind may see only confusion and a maze of unconnected words, another may discern order and light and the outline of a definite and consecutive chain of pathological processes, and, consequently, a clear indication for the use of the drugs in the treatment of the sick.

For, while the materia medica, in the books, is a simple record of observed facts, in the mind of the practitioner it becomes the subject of reflection, of comparison and of hypothetical reasoning, which will be more or less just and valuable according to the measure of the practitioner's natural ability and of his intellectual culture. For, as has been already said, "the significance of a fact is measured by the capacity of the observer."

It follows, from this, that each practitioner sees, in every drug of the materia medica, some properties and capabilities different in degree, and perhaps even in kind, from those which his neighbors see in it, inasmuch as his natural endowments and his acquirements differ from theirs.

The experience of all of us corroborates this statement. Where one practitioner perceives in the proving of Nux vomica an indication for its use in constipation alone, others see equally strong reasons for giving it in diarrhœa, in prolapsus uteri, and in hernia; while only a few, perhaps, would find in the proving grounds for believing Nux vomica to be, as it is, one of our very best remedies in strumous ophthalmia.

Many practitioners infer from the provings that Lycopodium is likely to be a good remedy for some forms of chronic constipation and of disease of the bladder and kidney. Not so many, perhaps, would discern its value, as Dr. Wilson did, in acute pneumonia, or, as others have done, in that painful form of acute duodenitis which is often loosely called bilious colic. Colocynth is universally recognized as a remedy for flatulent colic, for one form of dysentery, and for a variety of neuralgia. But how many practitioners have seen in the proving good reason for using Colocynth to cure a chronic ovarian tumor? It has cured one.

It were needless to multiply instances of this kind. Those already cited show that, while all practitioners read the same proving, they perceive each a somewhat peculiar significance in what they read. By interchange of ideas on these subjects, physicians may be mutually benefited and their capacities for usefulness greatly enlarged. It would appear, then, that while the text of our materia medica should be sedulously kept "pure," as we have defined its purity, we may, with profit, interchange our deductions from what we read therein and our views of its practical application.

And there would seem to be not only room, but a legitimate demand, for essays, or still better, for systematic works on the drugs, studied from a therapeutical and clinical point of view, as a sort of complement to our materia medica pura, which very properly regards the remedies strictly from a pathogenetic stand-point. Such works would necessarily be of a transient nature and have only an ephemeral value, since they would group symptoms and would necessarily interpret them in accordance with the physiological and pathological notions of the day. But they might be of none the less service to the physician of the generation in which they appear, since it is by the light of such notions, transitory as they are, that he gropes his way among the difficulties and obstacles of his professional path.

Considerations of this kind have emboldened us to lay before our colleagues, hitherto always kindly indulgent of such efforts, a series of studies and reflections upon portions of the materia medica. They are avowedly fragmentary, and are devoid of all claim to other authority than such as may come from their intrinsic reasonableness.

In the form of these observations, we propose to follow, in a general way, the *schema* contained in a paper called "Homœopathy the Science of Terapeutics" published in another volume,[1] although in the remarks on Aconite we prefer to change the order there given, making the special analysis precede, instead of follow, the general analysis.

[1] Homœopathy the Science of Therapeutics.

ACONITUM NAPELLUS.

REGARDING each drug of the materia medica as possessed of individual specific properties peculiar to itself, and which preclude its being a substitute for, or being superseded by, any other drug, it is not material with which drug we begin our special course.

Aconitum napellus, known as monkshood, from the shape of its flowers, and as wolfsbane, from the use made of its poisonous juice to exterminate obnoxious animals, was known to the ancients as an active poison, but was first proved by Stoerck in 1761. A proving of it was published by Hahnemann in the "Materia Medica Pura," vol. II. A valuable essay was published by Dr. Fleming, of Edinburgh, in 1844, which did much to cause the drug to be used by allopaths. There is no doubt that Dr. Fleming derived many of his ideas on the subject from the homœopathicians of his vicinity, although he does not allude to their use of Aconite.

It happens that Aconite is frequently indicated at the very beginning of some acute diseases and that, if properly used in such cases, it will often cut short the career of the disease. From these facts has arisen a fashion of giving Aconite almost as a routine prescription in the beginning of all acute cases indiscriminately; particularly if the cases are supposed to be characterized by that Protean phantom of the pathologist, inflammation.

Great mischief often results from this practice; negatively, inasmuch as it causes the loss of valuable time, during which the true specific remedy which should have been given at the very first, might have been acting; and, positively, inasmuch as the Aconite often, when inappropriately administered, does real mischief, exhausting the nervous power of the patient and adding to a prostration which is already, probably, the great source of danger.

From experiments upon animals and men, Drs. Pereira and Stillé, of the allopathic school, conclude that Aconite is a "cerebro-spinant," a "nervous sedative." Its first action is to benumb the nerves of sensation. This it does when taken internally; producing first, a sensation of warmth in the fauces, then, a rough prickling or smarting, and then, a want of sensibility and an absence of the sense of taste. When applied locally to the external skin, it produces anæsthesia, without, at first, impairing the motive power. It does not affect the consciousness and intelligence until its action is carried to a very considerable extent. (In this respect it is in direct opposition to Cocculus.) Preceding the anæsthesia, are observed all the sensations which characterize incomplete anæsthesia, such as tingling and pricking of the fingers and toes, numbness, etc.

A gentle feeling of warmth is diffiused throughout the body. This soon becomes increased to a disagreeable sense of internal heat with distention of the brain, lips and face, along with a very profuse perspiration over the whole body, itching and a miliary eruption. (Pereira, Stillé, Wood, Sturm.)

Dr. Fleming describes, in addition, nausea and oppression at the stomach, and a peculiar tingling sensation at the roots of the teeth. The pulse and respiration, which were at first markedly accelerated, become, after a time, retarded and enfeebled. When pushed to extremes, the cases of Aconite poisoning prove fatal with the usual symptoms of narcotico-sedative poisoning. They furnish no distinctive characteristic symptoms.

The proving by Hahnemann was corroborated in a remarkable degree by a proving conducted in Vienna, in 1847, by the Homœopathic Society of that city, under the guidance of Dr. Gerstel. From these combined provings we derive the following portrait of the action of Aconite, in which we shall follow the anatomical order adopted by Hahnemann.

SPECIAL ANALYSIS.

Sensorium. Aconite produces a well-marked vertigo, a sensation as of a swaying to and fro in the brain. This is increased by stooping and by motion generally, especially by suddenly rising from a recumbent posture. Sometimes vision is obscured by it. In connection with these symptoms, a bursting headache, accelerated pulse, and internal heat of the head, with, at the same time, perspiration of the head and thorax. The character of the vertigo resembles that of Glonoine and Bryonia, and is the opposite of the vertigo produced by China, Ferrum and Theridion.

The mind is distraught, the thoughts confused, memory weakened.

Head. Heaviness and pressure in the forehead, as if there were a load there pressing outward, and as if all would come out there; pressive pains in the temples. Headache, as if the brain were pressed outward. Throbbing and internal soreness. Stitching and pressing headache, involving the eyes; also extending down into the upper jaw bone, with nausea.

The headache is characteristic,—pressing from within outward, sometimes throbbing. Its location is the forehead and temples, involving the eyes and upper jaw. It is aggravated by motion, stooping and noise, and relieved by repose. Head and face are hot, especially internally, and covered with hot perspiration.

Eyes. A sharp, anxious expression. They become distorted. Sharp, darting pain in the supraorbital region. The pupils are, at first, dilated. The globe of the eye and the lids feel very dry. Subsequently, there is a feeling of pressure in the eye, and pain when the ball revolves in the orbit.

Severe inflammation and chemosis are recorded. Pressure and burning in the eye and over the brow. Moderate photophobia.

Ears. Indefinite pains and pressure.

Face. Tingling in the cheeks. Sweat covers the cheeks. The face is red and hot, cheeks glow. A sensation as if the face were growing large.

Nose. Nose-bleeding.

Mouth. The lips burn and feel swollen. Mouth dry with thirst.

Teeth. Sensitive to cool air.

Tongue. Burning, tingling and pricking. Feels as if it were swollen.

Throat. Rough and scraped sensation.

Gastric Symptoms. Bitter, flat taste. Loss of appetite, salivation, great thirst, discomfort after food, nausea and vomiting. Burning in stomach and œsophagus.

Stomach. Pressure in the stomach and both hypochondria as if a stone lay there (resembles Bryonia, Arnica) extending through to the back.

Heaviness in stomach and hypochondria. After repeated vomitings there still remains a sensation as if a cold stone lay in the stomach. (Compare Colchicum.)

Burning in the stomach and umbilical region extending to the epigastrium with throbbing, at length a shivering followed by heat.

Abdomen. Pinching pain in various parts of the abdomen. Very sensitive to touch and pressure. Distended as in dropsy.

ACONITUM NAPELLUS. 71

Stool. Fluid, rather watery. Sometimes greenish, with some pain and flatulence. Generally fœcal. Irritation of the hæmorrhoidal vessels.

Anus. Sensation as of a discharge of warm fluid from the anus.

Urine. High colored, strong in odor and scanty, without sediment. It is passed frequently. Upon the sexual organs no definite effect is noticed.

Respiratory organs. Sense of smell unnaturally acute. Nasal membrane dry and irritable. Sneezing frequent and violent, though often restrained because of the pain which it produces in the walls of the abdomen or of the stitch in the left side of the thorax, which it often provokes.

Larynx and Trachea. Larynx very painful. Sensitive to inhaled air, as if it were deprived of its outer covering. This is an intense degree of the sensation of rawness, roughness, etc., in the larynx, of which every prover complains.

Sensation as if the larynx were compressed from all sides. Sensation of dryness and roughness in the larynx and all along the trachea. This sensation often gives rise to a little hacking cough.

Irritation (provoking a cough) in the larynx, on coming from the open air into a warm room. (Ranunculus bulbosus, the same. Rumex, Squilla, Ipecacuanha and Bryonia, have cough provoked by change from cold to warm air.)

Cough. Dry, hacking, from rawness in larynx and trachea. Or a forcible cough, producing a taste like that of blood.

Cough always dry, except when attended by clear bloody expectoration.

Cough accompanied by excoriated sore pains in the thorax.

Cough relieved when lying on the back, worse when lying on the sides.

Expectoration bloody, or consisting of clear blood.

Thorax. Much dyspnœa. Frequent deep sighing respiration. One prover, Zlatarovich, says:

"Frequent deep inspiration, not sighing, but like a desire to accelerate the course of the blood through the lungs."

Heaviness and fullness upon the chest, as though one could not dilate the thorax, compelling deep inspirations, conjoined with restlessness, anxiety and palpitation. Audible (subjectively) crepitation. Accelerated breathing.

Besides the heaviness, there are ill-defined stitches in the intercostal spaces, generally low on the right side, aggravated by deep inspiration.

Heat and burning in the lungs.

Heart. Movements irregular and inharmonious. Palpitation, which is worse when walking. Violent palpitation, with great anxiety, during repose as well as in motion. Anguish in the region of the heart, with rapid and powerful action of that organ.

Oppression, especially in the region of the heart. A pressing-in pain in the region of the heart.

The following remarkable symptom is reported by Zlatarovich, a keen and daring prover: Lancinating stitches in the region of the heart, feeling as if they were in the costal pleura, and which prevent the erect posture and deep inspiration, with disposition to cough; relieved by friction and by occasional deep inspiration; but the part remains sore.

Back. Pressive, drawing, tearing and numb sensations in various parts of the back. Sensitiveness in the region of the kidneys. Particularly a weariness and soreness in the lumbar and sacral region.

Upper Extremities. The same creeping, tingling, paralytic sensations in these parts as in the skin generally. Drawing, tearing pains in the joints of the hands and fingers.

Lower Extremities. Great lassitude of the legs, and weariness and heaviness of the feet. They refuse to perform their function. Drawing pains in the hip-joint on motion. Drawing and tearing in the tendinous expansion of the legs and feet. Drawing and pain in the tendo Achillis.

Sleep. Great sleepiness, as if from exhaustion, during the day. Nights are very restless. Patients sleep lightly; are too wide awake to sleep; restless and full of dreams.

Restless, alternating cold and heat, thirst and anguish.

Dreams terrifying and very vivid.

Skin. Itching, tingling, prickling, and paralytic, and all degrees of commencing and incomplete anæsthesia.

Reddish papules, filled with acrid moisture. Broad, red itching papules on the whole body, spots like flea-bites on the hands, face, etc.

General Condition. Whole body sensitive to touch.

Sensibility as after a long fit of sickness.

Paralytic sensation and lassitude in the whole body, especially in the arms and feet, with trembling of the whole body, and especially of the extremities,—one can hardly walk,—with very pale face, dilated pupils, faintness, palpitation, cold sweat on the back, and a bursting asunder headache in the temples. Soon after this comes burning heat in the face, with sensation of distention, redness of the face and sleepiness.

Joints. Pains in all the joints. Weakness of the joints, especially of the knees and feet. Weakness and laxity of the ligaments of all the joints.

Fever Chilliness, especially over the back and abdomen. Fugitive chills from the middle of the spine down the loins on each side.

Chilliness and formication between the shoulders and down the back. Shivering.

These symptoms at first alternate with heat, and are, finally, followed, as the Austrian provings show, by general and constant heat; dry heat of the whole body; burning heat; heat with moderate sweat.

Heat, with contracted, full, strong pulse, about 100 per minute in the adult.

Copious sweat, especially at night. Special and

general senses unnaturally acute. Noise, light, odor and touch are unpleasant.

Disposition. Very anxious, restless, full of forebodings, either ill-defined forebodings, or, sometimes, a definite anticipation or prediction of the day of death.

If we now review the symptoms of Aconite, as they have been detailed, for the purpose of making a general analysis of the action of that drug upon the organism, we find,

1. The action on the vital power is of such a nature that while the nerves of sensation are more or less benumbed (by large doses), the voluntary and involuntary muscles and the power of locomotion are but little affected. The action on the sensorium and on the special senses may, perhaps, be accounted for by that which is the most marked effect of Aconite, viz., the exalted activity which it produces in the arterial circulation.

The brain is congested; so are the lungs and the kidneys (as, indeed, the autopsies plainly show). The susceptibility of the special senses is greatly exalted.

2. *Action on the Organic Substance.* Of very few drugs, so powerfully poisonous as Aconite is, even in moderate doses, can it be said, as of Aconite, that they produce hardly any appreciable effect upon the organic substance,—hardly any change in the tissues or fluids of the body. The records of fatal cases of poisoning, as well as our provings, bear witness to this fact.

The complexion is affected only in so far as the capillary blood-vessels are contracted, producing paleness, and then congested, with redness and heat.

The evacuations can hardly be called abnormal, the urine being merely high-colored, inasmuch as it is concentrated. It is a peculiarity of Aconite that urine secreted under its influence has no sediment.

The cutaneous eruption furnishes the only modification to the above statement. It is of such a character as led Hahnemann to recommend Aconite in some cases of measles and miliary rash. There is no resemblance in the symptoms of Aconite to the features of any dyscrasia.

3. *Sphere of Action.* The head, the respiratory organs, the heart and the joints, seem to be the parts most markedly the seat of the local action of Aconite. In all of these, except, perhaps, the joints, the symptoms point rather to arterial excitement than to definite organic change, involving alteration of existing tissues or formation or deposit of new substances.

4. *Sensations.* These are mostly drawing pains,—or the various grades of anæsthesia,—from sticking, prickling, tingling, etc., down to absolute default of sensation.

5. *Periodicity.* None at all.

6. *Peculiarities.* The symptoms of Aconite are generally aggravated by warmth and motion, and also at night.

ACONITUM NAPELLUS. 77

There is one group of symptoms so characteristic of Aconite that Hahnemann said, "Aconite should not be given in any case which does not present a similar group of symptoms." These are the symptoms of the mind and disposition, viz.: Restlessness, anxiety and uneasiness of mind and body, causing tossing and sighing and frequent change of posture; forebodings, anticipations of evil, anguish of mind, dread of death, and even distinct anticipations of its occurrence.

Turning now to consider the kind of cases in which Aconite is most likely to be indicated by the similarity of its symptoms, we cannot do better than carefully ponder Hahnemann's most excellent cautions, contained in the introduction to the proving of Aconite. "In order to banish from our conscientious mode of treatment all of that quackery which is only too glad, in selecting its remedy, to be guided by the name of the disease, we must take care that whenever we give Aconite the chief symptoms of the malady, that is, of the acute disease, shall be such as are to be found in the strongest similarity among those of Aconite!"

This is the whole secret of a successful prescription of any drug under any circumstances, viz.: that whatever name we may choose to give to the patient's malady we shall select for its cure that drug which presents symptoms most similar, not to those which we regard as pathognomonic of the disease so named, but to those of that very patient, at the time of the prescription. "Then," as Hahnemann truly says, "then is the result most wonderful."

Hahnemann speaks of Aconite as likely to be of service "in those cases in which medicine has hitherto employed the most dangerous methods,—for example, copious blood-letting, the entire antiphlogistic apparatus,—and, too often, in vain and with the saddest results. I mean the so-called inflammatory fever in which the smallest dose of Aconite makes the entire antipathic methods of treatment altogether superfluous, and helps quickly and without sequelæ. In measles and miliary fever and in inflammatory pleuritic fevers, its power to help approaches the marvelous, when, the patient being kept somewhat cool, Aconite is given alone, all other medicinal substances being carefully avoided, even including vegetable acids." He then cautions us to avoid prescribing Aconite for a patient simply because we have given to his malady one of the above names, and enjoins us to be sure that the patient's symptoms closely correspond with those of Aconite.

"Exactly in those cases," he proceeds, "in which allopathy is most accustomed to regard herself as the only possible savior, in severe, acute, inflammatory fevers, in which she resorts to copious and frequent bleedings, and thereby imagines she far surpasses all homœopathic treatment in the help she affords exactly here, is she most in the wrong. Precisely in this is the infinite superiority of homœopathy displayed; that she has no need to spill a drop of blood, that precious vital fluid (which the allopaths so ruthlessly set streaming), in order to convert this dangerous fever into health again in just as many hours as the allopathist's life-exhausting treatment often requires months for a complete restoration; if indeed death shall not have rendered this impossible, or if it have not been supplanted by artificially produced chronic sequelæ."

"Sometimes," Hahnemann observes, "after Aconite has acted for several hours, a change in the symptoms may call for some other remedy; and," he adds, "it is extremely seldom that, after this, a second dose of Aconite is called for." It is manifest that the too frequent practice of giving in alternation repeated doses of Aconite and Belladonna, or Aconite and Bryonia, or Aconite and some other remedy, did not originate, and would not have found favor with Hahnemann.

Hahnemann continues: "In as short a time as four hours after the first dose of Aconite, thus carefully administered in the above-named diseases, all danger to life will have passed and the excited circulation will then, hour by hour, gradually return to its wonted course.

"So, likewise, Aconite, in the above-named small dose, is the first and chief remedy in the inflammation of the trachea (croup); in several kinds of inflammation of the throat and fauces; as well as in local acute inflammations of all other parts, especially where, in conjunction with thirst and a rapid pulse there are present in anxious impatience, a restlessness not to be quieted, distress and an agonized tossing about.

"Aconite produces all the morbid symptoms, the like of which are wont to appear in persons who have had a fright, combined with vexation; and for these symptoms it is the best remedy.

"Always, in choosing Aconite, as the homœopathic remedy, especial regard must be paid to the symptoms of the disposition and mind, for these, above all, must be similar.

"Hence, Aconite is indispensable to women after fright and vexation, during menstruation, which, without this soothing remedy, is often instantaneously suppressed by such moral shocks."

If we add to these practical directions of Hahnemann, the conclusions to which our analysis of the sphere of action of Aconite has led us, we shall begin to comprehend a large variety, at least, of the cases which call for Aconite.

As we have seen, Aconite, when given in moderate doses, excites the circulation, increases the heat of the surface and produces perspiration; it affects the innervation, producing extreme sensitiveness of the surface of the body to contact and the correlative sensation of tingling, etc.; in short, an incomplete anæsthesia. But it does not alter (in kind) the function of any organ, nor does it set up any new action in any organ to tissue.

Aconite produces, so far as we know, almost no localized diseased condition.

Even when given in large and fatal doses, it

ACONITUM NAPELLUS. 81

acts as a depressant, paralyzing the cerebro-spinal nervous system; but it produces death by this paralysis and without previously localizing its action in any organ or system. It gives evidence of no dyscrasia. Its action bears no resemblance to that of the poison which produces any of the miasmatic diseases—such as the exanthemata, or typhus or intermittent, remittent or continued fevers. Neither does its action, from beginning to end of a fatal case of poisoning, resemble the well-defined course of any local, acute inflammation—as of the brain, heart, lungs, pleura, etc.

For these reasons, Aconite can never come into requisition (save possibly (?) as a rare and temporary intermittent in some complication) for any of the miasmatic fevers or dyscratic diseases; because, in these the dyscrasia precedes and gives its features to the acute manifestations of the disease (and, therefore, the symptoms cannot find their analogue in those of Aconite).

Moreover, Aconite can never be the single remedy by the influence of which a patient may be safely carried through a complete course of pure, acute inflammation of any organ or system; because, in the action of Aconite, that localization is lacking which is the essential feature of these diseases. Yet in all of these pure inflammations, there is a period in which Aconite may be indicated and may do an heroic work. For every one of these inflammations which eventually become localized has a first stage which consists of arterial excitement; and which is prior to that stage that is characterized by change of function and of tissue and by local deposit. This stage is that in which Aconite plays so important a part and in which, if promptly and judiciously employed, it may arrest and cut short the entire disease.

Thus it may be employed in meningitis, ophthalmia, tonsillitis, croup, bronchial catarrh, pneumonia, pulmonary congestion and hæmoptysis, pleuritis, pericarditis and endocarditis (and as a palliative in hypertrophy), gastritis, peritonitis, acute rheumatism, neuralgia super-orbitalis; but only when the moral symptoms named by Hahnemann are present.

It is to such a use of Aconite in acute inflammations that Hahnemann undoubtedly refers when he speaks of its ability to restore to health in a few hours, saying: "In as short a time as a few hours, after the first dose of Aconite, thus carefully administered * * all danger to life will have passed and the excited circulation will then, hour by hour, gradually return to its wonted course." So rapid a change as this would be very possible and easily conceivable in the first stage of acute pneumonia before hepatization has taken place; whereas, after hepatization has become established, it would not be conceivable and we have no reason to suppose it ever takes place. Hence the propriety of Hahnemann's caution, in the following words: "Sometimes after the Aconite has acted for several hours, a change in the symptoms may call for some other drug; and it is extremely seldom that, after this, a second dose of Aconite is called for." Why? Because, probably, the inflammation has passed from the stage of arterial excitement to that of organic localization, and Aconite no longer corresponds. And, probably, that very "change in the symptoms" which called "for some other drug," was a sign that localization had taken place.

This view is in entire harmony with Hahnemann's urgent admonition to heed what he regarded as the great characteristic indication of Aconite: "the anguish of mind and body, the restlessness, the disquiet not to be allayed." This state of mind and body accords precisely with the general phenomena of that arterial excitement which attends the invasion of an acute inflammation, while the localization of the inflammation and the occurrence of exudation are marked by a subsidence of this general anguish; symptoms of local organic embarrassment being substituted for it; and the general constitutional symptoms being rather those of exhaustion and a depressed condition. Whoever has closely watched a number of cases of pneumonia through the first and second stages will, I think, corroborate these views.

Here, then, we have again an example of what the student of materia medica so often meets,— the entire coincidence of the teachings of a sound pathology with the results of an intelligent and discriminating application of the law of the selection of the drug by the correspondence of characteristic symptoms.

Though it is always hazardous to undertake the illustration of a scientific point by a rhetorical simile, we may venture to liken the action of Aconite and cognate remedies to the onset and effects of a tempest. Whoever is familiar with the general character of North America from the Alleghanies to the Atlantic, must have had opportunity to overlook some fertile valley in the luxuriance of its midsummer vegetation. As he enjoys the prospect, the breeze subsides, and the sunlight becomes obscured. The cattle cease to graze; they move uneasily through the field and snuff the air as if in dread. Soon the incongruous swayings of the foliage in different parts of the valley make it evident that the air is agitated by varying eddies and currents. To the same cause are due the variations in the sounds of the murmur of the brook and the hum of insects and the chitter of birds, that are brought to the ear at successive moments. Clouds of dust rise from portions of the winding road and are borne whirling along and upward. The cattle become more and more uneasy; they rush wildly to and fro through the meadows. A sound as of rushing waters comes up the valley, with a blast of cool air having an odor of freshly cut herbage, or faintly ammoniacal; clouds of dust envelop the spectator; the tempest breaks upon him and for a time he realizes nothing but wild confusion, and the crash and roaring of the elements in unrestrained collision.

After a short time the winds abate; the atmos-

ACONITUM NAPELLUS. 85

phere becomes clear and quiet prevails again. All things have resumed their normal state. Nature, animate and inanimate, has come to her former condition of repose. The violence of the tempest has swept past,—to spend itself in permanent effects elsewhere.

This represents, well enough the action of Aconite, which raises an arterial and nervous storm, and, though in fatal cases its fury may be great enough to induce chaos, that is, death, yet it does not localize itself in organic changes. Or, if the tempest be considered as representing disease, then Aconite is a happy influence (we know of none such in inanimate nature) which turns aside its force and sends it to expend its energies in material changes elsewhere.

But, the tempest does not always pass thus lightly over the valley. It too often happens, that when the calm that follows its outbreak permits the spectator again to survey the region, he looks upon a scene wholly changed. Trees have been prostrated, perhaps, and buildings overturned. The mill has been carried away, the dam has failed to resist the sudden increase of the stream; where was once a broad expanse of tranquil water is now an oozing waste, threaded by a narrow creek. The cattle are scattered and the crops destroyed. Havoc has been made and desolation reigns. The processes of nature still go on, but in every condition how changed!

This represents, in some sort, the action of

drugs which, like Aconite, produce a storm of general vascular and nervous excitement, but which, unlike Aconite, produce, after this storm, as a sort of sequel of it, a definite localization of pathogenetic action, viz., changes of function and tissues.

Such a remedy is Bryonia, in its action on the lungs and pleura, and Belladonna, in its action on the brain and lungs; such, indeed, are most of our remedies. For there are few storms which do not make more or less of local havoc.

With a few disconnected remarks, we may close these desultory observations.

It is clear that Aconite may be given in acute inflammation of every organ of the body, but only in a certain stage of a certain form of inflammation. How shall we know when this stage and form are before us? When, in addition to whatever signs there may be which designate the organ which is affected, the symptoms which have been called characteristic of Aconite are present; the heat of surface, or external cold and internal heat, thirst, quick, excited but not hard pulse, copious sweat with burning heat; and, above all, anguish and restlessness of mind and body, tossing which will not be quieted, foreboding and anticipation of death.

So, then, after all this talk, involving the terms and speculations of pathology, the selection of the remedy comes down again to a comparison of symptoms.

Yes! for the sagacity of the master led him to see clearly that the symptoms of the patient are the only facts of which we have absolute knowl-

ACONITUM NAPELLUS. 87

edge as concerns the patient; and the symptoms of the drug are the only facts that we absolutely know respecting it, and the relation in which they must be placed to neutralize each other, if it be found, must be such as to satisfy every sound hypothesis constructed on these facts. It must, consequently, harmonize with sound pathology. And many times this volume of talk will have been well bestowed if it shall convince any thoughtful mind that, first and most important, stands the correspondence of symptoms according to their rank, and that to this same result all sound hypotheses must lead.

Aconite is never to be given "first to subdue the fever," and then some other remedy to "meet the case;" never to be alternated with other drugs for the purpose, as is often alleged, of "controlling fever." If the fever be such as to require Aconite, no other drug is needed. If other drugs seem indicated, one should be sought which meets the fever as well; for many drugs besides Aconite produce fever, each after his kind.

Aconite may be called for, if the symptoms correspond, in the first stage of every acute inflammation, but remove from the mind the idea that it cures all inflammations; *e. g.,* in the second stage of pneumonia it is good for nothing.

It is a remedy of unspeakable value in a vast many cases of acute hæmoptysis, which present the general symptoms as above detailed, characteristic of Aconite, and yet the pathological origin of which, and their ultimate nature, if not controlled, are involved in obscurity. The blood is florid. (Spitting of florid blood, without the restless anguish of Aconite, calls for Millefolium.)

Aconite should never be given to "save time" while the physician goes home to study up the case. This is slovenly practice; it were better to give nothing, because Aconite, if given in a case which does not call for it, may do mischief; as, for example, in the commencement of typhoid fever, in which it will unfavorably influence the entire course of the disease, unless symptoms call for it, which they rarely if ever can do.

Notwithstanding this fact, so wide-spread has the notion become that Aconite is the remedy for fever, that the allopaths have adopted and are now using it as the stock remedy for typhoid fever in Bellevue Hospital (1864). The death rate does not lessen. Prescribing on a single symptom (it reduces the pulse in large doses) they give it in typhoid, overlooking the great pathological fact of the dyscrasia, to which Aconite has no relation whatever. Had they adopted Arsenic for typhoid, there would have been good pathological defense for them.

There are writers on the homœopathic materia medica who create a theory of the action of Aconite, and make it the great antiphlogistic. Hence they are compelled by logical consistency to recommend Aconite in all diseases, a flagrant illustration of the folly of prescribing on a pathological theory.

BRYONIA ALBA.

THE tincture of the root of *Bryonia alba,* or dilutions made from it, were used by Hahnemann in his provings. The root of this vine, which grows in hedge-rows and along fences in England and on the continent of Europe, furnishes us the tincture from which our preparations are made.

Pereira calls Bryonia a violent emetic and purgative. Trousseau and Pidoux speak of it as an active purgative, to be used like Colocynth and Elaterium. But Hermand de Montgomery declared that he had frequently cured vomiting, colic, diarrhœa and dysentery, with Bryonia,—an illustration, from allopathic sources, of the homœopathic curative action of this drug.

In the majority of modern works on materia medica, of the allopathic school, Bryonia is not mentioned. Yet it has for centuries been recognized, among the people of Europe, as a specific for certain ailments, and eminent physicians of earlier ages have recorded many cures by it. Cataplasms of the root were successfully used to scatter inflammatory swellings of the joints. This was a homœopathic prescription in so far as the selection of the drug was concerned. The ancients cured dropsy with it, and especially hydrothorax (and we use it for pleurisy with fluid exudation). Sydenham used Bryonia as a remedy for intermittent fever. Tests says the French peasants of Lorraine use the root as a specific remedy for hernia. I learned from observation that among the peasants residing in the Maremma, on the shores of the Mediterranean, north of the Pontine marshes, Bryonia is commonly (and successfully) used as a remedy for the peculiar type of intermittent and remittent fever which is endemic there. We shall see how these instances confirm the law of *Similia similibus curantur*.

Our entire knowledge of the action of Bryonia on the healthy subject is derived from the proving by Hahnemann and his pupils,[1] and from the Austrian provings, arranged by Professor Zlatarovich.[2] From these sources we construct the following *résumé* in which, as before, we follow the anatomical order:

Sensorium. The action of Bryonia is well defined and constant. Every prover describes, in language more or less emphatic, a "confusion of the head," a "distracted state of the sensorium." When we consider this symptom in conjunction with the peculiar febrile symptoms, the lassitude,

---

[1] "Materia Medica Pura," vol. ii. "Zeitschrift," vol. iii., 1857. "Œs-
[2] "Œstliche Homœopathische terreichische," 1847, vol. iii.

etc., we shall perceive its significance. Great heaviness of the whole head. Weight upon the vertex. Vertigo, when fasting, when standing, and especially on first rising from a seat, compelling to sit; often conjoined with headache in the occiput, aggravated by motion.

Headache. Dull, pressing headache in the forehead and temples; drawing and tensive headache in the temporal region; drawing and tearing pain from the temple down to the malar bone and to the lower jaw (this symptom promises aid from Bryonia in prosopalgia). Sticking, jerking, throbbing headache from the forehead backward to the occiput. (This symptom is characteristic, being paralleled in no other drug. Spigelia has pain darting from behind forward through the left eyeball. Silicea has pain coming up from the nape of the neck, through the occiput and over the vertex, and so down upon the forehead. Carbo vegetabilis has dull, heavy pain extending through the base of the brain, from the occiput to the supra-orbital region.)

The majority of the head-symptoms of Bryonia refer to the occiput, and we shall find it more frequently called for in headache involving the occiput In this respect it may be compared with Petroleum.

The sensorium is blunted.

All the symptoms of the head are aggravated by motion and exertion.

The pathologico-anatomical results of Bryonia poisoning are: "Redness of the diploe, injection of the inner surface of the cranium. Congestion of the membranes. A section of the cerebral substances is dotted here and there with blood."

Zlatarovich says: "The head-symptoms point to congestion and inflammation of the brain;" but, I think, the character of the fever and of the affection of the sensorium is such as to show that it is not likely to be a remedy in pure idiopathic encephalitis. If a remedy in encephalitis at all, it must be in those cases in which meningitis has supervened, by metastasis or otherwise, upon some previously existing miasmatic or other disease, *e.g.*, one of the exanthemata. The pains and perverted function of the two upper branches of the fifth pair of nerves call to mind prosopalgia.

The affections of the head and sensorium are worse in the morning; not immediately on awaking (as with Lachesis), but after waking and moving the eyes and head (see stool—diarrhœa).

Face. Red, hot and puffed. Red spots on the face and neck. The face is swollen; sometimes so much so as to close the eye. The pains are those that have been described as extending between the temple and the malar bone, and are of a tearing, drawing character.

Eyes. Lids swollen and puffed. A sensation of pressure from within outward in the globe of the eye, a kind of distention. The conjunctiva seems to be moderately inflamed, judging from these symptoms: sensation as if there were sand in the eyes; increased secretion of tears; discharge of muco-pus from the eye, obstructing vision; itching and burning of the margin of the lids. The right eye is most affected.

Contrary to the general rule with Bryonia, the eye symptoms are aggravated by warmth. The special sense of vision is not affected in Hahnemann's proving, but Zlatarovich mentions a play of colors.

Ears. Sensation of obstruction in the external meatus and noises in the ears are the chief symptoms. Discharge of blood from the ear is mentioned; this may possibly be accounted for as an instance of vicarious menstruation.

Nose. Often swollen at the extremity, with a sharp pain and sensitiveness to the touch. Frequent and repeated epistaxis,—a symptom recorded by many provers. It occurs in the morning, sometimes awaking the prover from sleep. The blood is florid. Nose-bleeding after the sudden suspension of menses has been observed under the action of Bryonia. It is probably this symptom which has induced the use of Bryonia in vicarious menstruation.

Mouth. The lips are swollen, with a biting, burning eruption. Aphthous patches appear on the lining membrane of the mouth and fauces. Dr. Huber, of Lenz, one of the Austrian provers, states that his proving of Bryonia cured him of a constitutional tendency to aphthous formations in the throat. The tongue is dry.

The teeth feel long and loose; drawing or

jumping toothache when eating or just after eating, or in the evening in bed ; aggravated by warmth, contrary to the general rule with Bryonia. Teeth and gums are sore.

Throat. Sticking pain on swallowing, on feeling of the throat and on bending the neck. Sensation of pressure or fullness. Great dryness in the throat.

Digestive Organs. Taste unpleasant, flat, even with good appetite; sometimes bitter, sometimes putrid, with offensive breath; appetite generally diminished or destroyed, with aversion to food. One prover (Fr. H.) records an excessive desire for good, which, however, ceased as soon as the prover began to eat.

Thirst increased.

After eating, eructations, sometimes tasting of the food but generally bitter or sour, with an accumulation of sour water, sometimes tasteless, in the mouth.

Hiccough is a frequent symptom.

Nausea after a meal, although the food tasted well and was eaten with relish.

Nausea and vomiting, morning and evening, chiefly of water and mucus. Also, vomiting of food and of a fluid consisting of mucus and bile, and very bitter.

Food oppresses the stomach, is felt like a load at the epigastrium, and is often regurgitated.

Stomach and Abdomen. Pressure in the epigastrium, worse after eating and when walking. This pain sometimes extends down to the umbilical region; sometimes even to the bladder and perinæum.

After eating, there is often a constricting pain in the stomach, then a cutting in the epigastrium and then vomiting of food. The pains are worse during motion as is the general rule with Bryonia pains.

Sensation of distention, and sometimes actual swelling in the umbilical region.

Pains, sticking and shooting in both sides of the abdomen, aggravated by motion and sometimes changing into stitches from the abdomen into the stomach. The stitches the most frequent in the region of the spleen.

In the hepatic region, on the contrary, we find a tensive, burning pain; with a stitch which occurs only when the region is pressed upon, or when the prover coughs or takes a deep inspiration.

Flatulence moderate. Its movements occasionally produce pain.

Stool. It is a peculiarity of Bryonia that, in moderate doses, it produces, in the healthy prover, retention of stool; the stool is infrequent, large in form, solid and evacuated with difficulty and attended by prolapsus of the rectum and burning sensation. Besides this characteristic action, Bryonia produces also, as an alternate action, a kind of diarrhœa preceded by colic, occurring especially at night (or early morning as soon as the patient rises and begins to walk about), and coming on so suddenly that the prover can hardly prevent an involuntary evacuation.[1]

Zlatarovich calls especial attention to the tenderness of the abdominal walls generally; to the burning pains along the anterior connection of the diaphragm with the ribs; to the sensitiveness of the hepatic region to touch and on deep inspiration; also to the fact that Bryonia diminishes the intestinal excretions, weakens the peristaltic action of the bowels, and retards the stool. It produces diarrhœa, he thinks, only when taken in very large doses.

Urine. The urine is high-colored, concentrated; passed frequently, sometimes with pain. Occasionally, during exertion, it is passed involuntarily.

Menstruation. Bryonia uniformly hastens the coming on of the menses, and increases the flow. It may, therefore, as experience has shown, be a valuable remedy in too frequent and too copious menstruation.

Respiratory Organs. The action of Bryonia on this region of the body is well marked, and has enabled us to make many brilliant cures.

Nasal Membrane. Fluent coryza, beginning with violent and frequent sneezing, accompanied by stitching headache, when the prover stoops, and by hoarseness and an altered tone of voice.

[1] For a comparative notice of the diarrhœa of Bryonia, Sulphur, Thuja, and Podophyllum, see Dr. Lippe's lecture, "American Homœopathic Review," vol. v., p. 441.

Cough. Generally dry; it seems to come from the region of the stomach, and is preceded by a crawling and tickling sensation in the epigastrium. This is the general characteristic; sometimes there is a crawling sensation in the throat also, inducing a cough, followed by mucous sputa.

Hacking cough, as if caused by something (mucus?) at a definite spot in the trachea; after coughing for some time this spot becomes very sensitive, and it is worse from talking and smoking.

Cough induced by coming from the open air into a warm room; from a sensation as of a vapor in the trachea, which prevents the prover getting air enough.

Concomitants. The cough is accompanied by stitching pains in the brain; by rawness in the larynx; by stitches in the intercostal spaces and in the sternum; by soreness in the epigastrium; by gagging, without nausea; by vomiting of food when coughing.

It is very characteristic of the Bryonia cough that, while coughing, the patient presses with his hand upon the sternum, as though he needed to support the chest during the violent exertion. Also, that the parts which are the seat of subjective pain become subsequently sensitive to external pressure; *e.g.,* the sternum. (So also the joints.)

The expectoration, which is infrequent and scanty, is tough and sometimes bloody.

Respiration is impeded, as though by a pressure on the epigastrium, and is accelerated, as though by a feeling of heat in the epigastrium and chest. The prover feels a desire to take a deep inspiration, but when he attempts to do so he experiences a pain which does not allow him to expand the chest. Thoracic respiration is often almost impossible, by reason of the stitching pains in the sides of the thorax. These symptoms might call our attention to Bryonia in pleurisy, pneumonia and asthma. Ranunculus bulbosus has similar symptoms which, equally with the Bryonia pains, impede thoracic respiration; but the sitches are not so sharp and knife-like as those of Bryonia.

Thorax. Pressing pains, sometimes just above the epigastrium, sometimes over the whole chest, or on the sternum, impeding respiration. Stitching, lancinating pains are, however, more frequent. They occur on inspiration, or on turning around in bed; they are situated sometimes in the sides of the thorax, and sometimes they extend through the thorax from the front to the scapulæ; generally the seat of the pain is sensitive to pressure, and when the arms are moved.

Back. Here we meet a new variety of symptoms. Sticking and jerking pains pressing between the scapulæ and extending thence through to the epigastrium, when sitting; pain in the lumbar and sacral region, as if beaten; stiffness, tearing and tenderness in the joints and muscles of the lumbar region, which prevent motion and stooping; these are felt most when standing or sitting, and not so much when lying.

BRYONIA ALBA.

Extremities. In the extremities we have stitching pains in the region of the large joints, as in the shoulder, over the trochanter, and at the knee, —all greatly aggravated by motion, touch, or any jark or shock. Drawing and pain, as if luxated, in the medium and smaller joints. The limbs and the joints swell, become red, and are very sensitive to touch or motion. The pains are relieved by warmth.

Skin. Various eruptions. Small red spots on various parts of the body; some with sensibility, and not disappearing on pressure; some burning, and disappearing on pressure.

Sleep. Great sleepiness by day, with yawning, lassitude, stretching, etc. Yet, at night, the prover cannot sleep, because of the tumultuous course of the blood, anxiety and heat. A concourse of anxious thoughts keeps the prover awake till three or four A. M. Sleep full of dreams. Often a prattling and muttering delirium. Also, sleep-walking has been observed under the action of Bryonia, and has been cured by it.

Fever. In the fever which Bryonia produces, cold predominates. Coldness and shivering over the whole body. Heat often only internal, or on single parts of the body, and it is conjoined with great thirst. So, indeed, is the chill. Sweat on slight exertion, even when walking in the cool air. It is frequent at night, and is often sour.

Disposition. Anxious, peevish and hasty.

GENERAL ANALYSIS.

1. *Vital Force.* That Bryonia exerts, in some respects, a depressing action on the vital force, appears from its effect on the sensorium, which is depressed and benumbed; there is a decided sensation of weaknss and lassitude; the arms incline to sink by one's side; the limbs move but sluggishly. This sensation of lassitude is most marked early in the morning, as though the night's sleep had brought no refreshment. The least exertion seems to use up the forces of the body.

Nevertheless, this prostration is not excessive, nor is it universal. For the disposition is not indifferent, as might have been expected; on the contrary, the prover is hasty and peevish. Again, the special senses are not materially affected; the sphincters are not relaxed, nor do any involuntary muscles seem to be greatly embarrassed in the exercise of their functions. There is no laxity of fiber, such as is shown by the occurrence of involuntary excretions.

The depressing effect seems to be confined to that part of the nervous system which presides over voluntary motion, and over the operations of the mind.

2. The *Organic Substance* of the body is affected as follows: The secretions from the intestinal surfaces are diminished; the capillary circulation appears to be somewhat impeded in the mucous membranes, but is particularly so in the serous

membranes which line the closed cavities of the pleura, peritoneum, pericardium, and joints. As a sequel of this impediment we have effusion (so called) into these cavities.

3. *Sphere of Action.* The action of Bryonia, as appears from the proving, is exerted chiefly upon the nervous system of animal life, presiding over ratiocination and voluntary motion; upon the gastro-intestinal region, producing various perversions of digestion, a deficient intestinal secretion and a form of constipation, and, moreover, the symptoms of a well-marked hepatitis,. Upon the respiratory mucous membrane, the action of Bryonia, though evident, is subordinate. The serous membranes of the large cavities, and of the joints and the ligaments, are eminently affected. Finally, the female sexual organs are in such wise affected that menorrhagia is produced, the discharge being florid.

4. *Sensations.* The sensations peculiar to Bryonia are stitching, lancinating pains,—such pains, in fact, as usually attend and characterize acute affections of the serous and fibrous tissues. Drawing pains are analogous to these. In addition, we note the peculiar sensations of lassitude in the limbs that have been already described. It must not be forgotten that many other remedies likewise produce stitching, lancinating pains,—as Squilla, Ranunculus bulbosus, Asclepias.

5. *Periodicity.* A disposition to a recurrence of the pains in the morning early, not immediately

on awaking (as with Lachesis), but on first moving after waking.

6. *Peculiarities.* The great feature characteristic of the Bryonia symptoms is their aggravation by motion and touch. This applies to all, except a few isolated symptoms, which it is evident, from the context, are purely nervous.

It is also noteworthy, that the seat of the subjective pain soon becomes objectively sore, and then swollen and red.

The pains of Bryonia are, in general, relieved by warmth and aggravated by cold.

They are aggrevated by mental excitement.

PRACTICAL APPLICATIONS.

Hahnemann mentions the importance of Bryonia in the treatment of various kinds of fevers, and refers to his treatment of a malignant typhus that was epidemic in Saxony in 1813, after the retreat of the French army. This will be spoken of when we treat of Rhus toxicodendron.

Hahnemann recommends Bryonia in certain kinds of abdominal cramps in women, of course, when the symptoms correspond.

Head. Seeing the action of the Bryonia on the serous membranes one might infer that it would occupy a prominent place in the treatment of meningitis. But this inference is not justified by the symptoms. They represent a fever too asthenic to correspond with any form of idiopathic meningitis.

In repercussed eruptions, however, as, for example, during the course of an exanthematous fever,—scarlatina or measles,—when the eruption has disappeared, and the sensorium becomes immediately affected, Bryonia has often done excellent service. The oppression of the senses, the general prostration, the peculiar form of fever, consisting of predominant coldness, first a chill and then a fever, mixed up of chill and heat, with a small pulse, and which never, even when the heat is greatest, becomes very full or hard,—these symptoms correspond well to the kind of case to which we refer.

But it is only in a certain class of cases of repercussed exanthemata that Bryonia is indicated and useful, viz., where the sensorium and the system of animal life are depressed, benumbed, but the functions not perverted. There is another class in which they are perverted, and in which, consequently, convulsions more or less complete occur. In such cases Cuprum aceticum (or metallicum) is likely to be indicated, a fact for the knowledge of which we are indebted to Dr. G. Schmidt, of Vienna. In other cases of this kind, without fever or disturbance of the general system, the entire sensorial life is suspended. Here Hellebore may be required, as Hahnemann has shown in his introduction to the proving of that drug. Or, again, together with this suspension of sensorial life, there may be signs of effusion within the cranium; the patient lies like an animate but not intelligent log; the pupils are dilated; the eyes converge or diverge; and here Zincum metallicum will sometimes save the patient. I made this observation in 1853, in a case of scarlatina. About the same time, and unknown to me, Dr. Elb, of Dresden, published some similar cases in the "Allgemeine Homœopathische Zeitung."

Under these circumstances the vital processes move very slowly, and I believe it is necessary to repeat the Zinc freqeuntly, and to continue it for many days.

Epistaxis. Bryonia has been named as a remedy. The blood is florid. The epistaxis occurs in the morning, often waking the patient from sleep. It is often a concomitant of suppressed menstruation, or where the symptom accompanies a case of typhoid fever.

Fevers. In the fevers marked by gastro-intestinal localizations, such as bilious remittent, some forms of intermittent and some forms of typhus fever, Bryonia has done good service. It compares with Eupatorium and Rhus toxicodendron, and with Nux vomica and Mercurius.

The fever is marked by gastro-hepatic complications, resembling the symptoms. The headache is a splitting pain through the temples, and at the same time, more severely, in the occiput. Oppression at the pit of the stomach and tenderness there; vomiting of food, mucus and bile, stitches in the hypochondria, and soreness and tension in the hepatic region, along with dry cough and decided constipation, without any desire for evacuation of the bowels. Together with these local symptoms there are frequent short chills, alternating or mixed up with heat of the body; a pulse small and frequent, but somewhat hard. Add to the above a slimy and bitter taste, aversion to food, eructations, pains in the back and limbs, much aggravated by touch and motion, together with dullness of the sensorium, and aversion to noise and to mental exertion, and we have a picture of the form of fever for which, whether remittent or intermittent, Bryonia is appropriate.

Similar symptoms often characterize what is popularly called "a bilious attack." These "attacks" are very common in persons who have for years been accustomed to take frequent doses of calomel or of blue mass for headache and "biliousness." And we are often called upon to supply a substitute for these drugs. In the majority of these cases Bryonia is the remedy. If early restorted to, it will generally break up the attack; and a repetition of this treatment rarely fails to destroy a tendency to its recurrence.

Bœnninghausen gives the following picture of the Bryonia fever: "Pulse hard, frequent and tense. Chill and coldness predominate, often with heat of the head, red cheeks and thirst. Chill, with external coldness of the body. Chill and coldness most at evening, or on the right side of the body. Chill more in the room than in the open air.

"Dry, burning heat, for the most part only internally, and as if the blood burned in the veins. All the symptoms are aggravated during the heat.

"Much sweat. Easy sweating, even from walking slowly in the cold, open air. Copious night and morning sweats. Sweat sour, or oily."

Hahnemann gives the following groups of symptoms, as characterizing those cases of typhus for which he gave Bryonia so successfully:

"The patient complains of dizziness, shooting (or jerking-tearing) pains in the head, throat, chest, abdomen, etc., which are felt particularly on moving the part, in addition to the other symptoms, the hæmorrhages, the vomiting, the heat, the thirst, the nocturnal restlessness," etc.

In acute hepatitis it is very evident, from the symptoms, that Bryonia may be a most valuable remedy. Experience has confirmed the indication.

Bryonia is also a remedy for constipation, being, as Hahnemann remarks, one of the few remedies of which the primary action is to diminish the intestinal excretion, and likewise the peristaltic action of the intestine.

It differs from Nux vomica, as we shall see, in this respect, that the action of the intestine is diminished. Nux vomica does not diminish the action of the intestine. It rather increases it, but at the same time renders it inharmonious and spasmodic, a hindrance, therefore, and not a help to evacuation. This is the reason why the constipation characteristic of Nux vomica is accompanied by frequent ineffectual desire for stool, the action of the intestine being irregular and spasmodic, and the constipations resulting from this irregularity of action, and not from inaction. Bryonia has nothing of this. Under its influence the intestinal activity is really diminished,—there is no desire for stool. As a remedy for constipation, Bryonia is analogous to that other valuable remedy for the same trouble— Veratrum.

It has been already remarked that Bryonia is our great remedy in the treatment of vicarious menstruation—a perversion of function which is not so rare as has been supposed. At the period when the menstrual discharge should naturally take place, there occur hæmorrhages from some other parts of the body, as from the nose, mouth or lungs. I have seen, under such circumstances, likewise, hæmorrhage from the eye, the ear, and once from the nipple. These vicarious discharges are not difficult to distinguish from hæmorrhage attending and consequent upon diseased conditions of these organs themselves. If, for example, about the time of menstruation, this phenomenon not occurring, a copious expectoration or vomiting of blood take place, without any other symptoms of disease of the lung or stomach,—if it last two or three days, with no greater disturbance of the general health than commonly attends menstruation,— if it then cease, leaving no sign of disease in the organ apparently affected, and, if it recur again after the usual menstrual interval, there can be no reasonable doubt of the nature of the trouble.

Clinical experience has shown that Bryonia generally cures these cases.

About the third day after confinement, women are liable to chill and an access of fever, just when the mamma begins in earnest the performance of its peculiar function. Experience has shown Bryonia to be one of our most valuable remedies in this condition. The correspondence of symptoms indicates this; for, the "milk fever" is one in which chill predominates; it is a mixture of chill and fever, the former much in excess, and, moreover, the gland, which is the seat of pain, becomes rapidly sore and sensitive to touch or motion. In addition, there are drawing tearing pains in the limbs and a headache resembling that of Bryonia. Bryonia is likewise our foremost remedy in inflammation of the mammæ during lactation.

A word of caution, bearing on the diagnosis of the latter affection, may not here be inappropriate. It is of the utmost importance to avoid mistaking symptoms of exhaustion of the supply of milk in the gland for symptoms of commencing inflammation, and treating, with medicine, a condition which should be met by rest of the organ and an appropriate diet.

In primiparæ the secretion is often established tardily, and the milk fever is severe. For this reason the patient is apt to be kept on a very low diet, with a view of preventing inflammation of the mamma and, for the same object, the child is applied to the breast at very short intervals, in order to prevent "accumulation of milk in the gland," "to keep it free." Under these circumstances, the supply of milk is apt to be scanty. If, now, the child be vigorous, the supply will soon be exhausted, and the child will "draw upon a vacuum." Very soon an acute dragging pain is experienced by the mother, extending from the nipple through the gland and the thorax to the scapula. It would be a sad mistake to regard this as always a sign of existing inflammation, to still farther curtail the diet and to resort to medication. It is not always a sign of inflammation, it is a "dragging on the milk-tubes." The diet should be increased in its nutritive qualities, and directions given to apply the child less frequently to the breast, and to remove it as soon as this peculiar pain begins to be felt. This is very important; for, if the "dragging" be allowed to continue long, and be often repeated, it will produce inflammation, first of the nipple and subsequently of the gland. This is the origin of perhaps a majority of the cases of "sore nipples" met with in practice, and attenion to these precautions constitutes one of the best preventives of that distressing affection.

It should be observed, however, that cases sometimes occur, in which, as soon as the infant begins to nurse, the patient experiences severe acute dragging and stitching pain, extending from the extremity of the nipple to the scapula, and rendering the pain of nursing almost unendurable, and this, too, when there can be no reason to suspect a deficiency of milk. Indeed, the pains set in as soon as the child begins to nurse, and not, as in the case before described, after the child has already nursed, for a time, satisfactorily. These are cases of irritable nipple, and they often result in mammary abscess, because the mother cannot endure the pain of having the breast freed from the milk that is secreted. Such cases find their best remedy, as I learn from Professor Guernsey, of Philadelphia, in Croton tiglium. But if the pains come on and exist only or chiefly during the interval between nursing, they are relieved by Phellandrium aquaticum (Gross).

On the respiratory organs the action of Bryonia is very emphatic.

Dr. Wurmb says of it: "Although Bryonia be not so often administered in diseases of the mucous membranes as in those of the serous and fibrous tissues, it is, nevertheless, in the former, a very important remedy. Its action on all the membranes must be a very extensive one, because of its powerful influence upon the processes of secretion and absorption, and because the mucous membranes, in particular, belong to those organs by means of which these operations are, for the most part, carried on.

"The results of provings show that Bryonia produces powerful irritation in the mucous membrane of the respiratory organs. This condition is important, not only inasmuch as it enables us to designate Bryonia as an important remedy in acute bronchial catarrh, but also as giving us a *point d'appui* in studying the remedy. For experience teaches us, on the one hand, that the more violent forms of catarrh almost always involve the pleura, causing stitch in the side, and, on the other hand, that stitching pains almost always yield, and in a short time, to Bryonia.

"We lay great stress on the fact that in the Bryonia catarrh the mucous secretion is diminished, because a great majority of the symptoms which are considered to indicate Bryonia derive their significance from this fact, and it will serve to keep them in memory. They are: hoarseness, hacking cough, which sets in especially in the morning and evening, and is generally dry or yields but a little tenacious mucus (which is sometimes streaked with blood), and which sometimes, through its violence, causes retching and actual vomiting. As rarely failing concomitants of the Bryonia cough, we have stitching pains in the throat and chest, and pressing pains in the head."

In the bronchial catarrh, with scanty secretion, and attended by dyspnœa and nervous erethism, to which infants are subject, and which is often mistaken for true pneumonia, Bryonia is a most valuable remedy. In a subsequent stage of the same affection, when the secretion has become very abundant, every paroxysm of coughing producing nausea and copious vomiting of mucus, with dyspnœa, exhaustion and sweat, Ipecacuanha is likely to be required. In former days, before I learned to distinguish sharply between the indications for these remedies, I used to give them, as was and is so commonly advised and practiced, in alternation,—a slovenly practice which cannot be too strongly condemned. Each of the remedies has its place in the appropriate stage of the malady.

In the pneumonia of adults, especially in that form in which the deposit or exudation is scanty and fibrinous, Bryonia is the remedy most frequently required. So true is this, and so valuable is Bryonia in this case, when indicated, that some practitioners have not hesitated to say that Bryonia is the sole and all-sufficient remedy for pneumonia, and that they give nothing else. This view, however, restricts the idea of pneumonia to one pathological form, ignoring that form in which the exudation is not purely fibrinous, and in which Phosphorus or Tartar emetic is likely to be indicated, as we shall see when we come to Phosphorus.

A reference here may be permitted to the singular fact that whereas, in New England, where pneumonia is frequently met with, more than one busy practitioner places his whole reliance on Bryonia in pneumonia, and claims to cure every case with it; in Vienna, on the other hand, where pneumonia is still more common, Dr. Fleischmann regards Phosphorus as the specific, and uses it almost exclusively.

Admitting the looseness of the practice, which, in any locality, looks to one remedy exclusively as the specific for any disease whatever, may it not be that the character of the pneumonia, in the two regions, is radically different, depending on differences in the constitutions and habits of the races in the two countries? Be this as it may, the facts are a warning not to prescribe on the basis of the name of the disease.

Important as is the action of Bryonia on the regions already designated, it is still more marked in the serous and fibrous tissues.

The stitching pains in the thorax and abdomen, especially the stitch in the intercostal regions on taking a deep inspiration, all point to the efficacy of Bryonia in pleuritis, an indication which experience has confirmed. It is believed to be more suitable for pleurisy of the right side.

In pericarditis, also, it is valuable, though perhaps less frequently indicated than Spigelia. (Asclepias tuberosa.)

In its relations to affections of the pleura, Bryonia is resembled by Spigelia, Squilla, Ranunculus bulbosus and Kali carbonicum, and amongst the new remedies, Asclepias tuberosa.

In rheumatism, Bryonia is one of our most important remedies. Its symptoms of the extremities simulate a muscular rheumatism, with moderate fever; while the symptoms of the joints show it to be still more appropriate to articular rheumatism.

The joints are much swollen and are reddened; streaks of red extending up and down the limb. They are very sensitive to touch, and are especially painful during motion, the pain being less the more perfect the repose. Dr. Wurmb gives the following indications: "The fever not very violent, or, if so at first, much diminished; the rheumatism does not change its location; the local phenomena, especially the swelling and pain, very violent; the irritation of the skin but slight; the redness not very great." The aggravations as to time are in the morning some time after waking, and in the evening. The pain is of a sticking and tearing character.

EUPATORIUM.

THIS drug, which has hardly as yet an established place in the pharmacopœia, although it is a much used and highly prized "domestic" remedy, has been but imperfectly studied, and we have nothing approaching to an exhaustive knowledge of its properties and capabilities. Enough is known, however, to give it rank beside Bryonia in regard of its febrile and gastro-hepatic symptoms.

Eupatorium perfoliatum—thoroughwort or boneset—is popularly used as a diaphoretic (a hot infusion in frequent, moderate doses), or as an emetic (hot infusion, large doses), or as a tonic (cold infusion, small doses).

Its history and its uses by allopathic and eclectic physicians are well detailed in Dr. Hale's work.[1]

Eupatorium is said to have been a principal remedy for intermittent fever with the Indians.

Dr. Anderson, of New-York, in 1813, published a number of cases of intermittent fever successfully treated with it in the City Hospital. He proposed it, therefore, as a substitute for Cin-

[1] "New Remedies," etc., p. 159 *et seq.*

chona bark. Subsequent experiments with it in that hospital were not successful and the remedy fell into disrepute.

This is the history of every drug in the allopathic materia medica. There can be no doubt that the Eupatorium did really cure the cases which Dr. Anderson reported. But there was, assuredly, some peculiarity about these cases, by virtue of which they exactly corresponded to Eupatorium. The cases in which it was tried unsuccessfully, unquestionably, did not possess this peculiarity, whatever it was, and which must be the characteristic of Eupatorium. But the physicians who were testing the remedy took no note of this; they regarded all cases as virtually alike, because to all of them the name "intermittent" could be applied. So regarding them, and taking no note of any peculiarities wherein one case, differed from another, they could not of course perceive why Eupatorium might correspond to one case and cure it, and not to another.

The number of cases of intermittent fever to which Eupatorium is appropriate is not very large, except during certain seasons, when an epidemic requiring it may prevail (as was the case in some parts of the State of New-York, in the autumn of 1865).

The first proving of Eupatorium was made in Philadelphia, and was reported by Dr. W. Williamson to the American Institute of Homœopathy[1] in 1847. Its great action is upon the muscular

[1] "Transactions," vol. I.

EUPATORIUM.

system (or fibrous tissues), producing great soreness and aching, and upon the gastro-hepatic system, producing a condition resembling what is known as a "bilious state."

It produces intense headache, throbbing and great sense of internal soreness in the forehead and occiput, with a sensation of great weight in the occiput, distress and painful soreness in the top and back of the head.

Soreness of the eyeball; redness of the face, with dry skin.

Tongue coated whitish or yellow.

Loss of appetite; thirst for cold water.

Eructations tasteless or bitter.

Vomiting after drinking; vomiting of bile, with trembling and with pain in the epigastrium.

Nausea and sense of extreme prostration (this is not real prostration).

Soreness around the epigastric zone; soreness and fullness in the region of the liver.

Constipation; urine high-colored and scanty. Roughness and rawness in the trachea. Hacking, dry cough, with flushed face; the patient supports the chest with the hand (like Bryonia).

Weakness in the small of the back; deep-seated pain in the lions, with soreness on every motion; pain in the back and lower extremities.

Soreness and aching in hands and wrists, as if broken and dislocated; the same in arms. Stiffness and soreness of lower extremities, as if beaten, worse on motion and touch.

Fever, commensing generally in the morning; thirst begins several hours before the chill, and continues during chill and heat. There is vomiting of bile at the end of the chill.

During the heat the face is of a dull, mahogany-red color, and the eye glistens, the sclerotica being yellow.

It is a distinguishing peculiarity that little or no sweat follows the hot stage.

The peculiar headache, the soreness of the eyes and their yellowness, the yellowish-red face, the vomiting of bile, with nausea and prostration, the soreness in the region of the liver, the constipation, etc., are one group of symptoms. The internal soreness and the external soreness all over the body, from head to foot, constitute another group. These two groups together furnish an indication for Eupatorium in certain forms of "bilious fever" (in the first stage), too strong to be questioned.

The absence of much perspiration after the heat, showing an imperfect resolution, points to the type of fever as the remittent.

Experience has confirmed these views. I regard the severe bone pains and the absence of much sweat as especially characteristic.

The symptoms of the gastro-hepatic region, and the character and aggravations of the pains in the body and extremities, very closely resemble those of Bryonia. But a broad distinction at once appears when we consider the perspiration which, under Bryonia, is profuse and easily provoked, while, under Eupatorium, it is scanty or absent. Again, the Eupatorium pains make the patient restless; those of Bryonia make him keep very still.

Rhus toxicodendron produces pains and aching in the limbs; but these pains are worse during repose, and they keep the patient restless, constantly changing his position, whereas those of Eupatorium are not aggravated by repose.

R. D., a stout mechanic, thirty-five years old, of dark complexion, went into an ice-house one very warm morning in August, to get a piece of ice. Charmed with the coolness of the place, he foolishly remained there for a quarter hour or longer. Suddenly he felt chills creeping over him and became quite faint. He left the ice-house as quickly as he could and went home. In an hour he had an exceedingly severe chill, lasting several hours. This was followed by burning fever, which continued without abatement until the following morning, when it gave place to a severe chill. As this chill was passing away I first saw the patient.

He had already become hot externally; his face was of a dull, red color; the eyes glistened, and the scleroticæ were yellowish red. The tongue had a thick, yellowish fur; there was intense headache in the occiput—an insupportable heaviness. Nausea and frequent effort to vomit, extreme tenderness in the epigastrium, fullness and tenderness in the hepatic region, with stitches and soreness on moving and coughing; intolerable aching in the back and limbs, "as if the bones were broken." Urine scanty and of a dark mahogany colour; a hard, dry cough and some dyspnœa. The patient, although in great pain, lay quiet.

I had no Eupatorium, but there was a swamp near the house, and I soon found the plant. From the juice pressed from a few leave I prepared, with water, the third attenuation, and directed it to be taken in drop doses, every three hours until marked improvement was observed.

In about ten hours the fever was gone; the chill and fever never recurred, and next day the patient was free from pain. On the third day I found him convalescent.

In many cases of influenza, a review of the symptoms will show why Eupatorium proves, as it does, a speedy curative.

RHUS TOXICODENDRON;

OR, RHUS RADICANS.

THESE two plants are now regarded by botanists as identical, differing only in their modes of growth. The former was proved by Hahnemann; the latter by the late Dr. B. F. Joslin. I can perceive no essential differences in the symptoms ascribed to them by provers. For ten years I have used them interchangeably in my practice, and have seen no differences in their effects. I shall therefore treat them as identical substances.

This plant is a native of North America. It was known to the Indians as possessed of medicinal properties. Dufresnoy, a French army surgeon, published in 1788, "An account of its supposed virtues in the cure of cutaneous eruptions, and of nervous paralysis." He also, as well as the traveler Kalm, described its property of causing inflammatory swelling of the skin, followed by vesication, in persons who touch the leaves, and even in susceptible persons who are exposed to its exhalations at night.

Indeed, it is well known that contact with the leaves of the Rhus radicans or "poison vine" produces, not merely in the parts touched, but also often in other parts of the body, as the neck and face, a swelling, with redness, œdema and vesication, that bears a marvelous resemblance to vesicular erysipelas. This eruption is attended by constitutional symptoms which resemble those of erysipelas. It is well known, too, that in this form of vesicular erysipelas, homœopathicians long ago found reason to look upon Rhus toxicodendron or radicans as their most valuable remedy. The striking confirmation of the homœopathic law of cure which these facts afford, has caused some bitter opponents of homœopathy actually to thrust Rhus out from the materia medica. We find Dr. Stillé, after giving a very imperfect summary of the effects of Rhus and the opinions held respecting it, coolly remarking: "It, however, does not really appear to deserve sufficient confidence as a medicine to entitle it to retain a place in the materia medica."

Very different are the judgment and method of Prof. Trousseau, who, though no advocate or friend of homœopathy, is yet too wise and honest a man to refuse to learn from an opponent.

He relates an interesting proving of Rhus: "Dr. Savini applied two drops of the juice of Rhus radicans to the first phalanx of his forefinger; he left it there only two minutes, and yet, at the end of an hour, it has produced two black spots. Twenty-five days afterward, the following symptoms suddenly manifested themselves: great heat in the mouth and gullet; rapidly increasing swelling of the left cheek, of the upper lip and of the eyelids. The following night, sweelling of the forearm, which had acquired double its normal volume; the skin was rough, the itching intolerable, the heat very great, etc.

"This singular action of Rhus radicans," continues Trousseau, "upon the human economy, has induced the homœopathists to use it in skin diseases; but already before them, Dufresnoy, of Valenciennes, had published a pamphlet in which he extolled the virtues of this plant against cutaneous diseases, and subsequently against paralysis.

"Since that time a number of essays on this subject have appeared in medical periodicals, and many respectable physicians have confirmed Dufresnoy's experiments.

"We have ourselves," continues Trousseau, "often used Rhus radicans for paralysis; but the experiments we have made in skin diseases are too few and too little conclusive to admit of our referring to them here.

"The only forms of paralysis which we have seen treated by M. Bretonneau, of Tours, and which we have ourselves treated, are those of the lower extremities which succeeded a concussion of the spinal marrow, or a lesion of that organ, which did not destroy its tissue. On this point we have collected facts enough to place beyond a doubt the therapeutic efficacy of Rhus radicans."[1]

[1] Trousseau et Pidoux, "Traité de Therapeutique et Materia Medica," vol. i., 787, 788.

We shall see that the symptoms clearly point to the use of Rhus in paralysis of the lower extremities. The powerful testimony of Trousseau is an indorsement of our law for the selection of remedies.

Our knowledge of the positive effects of Rhus toxicodendron upon the human organism is derived from the proving by Hahnemann and his pupils, published in vol. II. of the "Materia Medica Pura," and from the proving of Rhus radicans conducted by the late Dr. Joslin, and published by him in the "Philadelphia Journal of Homœopathy," and in "Jahr's New Manual"; also later in the "American Homœopathic Review."

Hahnemann, in the introduction to his proving, remarks that a careful study of the symptoms will enable us to discover many characteristic peculiarities of this remarkable and very precious drug one of which (possessed by very few other drugs, and by none in so high a degree), he describes as follows: "It excites the strongest symptoms when the body or the limb in qestion is in the greatest repose and is kept as free as possible from all motion."

He further remarks that "whoever has studied the symptoms of Bryonia will observe a great similarity in them to the symptoms of Rhus toxicodendron, and at the same time a great contrariety. Thus, for example, how remarkable is the aggravation under Bryonia by motion, and the amelioration during repose, of the very same symptoms which under Rhus are ameliorated by motion and aggravated by repose."

Taking a general view of the action of Rhus before we proceed to examine its special action upon each apparatus and organ of the body, we find: The sphere of action of Rhus to be extensive. Upon the system of nutrition it acts as a depressent, retarding all the functions. The secretion of the mucous membranes is altered and increased, as is shown by diarrhœa and by the sputa attending the cough as well as by secretions from other mucous membranes. The lymphatic glands are affected throughout the body, as, for example, the cervical, the inguinal and the mesenteric, which are all enlarged and inflamed. Emaciation is produced. Perspiration is abundant and is sour.

From the character of the fever symptoms which it produces, it would be reasonable to infer that Rhus affects the composition of the blood.

But it acts quite as decidedly upon the system of animal life. The sensorium is depressed, and the capability of the mind for continuous though is absolutely destroyed, thus a patient meaning to write the number 12 will write the figure 1, but cannot recollect the figure 2 which should follow it. Like the typhus patient, who begins his sentence coherently and intelligibly, but allows it to dwindle away into an inarticulate murmur.

Listlessness and horrible depression possess the mind. This marks a more profound depression than that produced by **Bryonia**, for the latter results in fretful peevishness and irritability. Rhus has listlessness, a feeling of helplessness and profound despondency. A similar feeling pervades the whole apparatus of voluntary motion, expressing itself in a sense of physical prostration, of inability to move, of powerlessness, approaching paralysis. So great is this that, on first attempting to move after a repose of some length of time, the limbs tremble, the joints are stiff, and there seems to be actual inability to move. This condition is more pronounced in the lower extremities than in the upper.

The special senses are dulled, but not perverted.

The skin, as we shall see, is the theater on which are displayed some of the most powerful, characteristic and valuable properties of Rhus. Rhus, then, acts prominently on the mucous membranes, on the lymphatic glands, on the organs of animal life, and on the skin. To this list must be added the tissues which compose the joints.

The sensations which are characteristic of Rhus are:

Soreness, as if beaten; this is felt in the muscles and in the neighborhood of the joints.

Heaviness and pressure; this is felt in the head and eyes and eyelids and in the limbs.

Lassitude and langour and weight; felt in the extremities, especially the lower limbs.

The action of Rhus may be summed up as follows: It produces a kind of rheumatic affection of the muscles and ligaments, alleviated by motion; a paralysis aggravated by motion; an apparent passive congestion of head, relieved by repose; a debility of the organs of nutrition, marked by deficient and depraved appetite and by tympanitis; a serous infiltration of the cellular tissue in various parts, as face, fauces, genital organs, feet; a vesicular eruption generally; and acrid state of the secretions generally, as tears, nasal mucus, gastric mucus, intestinal mucus, urine, menstrual flow, contents of cutaneous vesicles; general depression of sensorium.

We shall gather evidence of these generalizations as we proceed.

Periodicity is not marked in the symptoms of Rhus.

Peculiarities. The great and characteristic peculiarity of the symptoms of Rhus is that, with few exceptions, they occur and are aggravated during repose and are ameliorated by motion.

This statement, however, requires some degree of explanation. In addition to the symptoms of Rhus which resemble paralysis, there are also groups of symptoms resembling muscular and articular rheumatism. These rheumatic symptoms come on with severity during repose and increase as long as the patient keeps quiet, until they compel him to move. Now, on first attempting to move, he finds himself very stiff, and the first movement is exceedingly painful. By continuing to move for a little while, however, the stiffness is relieved and the pains decidedly decrease, the patient feeling much better. But this improvement does not go on indefinitely. After moving continuously for a longer or shorter period and finding comfort therein, the paralytic symptoms interpose their exhausting protest, and the patient is compelled from a sensation of lassitude and powerlessness to suspend his movements and to come to repose. At first this repose after long-continued motion is grateful, since it relieves, not the aching and severe pains, but only the sense of prostration. Before long, the pains come on again during this repose and the patient is forced to move again as before.

This will explain seeming contradictions in the symptoms of Rhus.

The amount of it is that the pains of Rhus are aggravated by repose and relieved by motion. But the paralysis and languor of Rhus, like all such symptoms always, when real. are relieved by repose and aggravated by long-continued motion.

SPECIAL ANALYSIS.

The sensorium is affected as follows: There is vertigo, which occurs when standing and walking; but also when sitting and even comes on when lying down. In this particular it corresponds with the conditions of the rheumatic pains of Rhus toxicodendron. It is described as if something kept going around in the head; one feels as if drunken, as though one would fall forward or backward. On rising in the morning one can hardly support one's self. This is not only from dizziness but also from the paralytic condition and from the stiffness and lassitude which follow long repose.

Excessive vertigo on lying down, with fear of dying.

Memory is markedly impaired even for the most familiar facts. The thinking power almost suspended, with absence of mind. Head confused; he cannot write nor remember what it was he wished to write.

Headache. Among the pains in the head properly so called, we notice first pressure, both in the temples and in the forehead and behind the orbits, where it feels sometimes like a wearisome pressure downward; sometimes as if the eyes would be pressed outward; sometimes as if the brain were pressed together from both sides. Also a radiating pressure in the temples, worse during repose; sometimes a burning pressure in the temporal bone.

The sensation most closely allied to the above is heaviness, which is felt in this way: that when the patient stoops it seems as though he could not rise again. There is a sensation as if a quantity of blood shot into the brain; as if a weight fell forward in the forehead and drew the head downward, or as if the head were being pressed asunder.

Sometimes there is a tearing in the head in every part and direction; or on awaking and opening the eyes a violent headache, as if the brain were torn, worse on opening the eyes.

A singular sensation characteristic of Rhus is

noted on shaking the head and when walking, when jarring the body, etc., namely, a sensation of swashing and jarring in the brain, and each step concusses the brain. China has a similar symptom. Externally the scalp is sore to the touch. There is itching on the scalp, face and lips, and the formation of a vesicular eruption.

To recapitulate: The vertigo occurs when standing and walking; is worse when lying down, though there is a tottering when walking, with which, probably, the paralysis is connected.

The pains in the head are pressure, heaviness, tearing and swashing. They affect chiefly the forehead, temples and post-orbital regions, and, unlike the rheumatic pains, are generally worse on motion, although some are aggravated by repose.

Face. The face may be pale and sickly-looking, with the features distorted; or red, and covered with sweat without thirst. As regards the skin, there has been observed an erysipelatous redness of the face, swelling of the face and eyelids, with burning pain or itching. On this surface, after a few days, vesicles make their appearance, which discharge and leave a fine, mealy scale. This resembles so exactly the vesicular erysipelas of the face that it is often mistaken for it.

Eyes. In the eyes a burning pressing pain; they itch and bite. The white of the eye is reddened; they lachrymate and are agglutinated in the morning. The lids smart, as if excoriated by the tears, or else they have a sensation of dryness

There is often a sensation of heaviness or of paralysis in the lids, so that they can hardly be kept open.

As regards the sense of vision, there seems to be something like a veil before the eyes, preventing distinct vision.

Ears. Earache and a feeling as if some one were blowing into the ear. There is a whistling, a squealing noise heard, or a ringing when walking, which changes to a loud resonance when lying down, as if the membrana tympani were burst.

Nose. Nose-bleeding, the blood being dark; it occurs at night; also when stooping and when clearing the throat. A scabby eruption about the nares, with itching, burning pain.

Cheeks and Jaws. A peculiar phenomenon is noteworthy: A cramp-like pain in the maxillary joint, as if beaten, as if it would break, and on each motion of the jaw it cracks and snaps audibly. There is a constant desire to yawn, until it seems as though the jaw would break. (This corresponds with, and is analogous to, the stretching and twisting so characteristic of Rhus.)

The toothache of Rhus is a jerking pain extending into the head. It is relieved by applying the cold hand. The gums burn and are sore. The teeth are loose.

In the mouth a sensation of dryness, which persists notwithstanding all the patient may drink.

In the throat a sensation of swelling, with

aching pain when speaking, and independently, but attended by stitching on attempting to swallow. There are also sticking pains when swallowing saliva or food, sensations of soreness in the muscles of the root of the tongue and when yawning; pressure on empty swallowing.

The action of Rhus on the digestive organs is not very characteristic. It produces a bitter, sour or coppery taste, a total loss of appetite, a sensation as if the stomach were always full; nothing tastes good. Or, on the other hand, a kind of canine hunger, along with which there is a soapy, slimy condition of the mouth; everything tastes like straw, and there is an immediate feeling of fullness. Frequent eructations; occasional nausea, relieved by lying down and by eating; sometimes nausea and retching at night; pressure in the epigastrium, as if swollen; throbbing, cutting, pinching pains in the abdomen; great accumulation of flatus in the abdomen, with great distention.

Stool. As regards the stool, we notice: Constant tenesmus, with nausea, tearing and pinching in the intestines; the stool is scanty, consisting of mucus, or a watery, jelly-like substance, yellow or streaked with white, frothy, and often mixed with blood. Before stool a burning in the rectum. After stool all pains are relieved. Itching and burning in the rectum, with smarting, blind hæmorrhoids.

The urine is dark, soon becomes turbid, with a white sediment (probably urate of ammonia). It is evacuated frequently with sticking pain in the bladder.

With regard to the genital organs we find, as in various other distensible parts of the body, the characteristic effects of Rhus, viz.: Swelling, produced by serous infiltration of the cellular tissue, redness of the cutis, followed by vesicular eruption, which forms a light scab or small white scabs. The moisture exuded is limpid and acrid. Moreover, the natural secretions are acrid. Hence the menstrual flow which Rhus makes to appear earlier and more copiously than is normal, is acrid.

Respiratory Organs. Sneezing; free nasal secretion.

Hoarseness.

Respiration impeded. Cough, dry, hacking, worse evening and before midnight, or in the morning after waking.

Sensation of heat in the chest and of weakness there, hindering speech. Stitching pain here and there.

It cannot fail to be remarked how much less action on the respiratory organs Rhus has than Bryonia.

Sometimes violent palpitation, sometimes weakness in the cardiac region and a feeling of trembling in the heart.

Neck and Back. In the region of the neck and back we find stiffness of the nape and entire neck, with tensive pain and crying out on moving. The sacral region is stiff when he moves, but pains when sitting, as if he had been stooping and bending the back too much. Stitching and pressing pains.

In the extremities we have, most frequently, sticking pains. They may occur in all parts. Also tearing pains, aggravated by hard labor. When felt of, the bones feel sore. The salient osseous processes, condyles, olecranon, etc., are sore to pressure.

Drawing pains are frequent. They go from the elbow to the hand. In Dr. Joslin's proving of Rhus radicans a pain is described as following the ulnar nerve. I have twice met this in patients and relieved it permanently with a dose of Rhus radicans. Tensive pain; aching and pains as if luxated are common under Rhus. They affect all parts of the extremities and all the joints.

Besides the above pains and sensations there is a feeling of creeping, formication and numbness as if the fingers were asleep. This is allied to the paralysis.

Also a sensation of great weakness in the limbs; a trembling of the arms and fingers on moderate exertion; a heaviness and lassitude of the lower extremities so that one can hardly move.

There is painless swelling of the feet at evening, evidently œdematous.

Also swelling and pain of the axillary glands.

Sleep. There is great sleepiness during the day, and also early in the morning, with indisposition to rise and dress. Constant desire to lie

RHUS TOXICODENDRON. 135

down. Incessant yawning, spasmodic, fatiguing, and almost breaking the jaw. Yet the patient can't get asleep before midnight, partly from sheer wakefulness, partly from heat and restlessness or anxiety; tumultuous coursing of the blood, without thirst.

On going to sleep, shuddering and twitching in the body. The sleep is restless with tossing and unpleasant thoughts and dreams about the business of the day or of things recently done or heard, The gastric symptoms are apt to be felt or to be worse at night.

Fever. The proving of Rhus is rich in fever symptoms. The cold fresh air is not tolerated; it seems to make the skin painful. (This symptom is of inestimable value in treating rheumatic patients.)

The chill occurs early in the morning. It is characteristic of the chill that it is accompanied by cough, dry and fatiguing. I have often cured intermittent with Rhus, guided by this symptom alone. More frequently the paroxysm is mixed up. External chill with internal heat, without thirst, followed by general sweat. The sweat often appears on the whole body, except the head and face. In this respect the opposite of Silicea.

As regards the disposition, it is depressed and despondent, averse to all exertion, full of sad anxiety and care-taking, depressed, lonesome and prone to weep; anxiety is so great he thinks he shall die or lose his mind; the forces sink; he gets fits of trembling; then comes restlessness; the patient can't sit still but must always keep moving; becomes fearful, thinks he has been poisoned; the anxiety goes to such an extent that he feels as though he should take his own life; at the same time a sense of dyspnœa and yet relief from deep inspirations.

A better picture than this of the mental and moral condition which ushers in one form of typhoid or nervous fever—the erethistic as distinguished from the torpid form—could hardly be conceived.

We come now to the practical applications of Rhus, in which department, for lack of space, we shall restrict ourselves to its application in fevers, in rheumatism, in paralysis, and in cutaneous diseases, including the exanthemata and glandular affections.

PRACTICAL APPLICATIONS.

In fevers Rhus has had a most successful and extensive application. As the symptoms indicate, the forms of fever which require it can only be what used to be called the nervous fevers, and are now known as typhoid or typhus.

Comparing it with Bryonia and Eupatorium, we miss at once the whole train of gastro-hepatic symptoms, the vomiting of bile, soreness and pain at the pit of the stomach constriction around the epigastric zone, fullness and tenderness of the hepatic region, etc., which indicated those remedies in bilious remittent fevers. On the other hand, we

RHUS TOXICODENDRON. 137

find Rhus producing some degree of tenderness of the abdomen, great flatulent distention of the abdomen, amounting to tympanitis,—occasional watery or mucous diarrhœa,—symptoms which, though not so strongly pronounced as similar symptoms are under Phosphoric acid, yet decidedly resemble the symptoms of typhoid fever, or, as the Germans call it, abdominal typhus, and indicate the use of Rhus in that disease.

With this indication, the depressed and collapsed sensorium, the absent-mindedness, the inability to think of what one wishes to do or say, to remember even familiar circumstances, the depression of spirits, the lassitude and actual muscular feebleness, exactly coincide. So do the restless nights and sleepy days, the mixed-up fever and the partial sweats which give no relief.

Hahnemann, in writing of the epidemic of 1813, gave the following directions for selecting Rhus: "This fever has two principal stages: In the first period (which is all the shorter, the worse the disease is to be) there are present, full increased sensation of the pains usually present, with intolerably bad humor, sensation of heat in the body and especially in the head, dry feeling or actual dryness in the mouth, causing constant thirst, bruised feeling in the limbs, restlessness, etc.; but in the second period, that of delirium (a quasi metastasis of the whole disease upon the mental organs), no complaint is made of all those symptoms, the patient is hot, does not desire to drink, he knows not whether to take this or that, he does not know those about him, or he abuses them; he makes irrelevant answers, talks nonsense with his eyes open; does foolish things, wishes to run away, cries aloud or whines, without being able to say why he does so; has a rattling in the throat, the countenance is distorted, the eyes squinting; he plays with his hands, behaves like a madman, passes fæces and urine involuntarily, etc.

"In the first period of pain and consciousness, two remedies are of use and generally quite remove the disease at its commencement,—Bryonia alba and Rhus toxicodendron. If, for instance, the patient complain of dizziness, shooting pains in the head, throat, chest, abdomen, etc., which are felt particularly on moving the part; in addition to the other symptoms, the hæmorrhages, the vomiting, the heat, the thirst, the nocturnal restlessness, etc., we give him a dose of Bryonia, and give no other medicine, nor even repeat the same as long as he continues to improve.

"If now," he proceeds,—"if now, the amendment produced by the Bryonia goes off in the course of a few days; if the patient then complains of shooting pains in one or other part of the body while the part is at rest; if the prostration and anorexia are greater; if there is harassing cough, or such a debility of certain parts as to threaten paralysis, we give a single drop of the Rhus toxicodendron.

"Or the Rhus may be given at the very commencement, if the symptoms I have described occur at the commencement of the attack. * * * Indeed, Rhus is suitable more frequently than Bryonia in this disease, and hence can more frequently be used first and alone in treating it."

Observe, first, the clear and sharp distinction which Hahnemann draws between the indications for Bryonia and Rhus respectively; how carefully he advises us to give each remedy only when the symptoms which specially call for it are present in the case; and how different these symptoms are! Could you gather from this statement that Hahnemann advises the giving of Rhus and Bryonia, in alternation, in typhoid fever? It would seem to me impossible. And yet the majority of homœopathicians will tell you, and the majority of works on practice will teach you, that the standard prescription in typhoid fever is "Bryonia and Rhus in alternation," and that this was recommended and used by Hahnemann! There is no better foundation for alternation in any case than there is for this assertion.

Dr. Wurmb, in his "Clinical Studies of Typhoid Fever," has given us some exceedingly valuable summaries of the action of Rhus and its cognate remedies, so valuable that I cannot do better than to quote freely from his work. Speaking generally of the therapeutics of fevers, he says:

"In typhoid epidemics, inasmuch as the cases present at given times and in given localities, apart from all special peculiarities of individual cases, a determinate and distinct general character, and are thereby clearly distinguishable from those which occur at other periods and in other localities, we must regard it as our first problem to get an accurate knowledge of the character of the prevailing epidemic. * * * * *

"When we have done this, the second problem remains for solution, viz.: The discovery of the group of remedies which most closely corresponds in the similarity of their effects upon the healthy to the character of the epidemic. If we succeed in this, then is the most difficult part of our labor done; for the number of remedies contained in this group cannot be very large, and it cannot consequently be very difficult to select from it the most suitable remedy, that is to say, the remedy of which the individual peculiarities coincide most nearly with those of the case to be treated."

Acting upon this rule Dr. Wurmb has described the peculiarities of several groups of drugs and pointed out their adaptations to different forms of typhoid fever. The first of these groups consists of Rhus toxicodendron and phosphoric acid, the similarities and peculiar differences of which are finely depicted by him. He remarks first that the cases of fever in which these drugs are required and were used by him, are not very grave and severe forms,—the epidemic could not be called a malignant one. "The disturbances in the vascular and nervous systems, though often tolerably severe, were never excessive, and the tendency to decomposition of the organic substance, although it existed and was developed, was not very striking. The appropriate remedies, consequently, were such as, in large doses, in healthy subjects, act powerfully, it is true, on the life of blood and nerve; pervert the latter, but do not completely suspend it; cause disturbances in the vital chemistry but do not entirely supersede it!"

Rhus toxicodendron and Phosphoric acid, being drugs which act in an equal degree upon both the vital force and the organic substance, and which act powerfully but not destructively, were suitable to an epidemic of this character.

Now, the distinction between these two drugs may in a word be stated as follows: Rhus is characterized by symptoms of erethism, excitement, orgasm; Phosphoric acid by symptoms of torpor, collapse, sluggishness. This is the proposition which, in so far as Rhus is concerned, we proceed to elaborate in the words of Dr. Wurmb.

'*Indications for Rhus.* The patients are generally strongly built persons who have hitherto been healthy; the typhoid for the most part comes on suddenly, runs a rapid course, and reaches in the course of a few days a high degree of development. At the same time with the disturbances in the vascular system, there is felt a strong sensation of illness, which advances at a more rapid rate than the other symptoms do; for example, the actual debility is not so great as the sensation of debility, inasmuch as tolerably rapid and forcible motions are still capable of being made. (N. B.—During convalescence, the contrary condition obtains; the patients take themselves to be stronger than they really are.)

"Soon, however, the forces fail; movements become difficult and feeble and the patients are constrained to lie quietly in bed, in one place. They complain of aching in the limbs and, sometimes, of violent pain in some joint or other, as in rheumatism.

"These disturbances in the general condition do not long continue alone; there are soon associated with them irregularities in the vascular system, viz.: in the beginning, gentle, fugitive chills and heat, but especially heat of the head; at a later period the heat predominates, and at last it becomes continuous and is very violent; there is tendency to rush of blood to the head; roaring pains in the head; the temperature is elevated; the face is burning hot to the touch; the eyes shine and are moderately injected; the cheeks, lips and tongue are of a deep red color; the thirst is very great; the pulse 110-112 in a minute. Even at the very beginning of the vascular excitement hæmorrhages occur, especially from the nose, and in women, from the genitals. The former almost always afford relief, the latter, which are generally mistaken for the menstrual flow, last but a few hours, or, at the most a day, and produce no change in the condition of the patient.

"The symptoms of a change in the composition of the blood (of a sort of decomposition, being the first evidence of action upon the organic substance) appear in a moderate degree only and somewhat later. There appear upon the skin small ecchymoses; the expectoration has a bloody tinge; the stools rarely contain blood.

"The nervous functions are always powerfully affected; they are oppressed and restricted. The organs of sense are, in the beginning, in a condition of over-excitability. There is a great sensibility to light, noise, etc.

"At a later period the opposite condition obtains; the patients become insensible to external influences, complain of nothing whatever, and lie in a condition of atony.

"The sensorium is oppressed and ratiocination is difficult even in the very beginning of the disease. The patients are aware of this fact, but endeavor to prevent its being observed; and to this end, when a question is put to them, they evidently gather themselves up and reply hastily, but correctly; at a latter period, when their imagination has become too lively, they cannot quite succeed in this, and hence their answers are in part correct and in part incoherent; finally the incoherence increases; the patients murmur and keep talking to themselves, or they are disquieted by very lively phantasies of the most various sorts, especially at night. Sleep for the most part fails entirely; or when for a moment it visits the patient, there comes in its train a host of disquieting and burthensome dreams. * * * * *

"The abnormal condition of the vascular system is distinctly reflected upon the external skin. This is at first reddened, dry and hot; spots appear, resembling rubeola or measls, upon the thorax and abdomen; if the vascular excitement has subsided, copious sweats occur and along with them, almost always, a miliary eruption.

"The mucous membranes are always involved. The tongue is more or less coated, becomes rough, dry, cracked and woody; the lips and teeth are sometimes covered with brown sordes; the taste is gone. The condition of the gastric and intestinal mucous membrane is such as to produce want of appetite; aversion to food; nausea, retching, vomiting. Gases are developed in the intestinal canal, which distend the abdomen. The abdomen becomes sensitive to external pressure under the margins of the left ribs and in the right iliac region. The stools are at first scanty and infrequent, indeed there may be none for several days; generally, however, they soon become fluid and occur three or four times daily without tenesmus or other discomforts; and at a later period, when they are still more frequent, they pass involuntarily. They consist of serum and of a greenish-brown substance, which, at a later period of the disease, is mixed with white flocculi.

"Resulting from the affection of the mucous membrane of the aid passages, there is a sensation of dryness in the trachea; the somewhat accelerated respiration is, at first, somewhat louder, sharper, the expiration audible; at a later period, mucous râles set in, or large crepitation. The cough, which at first is moderate and dry, becomes gradually more violent and looser in sound, but accompanied by only a very little tenacious sputa, now and then streaked with blood.

"The parenchyma of the lungs is congested with blood, especially in the lower lobes, and pneumonic infiltrations often form there, which explain the following symptoms, not infrequent in typhoid: Constriction of the chest; short, anxious respiration; sticking pains in the sides, etc. The spleen is almost always enlarged. The urine is scanty; it is deficient in chloride of sodium and in urea; rich in sulphates, phosphates and other salts which are always abundant in diseases which are characterized by a tendency to decomposition of the blood. The urine, moreover, is turbid, looks like whey, deposits an abundant white sediment, and shows, by the albumen which it contains, the hyperæmic condition of the kidneys. * * *

"The condition above described may last many days. The patient may pass from it into a sate of health, or into a still higher grade of erethism, or into the opposite condition of torpor. * *

"In the former case, viz., that of a return to health, the febrile movements slacken; sleep again visits the patient; the sensorial phenomena become less abnormal; the patient gets his appetite again, and congratulates himself on his fine condition; the diarrhœa and tympanitis may last a few days longer than the other symptoms, but they then vanish and there remain only a moderate degree of weakness and emaciation, and paleness of the skin.

* * * * * *

"In the event, however, of the development of the disease to a still higher grade of erethism, we have not generally long to wait. In this case it is probable that Arsenicum will be our remedy."

For Arsenicum, as we shall see by and by, affects both the vascular and nervous life on the one hand, and the blood composition on the other hand; it acts, with almost equal energy, on the vital forces and on the organic substance. It is, hence, appropriate for such a form of fever as that described as requiring Rhus. But Arsenicum acts with greater energy, with a wider swing and deeper penetration than Rhus. It perverts more thoroughly, excites more profoundly the vital functions; it alters more extensively and more completely the blood and the organic substance than Rhus does. It is, therefore, appropriate for more malignant epidemics of fever, for more severe cases of the same form of fever than Rhus.

Thus, as regards the erethistic form of typhoid fever, a group is formed consisting of Rhus and Arsenic, which, instead of being contrasted as Rhus and Phosphoric acid were, are analogous and allied. They stand related to each other as less and greater, Rhus being the less and Arsenic the greater.

But if the fever change from the erethistic into the torpid form, then Phosphoric acid will probably be required as the correlative of Rhus; or if the torpor be extreme, Carbo vegetabilis may be required, as the correlative of Arsenic.

To show, now, the applicability of Rhus toxicodendron to the form of fever which has been described, Wurmb proceeds to say:

"If we hold up beside this picture of the disease, the picture of the action of Rhus toxicodendron, so striking is the similarity that it will not be easy to mistake it. They agree not alone in this, that in both, the same symptoms and groups of symptoms appear, but also that they have in both the same significance. The similarity is therefore not simply apparent, it is real. For, as in typhus, the blood-life is especially affected, the same is the case in the Rhus disease. As in typhus, by reason of the changes in the blood, a violent excitement occurs in the vascular system, the same is the case with Rhus; as in typhus, the sensorial functions are depressed, and in consequence of this depression the imagination is unchained and set loose to work its fancy, and the representations of the general perceptive faculty no longer correspond to the phenomena upon which this faculty is exercised; as in typhus, the mucous membranes, especially those of the intestinal canal, in which deposits and irritations never fail, are especially involved; in short, just as typhus, in spite of the erethism which is present, is an adynamic, morbid process, in the exact sense of the word, and tends to produce, even in the beginning, a decomposition of the blood and an exhaustion of the vital force; the very same is true in all these respects of the morbid affection produced in the healthy subject by Rhus toxicodendron.

Having thus treated very fully the subject of Rhus in fevers, I should, perhaps, in strict deference to the unity of subject, proceed to treat of Rhus in relation to other diseased conditions. But lectures of this kind are worth nothing if they are not practical. I cannot hope, in the short time accorded me, to treat of all the drugs in the materia medica, nor to treat fully of many, if indeed of any. The most I can hope for is to show you how to study drugs in a practical way, and how to reason upon and to apply the knowledge gained by study and observation. Now, the essence of the study of the materia medica is comparison,—the comparative study of one drug beside another drug, with a view of noting their resemblances and differences; the successive study of each drug of a group, in comparison with the picture of some disease to which you suppose the group, or some member of it, to be applicable as a remedy.

We have studied in detail a certain form of typhoid fever, and I have stated that the remedies most similar to that form and degree of intensity are Rhus toxicodendron and Phosphoric acid. I have stated the special similarity of Rhus, but the practical question for you is to know also what cases require Phosphoric acid, that you may be in a position when you meet this form of fever to discriminate between the indications for these two remedies respectively, and may be able to give each in just the case which requires it.

I shall help you then, I think, if now, while the subjects is fresh in your minds, I introduce into my lecture on Rhus an episode upon Phosphoric acid,—the correlative of Rhus toxicodendon,—and in this, as before, I shall follow my excellent friend and teacher, Dr. Wurmb.

Indications for Phosphoric acid in typhoid:

"The morbid condition corresponding to Phosphoric acid agrees in essential points with that which requires Rhus. In both we find the same relations to the blood and nerve life; the same tendency to decomposition of the blood and to a waste of the forces; the same changes in the mucous membranes generally, but especially in that of the intestinal canal, etc."

The difference between them consists in this, that in the Rhus affection there is more prominent an erethism of one portion of the vital phenomena and a depression of another portion, a one-sided excitement and a one-sided depression, whereas in the Phosphoric acid affection there is a general and simultaneous depression, letting down, atony of the entire series of vital phenomena. Whereas in the Rhus affection, we see excitement and overactivity in the functions of vegetable life, and simultaneous depression. in the functions of animal life; we see in the Phosphoric acid affection simultaneous and immediate depression in the functions of both of these departments of the patient's organism. Generally this depression appears in the very beginning of the sickness, though not always, for sometimes partial phenomena of excitement usher in the disease; these, however, are of short duration and very moderate intensity; and after their disappearance the torbid character of the attack is all the more distinctly perceptible.

Cases of this kind are most frequently observed in debilitated subjects who have passed the prime of life; they require a longer time for their development into a distinct form of disease. Thus, for example, there are often noticed loss of appetite, feeling of illness, and a host of other preliminary symptoms which indicate an impending illness but give no clue to its particular form and character,—these, for weeks together, before the peculiar and really important symptoms set in which assure the diagnosis. When these latter have at last made their appearance we observe the following:

The sensations of illness and prostration reach speedily a very high grade, and *pari passu* with these sensations goes an actual want of power, and hence the patients even in the very beginning of the malady are content to lie quiet, because every movement is a heavy tax upon them. The disturbances in the vascular system do not advance in the same ratio, but lag behind; the pulse is often accelerated, it is true, though sometimes it is not, and in the former case it is generally feeble and small. The temperature is but seldom elevated; indeed it sometimes sinks below the normal grade. If it is increased the increase is confined to isolated parts of the body, especially the head, while other parts, the extremities in particular, are cold to the touch; the patients hence are pale, or have only sometimes a flush of redness. Hæmorrhages, as for example from the nose, are much more frequent, but they afford no relief; nay, they commonly aggravate the condition of the patient. Ecchymoses are likewise common occurrences, and these are particularly apt to occur on the spots on which the patients lie,—livid spots, which at a later period become sloughing bed-sores.

The patients, for the most part, lie in a constant slumber, which is apt to pass into a higher grade of stupor; the expression of face is stupid; the sensorium is oppressed, the delirium, if it exist, is never lively or active; it takes only the form of an unintelligible murmuring. If the patient be aroused from this stupor it takes him a long time to come to his senses, he looks around him in a kind of dull, stupid wonder, answers slowly, even though it be correctly, and soon sinks back again into his former apathetic condition.

The special senses become dull, but especialy the sense of hearing. The patients are influenced and affected by nothing. They complain of nothing but weakness and confusion of the head.

The skin soon loses its plumpness, takes on a shriveled aspect and is loose and wrinkled; the cheeks become sunken; the nose pointed; the skin is constantly clammy, moist, and even often covered with a copious sweat and with countless miliary vesicles.

The affection of the mucous membrane is evidenced chiefly by increased secretions; the tongue is moist but pale.

In the thorax are heard large crepitation and rhonchus. Cough is rare, because the need to expel the mucus is not felt by the patient. A similar condition obtains in the mucous membrane of the stomatch and intestines; the stools are copious, often involuntary and passed unconsciously. They are very liquid, contain but little sediment and show sometimes traces of blood.

The pneumonic infiltration is not rare, but it is by no means so frequent as the hypostatic congestion.

Enlargement of the spleen never fails; the diarrhœa, even when it is ever so copious, has no influence upon this symptom.

The urine contains many protein compounds, much albumen, but few salts.

This state of things may pass off into health or may merge in a still higher grade of torpor. If the former change takes place, the recovery is a slow one and relapses commonly take place even when the improvement has been for some time in process.

If, however, the latter change takes place, and the state of things above described gives place to a still more complete and absolute torpor, then it is probable that Carbo vegetabilis will be the remedy indicated. For, just as we have seen that in the erethistic form of typhoid fever, Rhus and Arsenic bear to each other the relation of less and greater so in the torpid form of the disease do Phosphoric acid and Carbo vegetabilis bear to each other the same relation of less and greater. And the proving of Carbo vegetabilis, I may here remark, is the very type and representative of an asthenic and torpid pathogenesis.

These remarks will suffice to give an idea of the application of Rhus in fevers. They have included no name except that of typhoid fever— but surely, I need not at this hour remind you that, no matter how different may be the names that are applied to morbid conditions, if the conditions be similar the remedy may be the same. Now, it often happens that in the course of the exanthematous fevers, measles and scarlatina, a similar train of symptoms to those alrady described makes its appearance and calls for Rhus Especially is this the case in scarlatina, a disease in which the value of Rhus is not well understood by the profession. It will be more ably expounded than I can do it by Dr. Wells in some of the forthcoming numbers of the "American Homœopathic Review."

The indication for Rhus in scarlatina is still stronger if, in addition to symptoms already detailed, there be an œdematous condition of the fauces, soft palate and uvula, with vesicles upon these parts and a singularly annoying itching, smarting and burning. Independently of scarlatina, epidemics of influenza often occur presenting this œdematous condition of the soft parts of the fauces and pharynx, and even threatening œdema glottidis. The curtain of the palate is puffed and pink; the uvula is elongated, puffed, translucent, and the end is often nearly spherical, looking like a great drop of fluid or jelly just ready to fall off. Vesicles stud the pharynx. The rawness and roughness of pharynx and larynx are almost intolerable. Such an influenza is generally attended by symptoms of great debility; in any case, it finds a suitable and prompt remedy in Rhus, as I have often experienced.

In paralysis, especially of the lower extremities, Rhus is an important remedy. But the paralysis for which it is appropriate is not that form which results from a lesion of the spinal cord. It is rather of the motor than of the sensitive nerves; for I believe sensation is not much impaired. In the form known as rheumatic paralysis, where the paralysis supervenes upon rheumatism, Rhus is especially called for. So, likewise, as would be expected, in cases resulting from undue exposure to cold and dampness, especially exposure of the back or limbs.

This explains the value of Rhus in a form of paralysis not rare in very young children. It affects only the lower extremities, and comes, I am persuaded, though it is difficult to trace these things, from nurses allowing children to sit down on cold stone steps. If these paralyses last long they produce deformity by arrest of development. They are, in general, easily cured with Rhus and an occasional dose of Sulphur.

As regards the application of Rhus in rheumatism, I believe enough has been said of the characteristic action of Rhus to solve all doubts on this subject. Just as Rhus produces in the mucous membranes an inflammation which is not phlegmonous only inasmuch as it does not go on to suppuration, so does it act on the serous membranes of the joints and muscles. The serous secretions are increased and œdematous swellings are produced. The local manifestations, therefore, resemble those of rheumatism.

The fever has been described. The general condition must be of an erethistic typhoid character. The joints are swollen, œdematous, the pains worse during repose and stimulating the patient to constant exertion and motion of the part, both day and night (restlessness only at night requires Causticum).

The condyles and salient points of bone are sore. The pains and soreness are relieved by warmth. Perspiration is copious and does not relieve.

The skin is the part most obviously affected by Rhus. It produces a most remarkable imitation of vesicular erysipelas, and is our most valued remedy in this affection. Any one who has seen a case of Rhus-poisoning (for which, by the day, the best remedy is Sepia) will recognize the similarity to eczema, for which, in its various forms, Rhus is a most valuable remedy. But its grand rôle is in the treatment of the pustular form,—impetigo eczematodes or eczema impetiginodes, or baker's itch, as it is called.

COLCHICUM.

HAVING now studied the properties and uses of Bryonia, Aconite and Rhus, remedies which, in addition to their applicability in fevers and various other affections, are eminently adapted to the treatment of the general class of maladies grouped under the name of rheumatism, it seems to me most fitting to study now certain other drugs which are eminently anti-rheumatics, before proceeding to other groups of which the characteristic symptoms indicate a different variety of action upon different organs and tissues. These drugs are Colchicum, Ledum, Rhododendron, Kalmia, and Spigelia.

The autumn crocus, or meadow-saffron, is a beautiful flower, found in most parts of temperate Europe, and especially abundant and beautiful near the site of the ancient Alba Longa, not far from Rome. The parts used are the root and the seeds, and various opinions have been expressed by different authors respecting the relative activity of these portions of the plant. The majority of the provings made by homœopathists were made with a tincture of the freshly gathered root. Colchicum was well known to the ancients, as indeed its name implies (from the island Colchos, where it abounded), and very little has been added, even in our day, to the knowledge which the ancients possessed of its properties and uses. It was described by them as a violent emeto-cathartic, and on that account a dangerous remedy; as, however, a specific remedy for gout and rheumatism in which it gave magical relief. They considered its frequent and continued use in gout to be injurious, because of its action on the stomach and bowels, and Alexander of Tralles, in the fifth century, says that although it does speedily relieve the pain and soreness of an attack of gout, it nevertheless favors the frequent recurrence of these attacks,—an opinion which is repeated by Mr. Barwell, the most recent authority on "Diseases of the Joints." (Londone, 1860.)

In general, the effects ascribed to Colchicum are the following: in large doses it produces loss of muscular power, slow breathing, and slow and feeble pulse. The sensorium is but little disturbed.

Upon the digestive organs it acts with great energy, increasing and altering the secretion from some or all of their mucous surfaces. Sometimes profuse salivation results. More frequently, profuse secretion of urine. But bost frequently of all, nausea, eructations and copious vomiting of mucus and bile with frequent and abundant alvine evacuations, consisting of watery matters with white, skinny flocculi, or of yellowish and bloody matter. There is much tenesmus. The flatulent distention of the abdomen is sometimes enormous; when this is the case the stools are not so frequent nor so copious. Perfect loathing of food,—a symptom which led Dr. Hawley to give Colchicum successfully in an intermittent.

This action upon the intestines is observed not merely when the Colchicum is taken into the stomach, but also when it is injected into a vein or rubbed upon the external skin of the abdomen.

In addition to the above symptoms, the nervous system has been observed to be affected as follows: "Numbness of the hands and feet, with prickling as if they were asleep; painful flexure of the joints; pain in the shoulder and hip joints and in all the bones, with difficulty of moving the head and tongue." (Henderson.) The general loss of power is as remarkable as the fact that even in cases of extreme poisoning, the mind remains clear. Death probably results from paralysis of the heart.

Colchicum is one of many examples of the great difference in both the degree and kind of action which drugs exert on the organism of different animals. In very small doses it is fatal to dogs, producing violent emeto-cathartic action. Hence the French call it *tue-chien*. In cows it produces scanty urine, great distention of the abdomen, but no profuse diarrhœa. In rabbits it produces enuresis, but hardly any serious symptoms. A frog will take with impunity a dose that would speedily kill a large dog. This example shows the fallacy of deducing from experiments on animals rules for the use of drugs in diseases of the human organism.

The following summary of the action of Colchicum upon the healthy human subject is derived from Stapf's proving, in the "Archives of the Homœopathic Art," vol. vi., and from records of provings which are abundant in medical literature, and of which an excellent summary is given by Hartlaub, in the "Homœopathische Vierteljahrschrift," vol. viii. The provings are still very imperfect.

Sphere of Action. Taking a general view of the action of Colchicum, we find it to be exerted chiefly on the bones (or periosteum), on the synovial membranes of the joints, on the urinary and digestive organs, and upon that part of the nervous system which presides over the function of voluntary motion. It acts also somewhat upon the respiratory organs. It therefore acts with about equal scope upon both the vital force and the organic substance.

It is a remarkable fact that although the action of Colchicum upon the regions and tissues already named is very energetic, the drug being a poison of a speedy and fatal action, even in moderate doses, yet upon the sensorium it produces almost no effect, the mind remaining clear to the last.

COLCHICUM.

Sensations. The sensations which Colchicum produces are a shuddering and creeping in isolated parts of the body, such as are wont to be felt on getting cold from change of weather. Also, a tearing, tensive pain in small portions of the body at a time, and quickly changing its location from one part to another. Also, sudden tearing shocks or jerkings throughout one entire half of the body. Sometimes sticking or jerking drawings, or weak drawing and tearing in various muscles. The most distressing pains are the sticking shocks or jerks, which are felt deep in the soft parts, and, as it were, upon the periosteum.

Aggravation. They are worse at night, and deprive the patient of sleep.

Concomitants. They are attended by a symptom which is characteristic of Colchicum, viz., a feeling of muscular weakness or paralysis, and this feeling it is which interferes with the patient's locomotion. Finally, there are sticking pains in the joints.

The weakness is very great; the whole body is sore and sensitive; there is a sensation of trembling felt throughout the body; all the muscles of voluntary motion, but especially those of the arms and legs, are paralyzed. The knees strike together, and the patient can hardly walk.

Peculiarities. The pains are much aggravated at night, becoming intolerable, and they are aggravated also by any mental exertion or by emotion. There is great sleepiness during the day, with indisposition to exertion of any kind, and confusion and dullness of the head. At night, however, the sleep is disturbed or driven away by pains. If he sleep, the patient is wakened by frightful dreams.

As regards fever, we observe chilliness through the limbs or down the back, sometimes dry heat, especially at night. Sweat copious and sour. But in general the febrile symptoms are few and moderate in intensity.

The sensorium is no further affected than that it partakes, in some degree, of the general depressd condition. The memory is weakened, and the ideas are not so clear as is customary with the patient.

Coming now to the special analysis, we find:

Head. Pressing pains, above in small spots or very severely in the substance of the cerebellum, and occurring on the slightest intellectual exertion; a pressing heaviness in the cerebellum, especially on moving or stooping forward.

Tearing pains, sometimes in one-half of the head and sometimes in the occiput (the pains, as already stated, wander), sometimes in the temples, sometimes in the pericranium. A pressing tearing in the occiput, finally a very painful, drawing tearing in one-half of the head, beginning at the ball of the eye and extending to the occiput. (This reminds us of Spigelia, which has similar symptom on the left side, and of Silicea and Belladonna on the right side.)

Character. To recapitulate, the pains are tearing, drawing and pressing. They are most frequent in the occiput, and are often semi-lateral. The characteristic symptom is the severe pressing pain deep in the substance of the cerebellum, occurring on the slightest intellectual exertion.

Some remarkable symptoms are recorded of the *Eyes.* Drawing, digging pains deep in the orbit, resembling those of sclerotitis. Pressure and biting in the canthi with moderate lachrymation. Violent sharp tearing pains in the globe of the eye and around the orbit.

Face. The expression of the face is that of a chronic patient. There are tearing and tensive pains in the facial muscles, moving from one location to another. Likewise drawing in the bones of the face and nose, a sensation as if they were being rent asunder.

The teeth are very sensitive when pressed together, as in biting. Tearing in the jaws and gums; the teeth feel too long. The pains in the teeth are aggravated when, immediately after taking something warm into the mouth, the patient takes something cold.

In the tongue, tearing burning and sticking. Also a loss of sensibility in the tongue, the first symptom we encounter of the Colchicum paralysis.

In the throat, a tickling as if a coryza were setting in, which induces, the patient to cough and to clear the throat. The mucus is thin and greenish and comes sometimes involuntarily into the mouth. Externally, in the cervical muscles, sometimes a pressing pain, sometimes a tension, felt even when swallowing. The throat is dry, and yet there is a flow of watery saliva, accompanied by nausea, fullness and discomfort in the abdomen.

In the digestive apparatus, we find considerable thirst, but absence of appetite. Frequent and copious eructations of tasteless gas. Nausea with great restlessness and, on assuming the upright posture, a qualmishness in the stomach and inclination to vomit. Violent retching, followed by copious and forcible vomiting of food and then of bile. If the patient lie perfectly still, the disposition to vomit is less urgent. Every motion renews it. (This is characteristic also of Tabacum and Veratrum.)

The pit of the stomach becomes very sensitive to touch and pressure. Sometimes there is a burning sensation in the stomach, more frequently a feeling of icy coldness, accompanied by great pain and debility. (I cannot forbear remarking here the similarity of this symptom to one form of "retrocessed gout.")

Pressing, tearing, cutting and stitching pains in the abdomen. Great distention of the abdomen with gas, feeling as though the patient had eaten too much. This condition affects particularly the upper part, under the short ribs.

Tearing and burning at the orifice of the rectum are frequent symptoms, and prolapsus ani has been observed.

The symptoms of the stool present two characters depending on the magnitude of the dose and the period that has elapsed since the drug was taken, and also upon the extent to which other emunctories are affected. For, if there be copious salivation and copious secretion of urine, the stool will be scanty and attended by tenesmus, and *vice versa*. Thus, then, if the intestinal canal be the seat of the most powerful action of Colchicum, and if the symptoms be observed early, we have copious, frequent watery or bilious stools, often without pain, sometimes accompanied by cutting colic.

On the other hand, we observe scanty and difficult evacuation of a stool consisting of bloody mucus and shreds, with pains in the anus, great straining and a spasmodic action of the sphincter, and constant ineffectual effort to pass fæces. (Colchicum, taking these symptoms in connection with its rheumatic and semi-typhoid symptoms, will be, as it has proved itself, a valuable remedy in many cases of autumnal dysentery.)

Upon the urinary organs we have the same twofold action. The secretion is sometimes very copious, watery and frequent. But, generally in the human subject the secretion of urine is diminished; the urine is dark, turbid, and its evacaution is attended and followed by tenesmus of the bladder, and a burning pain in the urethra as if the urine were very warm.

Respiration. On the respiration organs the action of Colchium is a subject of dispute among old-school authorities. We find it produces a long-lasting coryza, which is never watery, but is characterized by secretion of abundant tenacious mucus, tickling in the trachea and a little cough.

It produces frequent oppression of the chest, dyspnœa, a tensive feeling in the chest, sometimes high in the chest, and sometimes low down. These symptoms point to the efficacy of Colchicum in some forms of asthma, a subject on which old-school doctors differ. Homœopathicians have often used it very successfully in asthma.

In the posterior part of the thorax, dull stitches, as much in the back as in the ribs. It is characteristic of of these stitches that they are chiefly felt during expiration and not during inspiration.

Back. In the back we note the various kinds of drawing tensive and stitching pains remarked elsewhere. They occur or are much aggravated on motion. On the sacrum, a spot as large as one's hand which feels sore, as if ulcerated, and is very sensitive to the touch.

Extremities. In the extremities, tearing pains in both muscles and joints, stitching pain in the joints. The pains wander from part to part. They are aggravated by motion and at night. They feel as if in the periosteum. Conjoined with the pains is a very distressing paralytic feeling, together with an actual loss of muscular power approximating paralysis. The action of Colchicum is more marked on the small joints than on the large.

Application. Colchium was regarded by the ancient Greek and Arabian physicians as a specific for gout, but a somewhat dangerous remedy. It fell into disuse until Stoerck, in Vienna, in the eighteenth century, called attention to it. He proved it in a rude way, and vaunted it as a remedy for gout, rheumatism, asthma and dropsies. Its efficacy in asthma, affirmed by many physicians, has been denied by others, except the asthma depend on hydro-thorax or hydro-pericardium, in which cases it is admitted Colchicum may relieve by removing the dropsical effusion. Stoerck's recommendation of Colchicum as a remedy in gout did not attract much attention until it was found that Colchicum was the chief ingredient of several famous nostrums for gout, as the *Eau médicinale* of Husson and the pills of Lartigue and others. At the present day its value is recognized and we all have opportunities to see the mischief inflicted by its improper uses.

Alexander of Tralles, in the fifth century, and Mr. Barwell, in 1860, affirm that it predisposes to relapses. In cases in which it does so it cannot be the true remedy.

It has been a subject of discussion whether it acts specifically in gout or only by virtue of its hydragogue properties. The question is settled by the fact that other hydragogues do not relieve gout as Calchicum does. Also by the fact which I have myself seen, and which is attested by many physicians, that its action is manifest in relieving the gout only or chiefly when means are taken to prevent its action on the bowels, as by combining Opium with it, or by copious draughts of rice-water.

Having alluded to injurious effects upon the use of Colchicum, I will quote a few sentences from "Barwell on the Joints," p. 176:

"Colchicum is a remedy whose value is undoubted, but its influences for evil are almost as certain; it is more powerful in gout than in rheumatism. It has a power in checking the pains, etc., of both rheumatic and gouty diseases, but it also has an effect in procuring relapses. Persons who have been treated with this remedy suffer from the return of the disease more rapidly than those treated by some other medicine."

Dr. Tod says the relapses are apt to assume an asthenic character, p. 224.

"Colchicum is a two-edged sword of considerable sharpness; there is no doubt of its great power in checking gouty and even rheumatic pains; but it is very questionable whether it does so in a beneficial manner. The late Dr. Tod believed that it changes the common acute form of gout into an asthenic condition which is less easy of management; and there is great reason to believe this idea correct. Any practical opinion which is the results of experience, not of mere *a priori* reasoning, deserves great attention; and we may be sure of this fact, that whatever the *modus operandi* of the drug may be, it hastens relapses, renders each one less amenable to treatment and requiring larger doses of the medicine (if treated with Colchicum) than its predecessors. Whether the remedy act simply as a purgative, or as stimulating the liver, or as causing a larger excretion of lithic acid, is not certain; but its use is permissible only when the constitution is vigorous, and it should not be given except when other means of procuring ease have failed."

I fancy that every one who has seen cases of gout or rheumatism treated by Colchicum will indorse the statements of Mr. Barwell and Dr. Tod. Yet they are wrong in banishing Colchicum from the list of remedies to be employed at the beginning of treatment. It has its place in the treatment of gout and rheumatism, and if properly employed in appropriate cases will do good, and good only. Allopathic authors are almost unanimous in recommending Colchicum as Mr. Barwell does, as suitable only in persons of vigorous constitution, and in whom the manifestations of the disease are acute and active or only approaching the sub-acut, and they caution us against using it in feeble cases and in asthenic conditions. Why? Because, as they tell us, its tendency is to produce an asthenic condition, and none but vigorous patients can bear it. Others would be reduced too low. Here we have the old idea of antagonism between the action of the drug and that of the morbid organism, the latter not being regarded (as I think it should be) as engaged in a struggle against the morbific influence, of which struggle the symptoms are the phenomena, and in which struggle the drug should act in co-operation with the organism and in the same direction as the symptoms.

If we look at the symptoms produced by Colchicum, we find the rheumatic or gouty symptoms characterized by a debility, a paralytic weakness, very suggestive of an asthenic type of disease. The fact that Dr. Tod and Mr. Barwell have observed the tendency of Colchicum to turn the active into the asthenic form of gout, furnishes additional evidence of this mode of action of Colchicum. Now, it is in precisely this form of asthenic sub-acute disease that Colchicum is truly indicated and does real service. But, what of the danger of reducing the patient? None whatever, provided we give doses so small as not to produce the physiological effects, but only the specific effects, which are known to be produced when the symptoms disappear. These doses, however, must be very small, and, noted as homœopathicians are for giving small doses, many of that school err in these cases in giving doses too large. I do not think it safe to give, in a well-marked Colochicum case, a larger dose than the 15th potency.

Dr. Wurmb speaks of Colchicum in its relations to rheumatism, as follows:

"This drug stands in close relation to the fibrous tissues; it produces, on the healthy, pains which are very similar to those of rheumatism; it excites a condition of irritation which is very closely allied to inflammation,—redness, swelling, heat, etc.; like rheumatic inflammation, this does not tend to suppuration, and it easily and quickly changes its location. In the Colchicum fever, as in the rheu-

COLCHICUM. 171

matic, the cold stage predominates, the sweat is very copious, etc., the urine and sweat have an acid smell and reaction.

"These features closely resemble those of a rheumatic attack. Yet, if we look at the entire action of Colchicum, we shall perceive that it cannot play an exceedingly important rôle in the treatment of rheumatism. For it produces another series of symptoms which would often contra-indicate it in rheumatism. For example, the muscular weakness, the paralytic symptoms, the diminution of vital heat, the capillary congestions, all which symptoms indicate a vital atony.

"Consequently, we should rarely find Colchicum indicated in the beginning of rheumatic disease, rather only when feeble, debilitated persons have suffered from it a long time."

It appears especially suitable to cases in which we perceive, on the one hand, an active excitement in the local symptoms, and, on the other, symptoms of torpor in the general condition of the patient.

Colchicum was recommended in 1833 against Asiatic cholera in England, and used successfully in eight cases. But as Dr. Stillé says, "notwithstanding its homœopathic appropriateness, it has not been used by others."

In autumnal dysenteries we have already alluded to its successful use.

It has been used as a diuretic and palliates dropsies. It may be useful in irritation of the bladder, and has been successfully employed in Bright's disease.

Ruckert reports its success in asthma. It quiets the heart's action. On the healthy it produces violent paliptation.

Bœnninghausen, whose veterinary practice was extensive, lauded Colchicum, as a specific for the excessive flatulent distention of the abdomen in cows who have been allowed to eat too freely of clover. This affection is very fatal. A single dose of Colchicum 200 gives prompt relief. This may direct our attention to Colchicum in tympanities after certain kinds of food in the human subject.

Before leaving the subject of Colchicum, I would call attention to the fact that in many cases of poisoning by it cataracts have formed before death in the eyes of the sufferers.

Professor Hoppe reports that with Colchicum he greatly benefited, though he failed to cure, three cases of soft cataract.

LEDUM PALUSTRE.

THE *Ledum palustre,* or marsh ledum, marsh tea, *Rosmarimum sylvestre,* a plant belonging to the heath family, is a native of northern Europe. It is also found in British America along the Canadian lakes. It can hardly be called a constituent of the allopathic materia medica; none to the standard works mention it.

Linnæus, in his "Flora Laponica," states that Ledum has been used by the inhabitants of northern Europe, especially Sweden, as a popular remedy against whooping cough, bilious attacks, etc. Odhelius recommends it in lepra, pemphigus and other skin diseases. The Swedes used a decoction of it to destroy vermin on sheep and swine. In Lapland branches of it are placed among the grain to keep away mice. It has been used in Switzerland to adulterate beer, but its rapidly acting intoxicating power was attended by the production of intense and obstinate headaches. The whole plant is used in medicine.

Our knowledge of the physiological properties of Ledum is derived from the proving by Hahnemann and his scholars, published in the "Materia Medica Pura," vol. iv. It is but a very fragmentary proving. The Provers' Society of Vienna are now engaged in a more extended proving of Ledum. The provings published are as yet too incomplete to be made the basis of a study.

In so far as our knowledge of Ledum will admit of our making a general analysis of its action, it may be said:

That Ledum acts on the vital force to this extent, that it interferes with and retards the capillary circulation, and particularly in the extremities and the external surface of the body. This is manifest by the coldness especially of the ends of the extremities, which characterizes the fever of Ledum and to which the heat of certain parts of the body at night form the only exception.

On the organic substance of the body Ledum acts extensively and peculiarly; witness the effect upon the skin, on which it produces eczema, lichen, pustular eruptions, pemphigus; and the action upon the small joints of the fingers and toes, in which enlargements, nodosities and deposits of inorganic matter do unquestionably occur.

The sphere of action of Ledum in so far as this is known to us embraces the sensorium, the digestive apparatus, the skin and the fibrous and serous tissues of the joints and their appendages.

The only periodicity remarked in the symptoms is this: that the pains in the joints are all aggravated at night and by the warmth of the bed; and that about midnight this aggravation becomes so great as to compel the subject to throw off the bed-covers.

As peculiarities attending the symptoms of Ledum, it is noted that the pains generally are aggravated by warmth at night, the joint pains (but not the others) are aggravated by motion; the itching of the skin attending the eruptions is aggravated by the warmth of the bed and is not relieved by scratching, until the part affected has been scratched raw.

The pains are in the joints, sticking, tearing or throbbing and a kind of paralytic pain. These pains in the joints are aggravated by motion, while other pains are not.

Ledum produces, moreover, hard and painful nodosities in the joints and then the warmth of the bed is intolerable, inasmuch as it causes heat and burning in the parts affected.

In the limbs, as considered apart from the joints, a feeling of numbness and torpidity.

A further peculiarity of Ledum is the general coldness and lack of animal heat which atends all the symptoms, with the exception of those above named.

Though sleepy and dull by day and in general not refreshed by sleep, the provers are sleepless at night, with restlessness, tossing, and dreams when they doze. On waking, a gentle sweat with itching of the whole body.

The fever consists almost entirely of coldness, shivering, here and there a little heat, as of the cheeks or forehead while the limbs are very cold, and a sour-smelling sweat, especially on the forehead; the sweat is often interspersed with shiverings.

SPECIAL ANALYSIS.

As regards the sensorium we find Ledum produces a feverish condition, a discontented and morose disposition, easily aroused to anger, with great intensity of feeling in whatever direction it may be aroused.

Vertigo is felt when walking and standing, even when sitting still, but is much more violent when stooping, when it is attended by a disposition to fall forward or backward; generally there is a constant sensation of unsteadiness and drunkenness in the head. This with the following symptoms should be remembered in connection with the adulteration of beer with Ledum already mentioned.

The head feels as if it were much affected and the brain is sore at every false step. (This is similar to Rhus toxicodendron.) The chief pain is a burdensome pressure in the forehead or over the entire head, with confusion and numb feeling. More rarely a sticking pain in the brain or a tearing in the head and in the eye (resembling Colchicum and Spigelia); at the same time the eyes are inflamed, the lids are agglutinated, and febrile movements occur in the evenings. Eruption and creeping sensation on the scalp.

Eyes. The pupils are dilated, the power of vision is diminished, with flashes before the eyes as after running violently. Lachrymation; the tears are acrid, the lids agglutinate, and yet there is no pain in them. In the eye a pressure or burning, but no inflammation. When inflammation does exist in the eye, the pain is tensive or tearing.

Ears. A kind of deafness as if something were laid before the ears. Noise of various kinds like the ringing of bells or the rushing of a gale of wind.

Nose. Burning internally in the nose, like coals of fire, and the nose is sore on pressure and on blowing it (a similar pain in the urethra).

Teeth. Pains in the teeth are violent, sticking; then attacks of intolerable tearing-outward pain on one side of the face, head and neck through the night, ending with shivering, deep sleep and lack of hunger and thirst.

In the throat sticking pains and sometimes a sensation as though there were a plug in the throat. (Sore throat with fine sticking pains.)

The stool is not well defined in the proving. Both constipation and a kind of dysenteric diarrhœa are described, yet no distinctive characteristics are given. It is not probable that Ledum is a remedy for either complaint.

Urine. As regards the urine the same twofold report is given; sometimes the evacuation is frequent and copious; sometimes it is infrequent and scanty. More careful provings on this subject are greatly to be desired, for the symptoms of the joints and the fevers would lead us to look upon Ledum as a valuable remedy in certain difficult forms of gout and of rheumatic gout; and in such diseases experience has shown it to be a most useful remedy. Pathology teaches us that in these affections the quality of the urinary secretion is much altered; and we should expect Ledum to produce analogous alterations in the healthy subject. It is probable that the Vienna provings now in progress will give us information on this subject.

The menses are hastened in their oncoming and are more copious than is usual, the flow being florid. In this respect, the action of Ledum upon the mucous membrane of the uterus is analogous to that upon the mucous membrane of the respiratory organs; for among the symptoms of the latter we find nose-bleeding, the blood being florid, and also spitting of florid blood frequently and in quantities; and in hæmoptysis Ledum is one of our most valuable remedies.

Respiratory Organs. Dyspnœa, constriction of the chest, worse on motion, walking, going upstairs; sometimes a tickling or creeping in the trachea and then embarrassed respiration. Cough, which sometimes takes away the breath. Remember that Ledum was a popular remedy for whooping cough. The cough is frequently attended with copious expectoration of florid blood, but especially at night and early in the morning, with purulent sputa.

Drawing and tearing stitches in the chest, which are felt on moving the arms and when sitting. Pressure on the chest, worse on expiration and on moving.

Back. Pain in back and loins, like a stiffness after sitting. Violent cramping pain over the hips. It occurs in the evening, and is so violent as to take away the breath, and that one cannot rise from a chair without aid. Also a drawing and tearing which extend from the loins into the occiput, and hot cheeks and inflammed eyes.

Extremities. In the upper extremities painful stitching about the shoulder on raising the arm; also in the hands, ankle, and in the toe and kneejoints, especially worse on moving.

Pressive pains in the shoulder and elbow-joints, more violent on motion, as likewise it is in the hip-joint. Beside this, there is sensation of heaviness in the arm, with a feeling of tenseness in the muscles of the forearm.

In addition to these symptoms, we have in the carpus and in the thigh a feeling as if the muscles had not their proper position. A similar sensation about the ankles, legs, the dorsum and margins of the feet, and in the toe-joints and on the soles of the feet; all worse from motion.

Also a tearing pressure from the hip-joint down to the angle; also from the shoulder-joint to the hand, worse on motion.

The limbs generally are languid, tried and lax. The small joints of the fingers, the knee-joint and the feet become the seat of nodosities, concretions or "gout stones."

The feet become and remain swollen. Ledum seems to act especially on the left shoulder and the right hip-joint.

PRACTICAL APPLICATIONS OF LEDUM.

Hahnemann observes that Ledum, from the symptoms which it produces, promises to be useful only in chronic affections, in which coldness and lack of animal heat predominate. This is not altogether justified by experience. It restricts too much the scope of the drug

In a number of cutaneous diseases, Ledum promises to be of service, and it has become an established remedy. Thus, according to Ruckert, "in pimples and pustules on the forehead, and in other parts of the body; in red blotches upon the face, which has a sticking pain when touched; in blotches on the forehead, like those to which brandy-drinkers are subject; biting itching on the chest, with red spots and miliary eruption."

In the proving, the eruption is described as: "Small round, red spots, insensible, on the inside of the arm, on the abdomen and on the feet;" "small pimples on the whole body (except face, neck and hands), with itching by day and only sometimes at night. Scratching relieves for a short time only." "Itching of the joints." "Tremendous gnawing-itching on the dorsum of both feet; after scratching it gets worse and worse; much more violent in the heat of the bed."

LEDUM PALUSTRE.

It will be applicable for various forms of lichen.

Teste, a more brilliant than trustworthy writer, says that Ledum is a specific cure for wounds with pointed instruments and for the evil effects of the sting of insects, from mosquitoes up to wasps. He applied locally a solution of the 15th dilution.

But the most interesting application of Ledum is in gout and rheumatism.

The characteristic indication is the aggravation by motion, and the midnight aggravation by heat, shown by throwing off the bedclothes. The febrile symptoms indicate that Ledum cannot be applicable in very severe acute cases; it would seem very appropriate to such cases as have been brought under the injudicious use of Colchicum to a low asthenic state.

It is in such cases that I have found Ledum a most serviceable remedy.

Also in hæmoptysis with florid blood and attended by rheumatic pain.

Its empirical domestic and allopathic use in whooping cough should not be forgotten, though Bœnninghausen says of it:

"This drug (used in some parts of Germany successfully in whooping cough as a domestic remedy) has never been given by me, and cannot, I think, be very often indicated."

RHODODENDRON CHRYSANTHUM.

SIBERIAN SNOW-ROSE. ALPINE ROSE.

THIS plant, which is most abundant in the Alpine regions of Siberia, but is found likewise in other mountainous and snowy regions of Asia and Europe, and perhaps (?) of North America, is not mentioned in the English and French works on materia medica. It is noticed in German works on the subject; by some of them a high value is set upon certain of its therapeutic properties.

Like most of our valuable remedies, it was successfully used by those pioneers of therapeutic science, "the old grandmothers," in domestic practice for centuries before it attracted the attention of scientific men.

The Cossacks and Mongolians used it as a specific for rheumatism and gout. The hunters and mountain rangers used to drink an infusion of it to remove the weariness and pains from their limbs after fatiguing expeditions. These facts were brought to the notice of Gmelin during his travels

RHODODENDRON CHRYSANTHUM.

in Siberia, and he was the first to recommend Rhododendron in Europe as a remedy for gout and rheumatism. The first publication on the subject was by Professor Kölpin, of Stettin, in 1779. It was used with greater or less success, and recommended accordingly by many German physicians.

Our knowledge of its physiological properties is derived chiefly from a proving published by Seidel. "Archiv," 10, 3, 137, in 1831.

Seidel introduces his provings with a general *résumé* of the action and character of Rhododendron, as follows:

"Although many remedies may produce effects that are in their general aspect quite similar, nevertheless each remedy possesses certain characteristic effects which belong to it alone, and which cannot be imitated, and for which no substitute will avail." It is these peculiarities of Rhododendron which he seeks to unfold to us.

"Turning vertigo. Early in the morning confusion of the head; drawing pressing pain in the forehead and temporal region, extending into the bones; headache very markedly increased by drinking wine; itching of the scalp in the evening; dry burning of the eyes; earache; early in the morning, obstruction of the nose, especially back in the left side of the nose; drawing tearing pain in the molar teeth, which is excited by uncertain (stormy) rainy weather; pressure in the epigastrium, and dyspnœa a kind of splenic stitch in the left hypochondrium; tardy evacuation of fæces, although the stool is normal; disposition to semi-fluid diarrhœa; itching, sweat and wrinkling up of the scrotum; soreness between the genitals and the thighs; swollen and hard testes; crushed pain and drawing in the testes; abundant offensive urine; the suppressed menses are brought on; coryza and other catarrhal difficulties; dyspnœo, rheumatic drawing pains in the muscles of the throat and nape of the neck; digging, drawing (gouty, rheumatic) pains in the extremities, especially in the bones of the forearms, hands, legs and feet; digging, drawing pains in the joints; occurrence or increase of the pains during repose; increase or re-appearance of the pains in unsettled, rough weather, and at the approach of storms; formication and itching in isolated spots on the limbs; weak, paralytic feeling in single limbs; the sleep is sound before midnight; toward morning it is disturbed; increased warmth in the hands; the disposition is indifferent, with disinclination to exertion.

"It is further to be noticed, that the symptoms often intermit for indefinite periods of time, sometimes longer sometimes shorter (two to twelve days), during which nothing will be felt of them; after which they will come again, and be felt for several days. They are most likely to come back when the weather becomes raw and unsettled, and a storm is threatening.

"The majority of the symptoms manifest themselves early in the morning though some are experienced only in afternoon or evening." Seidel, therefore, recommends giving Rhododendron in the evening, before the patient goes to sleep.

"The action of Rhododendron on the healthy extends over a period of three or four weeks."

To recapitulate, we find the action of Rhododendron to be eminently upon the fibrous and serous tissues. The pains in limbs and joints affect chiefly the forearm and hand and the leg and foot; they seem to have their seat in the bone or periosteum; they attack but a small extent of the limb at once; they disappear and re-appear as it were spontaneously and capriciously, nevertheless are always worse on the approach of bad weather. They are aggravated by motion and toward morning.

Rhododendron acts also upon the testes; and clinical experience has shown it serviceable in chronic enlargements and indurations of the testes and epididymis, and in hydrocele. * * *

PRACTICAL APPLICATIONS.

The only practical application to which I shall call your attention is that in chronic rheumatism of the smaller joints and their ligaments; to chronic periostitis, and especially to that form of chronic rheumatism which simulates rheumatic gout, but is distinct from it in this respect: that, as I believe, the enlargements of the joints are produced by fibrinous deposits and not by chalky excretions.

In the affection of the great toe joint, often mistaken for bunion, but which is really rheumatic,

Rhododendron is of great value. For true bunion from mechanical pressure Silicea is preferable.

The application to affections of the testes and to hydrocele is apparent.

It is analogous to and follows as regards the testes, Pulsatilla, Aurum. Spongia; as regards hydrocele, Clematis, Graphites.

KALMIA LATIFOLIA.

BROAD-LEAVED Kalmia, Calico-bush, Mountain-laurel, Spoonwood, a native of North America, not mentioned in allopathic works on materia medica. Bigelow, in his "Medical Botany," and Barton speak of poisonous effects from eating the flesh of game which has fed upon the berries of the Kalmia; and from eating honey supposed to have been gathered by the bees from the blossoms of the Kalmia.

The proving of Kalmia was made by Dr. Hering, of Philadelphia, and first published in the "Transactions of the American Institute of Homœopathy," vol. i., 1845. To this proving were subsequently added the results of further observations by Dr. Hering, a proving by Dr. J. Bucher, of Munich, and some clinical observations by Drs. Okie, of Providence, Williamson and Jeanes, of Philadelphia, and Gray, of New-York, and the whole was published in part v. of "Hering's Amerikanische Arzneiprufungen," 1., 1957.

In introducing his proving, Dr. Hering remarks: "Kalmia may be a very important remedy in acute as well as chronic diseases.

"As Ledum palustre finds its place in the swampy mountain meadows of Germany and northern Europe; as Rhododendron chrysanthum adorns with its yellow blossoms the elevated plains of Asia, so Kalmia latifolia displays itself in the narrow stony valleys of the brooks and smaller rivers of North America, and enlivens their banks with its evergreen foliage. In May and June it spreads out over them a rosy drapery, hanging down in such beauty from the rocky walls of the valleys, as to strike with wondering admiration even those who have been accustomed to the luxuriant glory of a tropical vegetation.

"As the mountain Rhododendron thrives in the home of the storms and under the Alpine mists, as Ledum flourishes in the regions of the swamp clouds of mountain ranges, so Kalmia prefers the fogs of the valleys. But all three have a mountain home. The entire family appears to correspond to those great families of diseases which we call rheumatisms and gout, and particularly to the northern forms of them. In intermittent and particularly in remittent fevers with a so-called gastric-nervous character, and which run a tedious course, all three remedies have shown themselves to be indispensable.

"There are but few remedies in the materia medica which have so great a mastery over the pulse and with so beneficial action diminish the too quick pulsations of the heart, as Kalmia and its cognates. Of course this is only in cases which

KALMIA LATIFOLIA.

in other respects correspond to the action of this family."

Kalmia, Rhododendron and Ledum act very often beneficially, when there is a very frequent pulse.

Next to this family stands the Colchicum family, which, singularly enough, is as often application in gout, and moderates the pulse as well as the Rhododendron family in rheumatism. But we must be careful nerver to give one after another, nerver to give Kalmia, Ledum and Rhododendron in succession, nor (of the Colchicum family) Colchicum, Veratrum and Sabadilla.

In heart diseases that alternate with rheumatism, or that have developed themselves out of rheumatisms, Kalmia promises to be a very important remedy.

(In a note Dr. Hering says: "This was written in 1843. This conjecture was brilliantly canfirmed. In 1853 Dr. Okie cured two cases with hypertrophy of the heart arising after acute rheumatism. In one of these cases auscultation showed thickening of the valves.")

The proving of Kalmia is as yet so fragmentary that nothing like a complete analysis can be made of it.

Its action upon the vital force is evidenced in the modification of the heart's action, which in small doses it accelerates, in large doses it moderates, reducing it almost to a minimum, producing at the same time spasm of the glottis, paleness of the face, nausea, obscure vision, coldness of the limbs, etc. The pulse is reduced to 35 or 40 beats.

The action upon the vital force is shown likewise by the pains, and still more by the excessive weariness, languor, lassitude in the limbs and especially in the lower extremities, a symptom which, unattended with any swelling or evidence of inflammation, is quite characteristic of Kalmia.

The action upon the organic substance is not so clearly shown in the proving. Yet so powerfully curative has Kalmia proved in grave organic affections of the heart and kidney that we cannot doubt its power to effect changes in the tissues of the body. It produces an itching, erysipelatous eruption something like that of Rhus, along with dangerous asthmatic symptoms. Also pimples and pustules in various parts of the body which itch very much, and after being scratched burn. The peculiarities of the action of Kalmia display themselves in the coldness and e imperfect reaction of the fever, in the very great reduction of the pulse from large doses, and in the serve pains and great lassitude felt in the extremities and particularly the lower. The pains extend through an entire limb, as, for example, from shoulder down to the fingers, from the hypochondrium to the hip and from the hip to the heel. These sensations indispose the prover to motion and exertion of any kind, and are greatly aggravated by moving.

SPECIAL ANALYSIS.

The vertigo is very marked. It accompanies every group of symptoms.

The sensorium is oppressed. Vision is obscured.

Head. In the head, pain in the vertex, which extends up from the cervical vertebræ (resembles Belladonna and Silicea). Headache in the forehead on waking in the morning; this is a frequent symptom.

Headache in the forehead and over the eyes and nose. The headache extends from forehead and temples down into the canine and molar teeth, into the face and the sides of the neck.

Eyes. In the eyes, pressure and aching, and stitches along with rheumatic pains in the limbs; vision obscured along with the vertigo; sticking pain under the left eye.

Face. Stitches and tearing in the bones of the jaw and face. (These symptoms might suggest facial neuralgia.)

The lassitude which characterizes Kalmia is first felt in the muscles of mastication.

Stomach. Eructations, nausea and vomiting from large doses; pressure in the epigastrium, relieved by sitting erect, worse when bent over; with the sensation as if something were being pressed under the epigastrium. (This symptom should be remembered in connection with heart disease.)

Respiratory Organs. Some degree of cough from a scratching in the throat, day and night, with mucous expectoration in the evening, of a saltish taste.

Dyspnœa, with a feeling as if there were a swelling in the throat. Dyspnœa, with pains in the limbs.

Heart. Palpitation of the heart. In large doses it diminishes the pulse, with great weakness in the arms and legs; vertigo on every attempt to move; pulse scarcely perceptible, very weak and thready. These are the effects of poisonous doses. The effects of small doses are to produce palpitation.

Trunk. Tearing in the nape of the neck; darting from nape into the head (Belladonna, Silicea); weak sensation from abdomen into neck.

Pain in right side of neck, also violent pressure. Pain and violent pressure on both sides of neck.

Violent pain in three upper dorsal vertebræ extending through the shoulders.

Constant pain in the spine, sometimes worse in the loins, with great heat and burning.

Sensation, as if the spine would break from within outward.

Violent pain down the spine.

Backache during the menses.

Aching across the loins; pains also during menses; feeling of paralysis in sacrum; also evening in bed, with heaviness in the head.

Upper Extremities. Pains in the scapulæ, going through shoulders; tearing pressing in right shoul-

KALMIA LATIFOLIA. 193

der; tearing from right shoulder down the arm; pressing below the left shoulder; drawing pain in the left arm at night; pains in the left arm.

Weakness in the arms, with slow pulse; tearing from left elbow along the index finger, which is spasmodically flexed; tearing from the knuckles of the left fingers to the elbow; repeated stitches in the hands; pains close on the wrist; a kind of paralysis in the hands; pains seem to paralyze the hand.

The pain seems worse in left arm; it moves and does not affect the joints particularly; it is characterized by weakness and a paralytic condition.

Lower Extremities. Stitches into the ossa ilii; tearing on the ossa ilii down the thighs into the feet.

Tearing in the flesh of the whole left limb.

Soreness of the left thigh down to the heel; pain in right glutei; in right limb; in thigh, before menses.

Pain in knees and feet; aching in calves; weakness in calves; paralytic sensation along shin-bone; aching in feet, in calves, with slow pulse; jerking in heel; stitches in toes and in soles of feet.

To recapitulate: We do not find any description of inflammation, swellings, redness of the joints, nor of deposits in them; nor is there pain which is confined to the joints, aggravated by touch, motion, heat, etc. On the contrary, the pains extend throughout a great portion of the limbs, move quickly throughout their province, and are attended by weakness and by some disturbance of the circulation. These paralytic sensations and great pains and achings in the limbs seem to be characteristic, for they accompany nearly every group of symptoms.

PRACTICAL APPLICATION.

It is evident that though Kalmia is similar in action to Colchicum, Ledum and Rhus, yet it is not so clearly called for in articular rheumatism or in gout. Its decided action on the heart led Dr. Hering to suspect its value in rheumatic heart affections, a value established by clinical experience.

In 1853, I had a most interesting case of this kind. A little girl of ten years had been ill ten days of what had been called "neuralgia of the chest." When I entered the room, her attitude, propped up in bed, her anxious expression of face, the lived hue of countenance and the visible, tumultuous and very rapid action of the heart, made it evident that she was suffering from violent acute endocarditis, —perhaps, also, pericarditis. She had just had acute rheumatism, great weakness of limbs, but no pain. I gave Kalmia latifolia, though her case was pronounced hopeless, and I had no hope of her. She recovered completely, continued to take the remedy, and, to my surprise, had no valvular murmur. She is now grown up and well.

Dr. Gray, of New-York, guided by a "medium," gave Kalmia in prosopalgia; the symptoms indicate its use in that affection.

Dr. B. C. Macy, of Dobb's Ferry, published in the "American Homœopathic Review" a most interesting case of Bright's disease of kidney cured by Kalmia. He was induced to give Kalmia by the great and persistent pains in the limbs.

This is especially interesting, because as yet we have no kideny symptoms that would suggest the use of Kalmia in Bright's disease.

SPIGELIA ANTHELMIA.

A NATIVE of the West Indies and of South America. It must not be confounded with the *Spigelia Marylandica,* a native of the United States and the officinal Spigelia of the United States Pharmacopœpia. The latter is a different species, is much less powerful in its action on the system, and is a well-known and very frequently employed anthelmintic, under the name of Pinkroot.

The *Spigelia anthelmia* is likewise a powerful anthelmintic, but it exerts also a powerful action on the nervous system, so much so that it is thought to have been a chief ingredient in the *"poudres de succession"* of the famous French poisoner, Madame de Brinvilliers.

Our knowledge of its physiological properties is derived from Hahnemann's proving in "Materia Medica Pura," vol. v.

The whole plant is used medicine. A general survey of the proving leads us to the following

GENERAL ANALYSIS.

The action of Spigelia is manifested chiefly upon the nervous system of animal life; and it is eminent among our remedies for the extent to which its action seems to be exerted upon the nerves themselves and their envelopes; upon the nervous centers, however, in so far as we are able to make the distinction, its action is probably very slight. The nerves of special sense are excited in a marked degree, and this without any well-defined lesion in the organs of special sense (except the eye); and even here the exception is more apparent than real, for the inflammation produced by Spigelia is in the sclerotic and choroid, while the functionary alteration of special sense is in the optic nerve and retina. In this regard, Spigelia differs from Belladonna, Rhus and other drugs which excite the animal nervous system. In the tissues of the eye it excites inflammation, giving a well-marked picture of rheumatic sclerotitis. It acts decidedly on the trifacial nerve; producing prosopalgia which involves the orbit, the zygoma and the superior maxilla; also on the nerves of the tongue; perhaps, also, on the portio dura.

The prosopalgia of Spigelia is distinguished by sticking burning pains, with subsequent swelling and soreness of the parts affected. In this respect it closely resembles the prosopalgia of Colchicum, from which, however, it is distinguished by the exaltation of the special senses and the general nervous erethism and excitement, and the intolerance of pain which characterize Spigelia; whereas Colchicum, on the other hand, is distinguished by an equally remarkable tolerance of pain and a patient, enduring disposition, and a general semi-paralytic condition.

Organic Substance. There is no evidence of definite modification of the organic substance of the body, unless the action on the pericardium and upon the fibrous tissues, which we infer *ex usu in morbis,* may be so regarded.

The sphere of action of Spigelia is not extensive. It embraces only the nerves of animal life and of special sense, and the fibrous and muscular tissues of the eye, heart, and perhaps of the extremities.

Upon the mucous membrane it produces no very definite action, save in the pharynx and posterior nares. The high repute of Spigelia as an anthelmintic might lead us to expect a more decided action on the apparatus of digestion. The absence of such decided action gives ground for supposing that in helminthiasis Spigelia acts rather as a palliative, killing and expelling the vermin, than as a radical curative remedy, modifying that condition of things in which they developed and flourished.

The pains of Spigelia are sticking, taring and burning-pressing. They are aggravated by motion, and in the afternoon and at evening, often preventing sleep.

SPIGELIA ANTHELMIA.

There is great lassitude and heaviness of the limbs; great restlessness; great sensibility of the whole body to touch. The least touch on any part of the body sends a shudder through the whole frame.

(This is different from the sensibility of China, which accompanies and characterizes only the parts which are already the seat of pain, and in which the sensibility is more in imagination and apprehension than in reality.)

There is no marked periodicity in the symptoms.

SPECIAL ANALYSIS.

The sources of knowledge of the pathogenesis of the drug are the provings of Hahnemann and his associates, in vol. v. of the "Materia Medica Pura."

Head. Vertigo, as if one should pitch forward; this occurs when looking down (as in Kalmia); or as if everything were going around when walking, relieved by standing still. (Arnica, Colchicum.)

Memory is weakened; intellectual effort is irksome.

Headache. The symptoms are well marked and characteristic, and present a good picture of one form of so-called "nervous headache." To take a general view of the head affections, before stating the parts especially acted upon and the varieties of sensations, we may say: There are dullness, heaviness and pain in the head; the pain is much increased by shaking and jarring the head, as when one walks, and especially by a false step, by coughing or sneezing, by moving the facial muscles, by speaking aloud, or by any loud noise, as well as by touch or bright light (increased sensibility of the special senses); these things increase the pain so that it seems as though the head would burst. There is a disposition to press upon and support the head with the hand, or to bind it around. See Apis. (Keep it warm is Silicea.)

The varieties of pain are, as affecting the whole head, chiefly heaviness or feeling as of a load or weight in the head; a pressing from without inward, much aggravated by stooping forward, unless the forehead be supported by the hand (Apis, China, Rhus); a sensation of swashing or surging of the brain within the cranium at every step or on the least motion or loud speaking; very severe when the head is concussed by a false step, much ameliorated by repose. (Rhus.) This swashing sensation is often attended by a tearing digging sensation in definite parts of the head, generally semi-lateral, as in the left parietal region, the left occiput and forehead.

As regards the localities particularly affected, it may be observed that the pain is generally circumscribed, is often confined to one side, more frequently the left. The occiput is the seat of many pains which extend into the nape, causing stiffness of the neck and at the same time restlessness. In the forehead, and especially in the frontal protuberances, we find: Pulsating stitches; pressure from without inward; boring and burning pain, the latter (burning) is probably superficial, and indicates an affection of the supra-orbital, nerve.

In the frontal protuberances, tearing pains extending into the eye, and aggravated by motion of the globe of the eye.

In the temporal region we find pulsating stitches; pressure inward, and burning extending into the zygoma. As to the time of their occurrence no special mention is made save once, when the pains for the most part occur in the evening and continue violent through the night.

The aggravations and ameliorations are uniform and as have been stated. The whole head is externally very sensitive to touch, and this is aggravated by motion of the scalp.

In the skin of the temples, forehead and eyebrows, a burning, tingling pain is felt, which extends down the cheek or into the eyes, and is aggravated by touch and motion. Near the orbit, swelling of the sub-cutaneous tissues occurs and of the skin, which is sore when touched.

The eyes also are affected in a special manner by Spigelia. Its action is exerted on all the tissues, but especially on the muscular and fibrous tissues and upon the function of special sense. In addition we have, especially in the left orbit, neuralgic pressing pains extending down to the zygoma and leaving, after the pain subsides, a tumor which is sensitive to the touch. (Colchicum.)

Compressive pain, generally in the orbits. The margins of the eyelids are sore, burning and painful. In the lids and their margins fine stitches, as from needles. In the margin of the left lower lid a fine cutting, as with a little knife. With these exceptions, which seem to imply an organic affection, the lids are not acted upon in their substance. On the other hand the innervation of their muscular tissue is modified as follows, along with the nervous affection of the pupil and retina: The upper lids are relaxed and paralyzed; they can be elevated only with the aid of the hand, the pupil being at the same time dilated.

The conjunctiva is moderately inflamed; we have pain as from sand in the eye, muco-pus and acrid lachrymation.

The globe of the eye is seriously involved, as we gather from the following symptoms: Dull and flat aspect of the eye; supra-orbital pains; redness and inflammation of the sclerotic with ptosis; pain in the eye and brow; the eye is painful when moved, and feels tense, as if it were too large for the orbit; sticking pain in the eye, also, when it is moved; digging pain in the middle of the eye (violent) with ptosis; pressure in the eye, from without inward; the eye is painful when moved in any direction; intolerable pressive pain in the eyeball, worse from moving the eye; in order to look around, rather than move the eye in the orbit, one moves the whole head; heat and burning pains in the eye, with perverted vision, occasional spasmodic, involuntary motions of the eyes.

As regards the secretions, we have moderate acrid lachrymation and a formation of muco-pus.

Vision. The special sense of the eye is exalted. The sensibility of the retina is increased, including photophobia, and perverted, causing illusions, as if hair or feathers were upon the lashes, aggravated by wiping the eyes, as if sparks or a sea of fire were before the eyes. The pupils are dilated. Vision is also impaired.

Ears. The ear, the zygomatic region, the maxillæ and the throat are involved in an affection, evidently neuralgic, characterized by pressing and occasional burning pain extending through these regions and aggravated by loud noise.

Beyond this, the ear is affected as follows: In the external ear, pinching, drawing, itching. In the meatus auditorious, pressure as from a pulg deep in the meatus, extending to the zygoma and molar teeth.

In the inner ear, occasional dull, boring stitches extending into the throat.

In the ear generally, sudden stitch extending to the eye, zygoma, throat, jaw, teeth.

The special sense of hearing is exalted, in connection with headache. Loud noises are painful. Otherwise we have deafness, sensation as if the ears were loosely stopped, with ringing and rustling sounds, and yet without deafness. When speaking, the sound of one's voice resounds like a bell through the brain.

Moreover, there are signs of catarrh, as sudden

obstruction of the ears on blowing the nose, relieved by working the finger into the meatus. Roaring before the ears, rustling and rushing as of wings, ringing of distant bells.

Itching of the alæ nasi of the nostrils, and of the dorsum of the nose. Unpleasant sense of obstruction at the root of the nose.

The part of the face chiefly affected is the zygomatic region. In preference, the left side is affected. The pains are burning or tearing-pressive, leaving a dull sensation of swelling when the pain abates. Stitches from the upper maxilla to the vertex and in the cheek and temple in front of the ear.

The facial muscles are distorted and swollen; the whole face is puffed in the morning, with a feeling of illness. (This and nose-itching signs of helminthiasis.)

Burning and tension in the upper lip.

Painless pustules upon the chin.

In the lower jaw, painful pressure upon the angle. In the articulation, pain as if dislocated only when chewing; otherwise a dull pain.

In the teeth, drawing, fine sticking or sudden jerking pains at short intervals in the moral teeth, generally in several or in all the teeth simultaneously, but most severe in the carious teeth. The toothache is worse at night and after eating, though not while eating; also by cold air and water, and particularly at night. It is accompanied by spasmodic closure of the jaw.

The tongue presents also neuralgic phenomena, confined chiefly to the right side; fine stitches, boring stitches from behind forward, with a sour taste.

The remaining symptoms belong rather to a gastric affection; the tongue is full of cracks, as if about to lose its epithelium. The tongue and palate have vesicles, which burn when touched. The tongue pains, as if swollen posteriorly. It is coated white.

Swelling in the fauces, with enlarged and painful cervical glands and pain on swallowing, with difficulty in opening the mouth. This affection is preceded by chill and shivering. Stitches in region of larynx, worse and worse, relieved by swallowing.

Mucus accumulates in the fauces. It is repulsive to the taste, and cannot be swallowed.

Offensive, putrid taste, and offensive odor from the mouth (helminthiasis), yet food has its natural good taste.

Great dryness of the mouth in the morning, as if full of pins, yet not really dry. No thirst.

Appetite sometimes gone, sometimes greatly increased (helminthiasis); great thirst.

Gastric Symptoms. Frequent eructations after a meal. Nausea, as from too long abstinence.

Epigastrium. Pressure, as from a load or ball, relieved by pressing with the hand; feeling as if it would be relieved by an eructation, which, however, is impossible.

Stitch in the epigastrium, with dyspnœa, aggravated by respiration, relieved by lying down.

Hypochondria. In the left hypochondrium, stitches compelling to bend forward, worse on inspiration; these are sharp, extending to the crista ilii, only on motion or inspiration.

In the right, deep inwardly; sharp stitches at regular intervals, relieved by full inspiration, recurring on expiration (evidently not inflammatory); stitch on making violent exertion only.

Abdomen. Flatulence; audible rumbling and gurgling, attended occasionally by pain, and preceding diarrhœa.

In the umbilical region, cutting pain with chill, diarrhœa. Pinching pain, as if all the intestines were twisted up, with dyspnœa and great anxiety. The abdomen is sensitive to touch. This group is attended by flatulence, and followed by diarrhœa.

In the abdominal ring, cutting and sticking, with protrusion of the old hernia.

Stool. Spigelia produces irritation in the rectum, much tenesmus, without or after stool, increased discharge of thick mucus; and occasional stools consisting first of fæces, solid or soft, and then of tough yellow mucus.

Urinary Organs. Frequent tenesmus of the bladder, and copious discharge of urine with white sediment. Also on externally pressing the bladder and on rising from a seat, incontinence of urine, followed by burning in the urethra.

Sexual Organs. Frequent erections with lustful

SPIGELIA ANTHELMIA.

thoughts, but no sexual instinct. Discharge of mucus from the urethra at stool.

Itching and burning in the right testis and in the penis. Tingling in the scrotum.

Respiratory Organs. Nasal catarrh, first dry, then fluent; discharge of bloody mucus from the nose.

Nasal catarrh, with hoarseness and heat of the body, without thirst or sweat. Profuse coryza, headache and depression.

The peculiarity of the Spigelia nasal catarrh is this: This discharge through the anterior nares is but slight, while through the posterior nares into the pharynx it is great and constant, and very sensibly felt. Sometimes it is quite liquid, but generally tough, stringy, and in such quantity as to threaten suffocation unless frequently removed by hawking. This prevents sleep at night; trickling into the larynx, also, it causes a kind of suffocative cough.

Cough. Spigelia is not prominent among the cough-producing drugs. It causes a spasmodic cough which stops the breath; is provoked by a tickling deep in the trachea, is violent, dry and hollow, and is excited especially by stooping forward.

Respiration. Several symptoms betray impeded respiration, the impediment seeming to result from sticking pains in various parts of the thorax, which are independent of respiration, though aggravated by it.

Chest. Pressure upon the chest in various localities, under the clavicle, over the center of the chest, over the whole chest, and over the xiphoid cartilage.

Stitches in various parts and on both sides, more frequent on the left side, from within outward; aggravated by inspiration and by motion.

The following symptoms deserve special notice Violent stitch in the left side, just under the heart, recurring periodically; stitch "in the diaphragm" on the left side, so violent as to arrest respiration; dull stitches (Colchicum) synchronous with the pulse in the region in which the heart's impulse is felt; stitches between this latter spot and the epigastrium. These symptoms, together with the following, which denote modified action of the heart, viz.: very violent pulsation of the heart, audible to the patient and visible to the by-stander; violent palpitation and anxiety; tremulous motion of the heart; palpitation increased by sitting down and bending forward, and by deep inspiration and retention of breath; palpitation as soon as he sits down after rising in the morning; and in the præcordial region a heavy, painful pressing load, causing constriction and anxiety, with cutting and griping, as from wind in the abdomen;—these two series of symptoms point clearly to an organic affection of the heart or pericardium, such as clinical experience has proved to find its curative agent in Spigelia.

Back. In the lumber, dorsal and scapular

regions various stitching pains are noted, generally worse on motion and inspiration, along with general lassitude.

Extremities. Pains, aching, restlessness, isolated tingling and numbness. Similar sensations to those already described in other parts of the body.

Upper Extremity. In the shoulder, arm and forearm, sticking and pressing pains, with a sensation of lassitude and weakness. The two spmptoms, sensation in the forearm, as if the bones were compressed by tongs and the pressing, cutting tearing pains in the wrist and finger joints, worse by motion, indicate the action of the drug upon the nervous and fibrous tissues respectively. The numbness and paleness of the hand (Symptom 381) does not indicate any variety of organic paralysis or depressed vegetation, but rather such a condition as results from pressure on a nerve, or when the hand, in popular phrase, "goes asleep."

Lower Extremity. The action of the lower extremity is more decided and more definite. As in the upper extremity, we have lassitude, fine sticking pains and spasmodic twitching of individual muscles. In addition, there is very great restlessness of the limbs, especially at night, preventing sleep and causing constant motion and flexion and extension of the limbs; this is attended by digging pain in the left knee (Aurum, Rhus toxicodendron, Taraxacum, Causticum). The knees are sensitive, and are painful when walking, and worse the longer the walk is continued. Luxated pain in knee, causing limping; sticking in the calf and pulsation in patella when knee is extended. Ankle; boring pain on flexion, as if tendons were too short; tearing stitches in the feet; soles sore when stepping.

Sleep. Frequent and great sleepiness, yet inability to fall asleep until very late in the evening; sometimes from great restlessness of limbs.

Sleep disturbed by lively dreams; he is fatigued on waking; more tired in the morning than on going to bed.

Fever. The entire paroxysm is often without thirst. Chill partial; frequent sensation of heat in the body; none external.

Chill generally in the morning, partial and wandering, often not followed by heat; it starts from the epigastrium and extends to the back, head and upper extremities.

During the heat, desire for external heat. The hands feel warm to each other but cold to the face; heat is partial.

Disposition. Irritable, excitable, with depressed anxiety for the future, and despondency.

PRACTICAL APPLICATIONS.

Hahnemann remarks in his introduction to the proving of Spigelia (A. M. S. R., 5,238):

"This annual plant, which was first used in South America as a domestic cure for lumbricoides, became known to our physicians about eighty years ago, who, however, have learned since that time to use it for nothing else than what the simple negroes of the Antilles first taught them, viz., to expel the lumbricoides.

"Yet let one only reflect that the accumulation of lumbricoides in the intestines is never an individual independent disease, but only a symptom of some other fundamental disease in man, and unless this be cured, the worms, although some may be driven away will yet perpetually re-appear in the intestines.

"It would therefore be foolish to use so extremely powerful a drug as Spigelia merely for the expulsion of worms, if this plant did not, at the same time, remove the disease which lies at the foundation of the existence of the worms. This it can do, as many cases show, in which the patients recover, even without having passed a single worm.

"Spigelia, however, has short-sightedly enough been regarded and used only as an anthelmintic. When people know not how to devote this most precious remedy to a more important use (a few cina-seeds would do for this), they act as inappropriately as they would do in applying a costly machine to do a trifling bit of work. The wonderful and many-sided power of this drug shows a much higher design for it than to bring few worms form the intestine."

1. The chief indications are in semi-lateral neuralgic headaches involving the eye, chiefly the left side.

2. In prosopalgia, involving the eye, the zygoma, the cheek, teeth and temple.

3. In rheumatic sclerotitis.

4. In pericarditis and endocarditis with stitches and violent pulsation.

It comes after Aconite; competes with Bryonia; precedes Spongia and Lachesis, Arsenicum and Lithium.

ATROPA BELLADONNA.

DEADLY NIGHTSHADE.

THE whole plant is used in medicine. It has always been known as a dangerous poison, classed among the "narcotics" or the "cerebral stimulants." In the seventeenth century first used in medicine to resolve tumors and "cure cancer."

The herbivorous animals devour Belladonna with impunity.

Cases of poisoning with Belladonna are abundant in medical literature. It is from a collation of these cases, along with a very thorough and exhaustive proving on the healthy subject by Hahnemann and his pupils, that we derive our knowledge of its physiological action.

As this drug is in very common use it may be well to make a minute and careful study of its action. As a preliminary, the following sketch of the action of a poisonous dose may be of interest:

"The eye became dry, the conjunctival vessels fully injected; there was a total absence of lachrymation, and motion was attended with a sense of dryness and stiffness. The face was red and turgid, and the temperature and color of the surface considerably augmented. The face, upper extremities and trunk exhibited a diffuse scarlet efflorescence, studded with innumerable papillæ very closely resembling the rash of scarlatina. The pulse was full, from 120 to 130. The feeling in the head was that of violent congestion, a full, tense, throbbing state of the cerebral vessels,—identically the same sensation that would be produced by a ligature thrown about the neck and impeding the return of the venous circulation. The tongue, mouth and fauces were as devoid of moisture as if they had been composed of burnt shoe-leather. The secretions of the glands of the mouth and of the saliva were entirely suspended. A draught of water, instead of giving relief, seemed only to increase the unctuous clammy state of the mucous membrane. About the pharynx this sensation was most distressing. It induced a constant attempt at deglutition, and finally excited suffocation and spasms of the fauces and glottis, renewed at every effort to swallow. A little saliva, white and round like a ball of cotton, was now and then spat up. The power of Belladonna over the secretion of urine seems very great. I am confident I passed in the course of an hour three pints of urine, accompanied by a slight strangury at the neck of the bladder."

This hasty description by an allopathic observer corroborates the observations of homœopathists.

GENERAL ANALYSIS.

The action of Belladonna on the system is so general and so complex as almost to defy analysis.

1. On the vital forces of animal life its action is preëminent. The special senses are all affected as regards the intensity, and perverted as regards the character, of their function. The voluntary muscular system is affected, tonic and clonic spasm being produced. They involuntary muscular fiber is affected, as we infer from relaxation or abnormal rigidity of the sphincters, dilatation of the iris, palpitation of the heart, etc., and throbbing of the arteries. The sensorium is eminently affected, delirium, illusions, exaltations, mania, stupor, being different phases of Belladonna poisonings.

Yet, violent as this action is, we see no permanent paralyses.

2. On the organic substance Belladonna acts less profoundly. No evidence of any dyscrasia. The skin is affected as by the scarlatinal eruption. The sub-cutaneous and sub-mucous cellular tissues are inflamed, as also the true skin,—witness the erysipelas. The bladder and the uterus, and also the lining membrane of the rectum, are structurally altered.

3. Sphere of action. Chiefly the skin and mucous membrane of mouth, fauces, genito-urinary organs and the eye; muscular system, nervous system in every branch. Digestive organs not affected, nor the serous and osseous and fibrous

tissues. Glands eminently affected; ovaries, parotid, lymphatic. Uterus and appendages also; skin, erysipelas.

Periodicity not marked; cough worse at night.

Characteristics. Pains gradually increase till intolerable; then suddenly decline and re-appear elsewhere. Painful spots, sore on gentle pressure, yet tolerating firm pressure, as ischia and ovary. Always attended by red face, full, hard pulse, throbbing carotids, wild delirium.

Head. Sensorium. 1. Dizziness, as if all things were going round and swimming before the eyes, such as one feels after whirling around, with a turning in the epigastrium. It occurs also while walking, with incoherent speech. It occurs on moving and when at rest; is better in the open air and worse in the chamber. It is conjoined with feeling of stupidity in the head.

2. Confusion of the senses a whole day; he knows not what he does; the whole head is confused. A feeling as if drunken; as during a debauch, immediately after a meal. Confusion and dullness, as if a pressing cloud were drawn over the forehead. These are aggravated by alcohol and by motion. As concomitant symptoms, are noted swelling of the cervical glands and swollen, red face.

3. Indisposed to mental labor, feels unstrung.

4. Perception confused; he knows not whether he is asleep or awake; still he dreams, though awake. Elevated, deceptive fantasies; he sees and hears objects not present, not existing.

ATROPA BELLADONNA.

Primary action, probably to excite and give fantasies.

5. Lies often unconscious; convulsions.
6. Memory enfeebled during the headache; generally enfeebled.

Headache distinctly marked.

I. Consider first the parts of the head affected:

1. The whole head, by a feeling of heaviness and pressure, as if drunken, or pressed by stone; a pressure as if the head were screwed together and made narrower, and a consequent feeling of pressure outward, as if the head would burst. Altogether the mass of symptoms, however, relate to the forehead, orbits and temples; the right orbit and supra-orbital region being especially attacked. We find:

2. In the forehead exclusively the heaviness and pressing pain. The pressing, as of a weight, is distinct and marked, pressing down so low as to hinder the opening of the eyes, with a feeling as if something had sunk down in the forehead. The pain affects the eyes also, which, from the intensity of the pain, are kept shut; they are painful to the touch. Pressing pain in the forehead and frontal eminences, ceasing occasionally only to return again with greater intensity. This pressing is from within outward in a majority of cases. This pain in the forehead is aggravated by motion, removed by lying down to recur on rising. Not affected by eating, etc.; made worse by the open air.

3. In the orbits. Just over the orbits and just

over the root of the nose, the pressing and pressing drawing pain is most intense (458). There is also a sticking and tearing and a drawing pressing from the temples to the orbits, especially on the right side.

4. In the vertex a single symptom, a digging and tearing pain and sensitiveness.

II. The kinds of pain are various, being movable and stationary; the latter predominate. They are heaviness and pressing, which are felt in the whole head, but especially in the forehead. Gnawing and throbbing, all felt more in the frontal than in other regions.

The former are sticking, tearing and jerking pains.

From within outword, as if the brain were too large.

As concomitant symptoms, are noted, acuteness of the senses, eyes must be kept closed; great irritability about trifles.

III. Conditions.

The symptoms are aggravated in general by—

1. Stooping forward, which causes a feeling as if all would pass out through the forehead.

2. Coughing or any sudden motion which shocks the head.

3. Stepping when walking, he feels the brain *quasi* rise and fall with every step.

4. Rising up, from sitting or reclining posture.

Ameliorated by lying down and by bending backward.

In addition to this, throbbing of the vessels is a marked symptom of Belladonna, occurring in the head and whole body simultaneously.

Heat in the head, redness of the face with the headaches.

Head. External. Heat of the head a constant symptom. The pains in the scalp and forehead are chiefly drawing and drawing together or contracting pain and a cramp-like, compressive pain. These occur chefly in the right side of the head. The compressive, cramp-like pain occurs in the frontal eminence and draws downward over the zygoma to the inferior maxilla (a kind of neuralgia).

The forehead itches and is sensitive to the lightest touch.

Pimples occur on the temples, and the head swells and the body is red.

Face. All symptoms agree; the face is red, hot and swollen.

The redness is of various degrees, from a scarlet, confined to a small part of the cheek, to a deep, livid, bluish-red, pervading the whole face and invading the chest. The heat is of various degrees, felt generally in the parts that are red, while in other parts, the cheeks especially, there is boring and throbbing pain.

The swelling may be scarcely perceptible, or intense, occupying cheeks, nose and lips; hard and hot. Aggravated by motion and touch, and accompained by violent headaches and by paleness and coolness of the rest of the body.

Eyes. The eyes appear protruding, with greatly dilated, insensible pupils; under still more powerful doses the eyes are distorted, with red and swollen face; they glisten and move convulsively with convulsive movements of the hands. Morbid changes are manifest. The eyes become injected, with pressing pains. They are inflamed, with enlarged veins and itching and sticking pains and increased lachrymation. The left caruncle is inflamed and suppurates, with burning pain, and a white vesicle forms on the left (much dilated) pupil.

The sensations vary from those of slight congestion to those of violent inflammation; pressing, as when hard spring water gets into the eye; pressing deep in the orbit when the eye is closed; these are attended by lachrymation. The pains are these sensations intensified, with the peculiar indications of inflammation superadded. Pressing pain, as if the eyes were full of sand, compelling to rub them; and heat, as if they were surrounded by vapor. Pain, as if the eyes were torn out; then, again, as if they were pressed into the head; and in addition, a pain pressing from the forehead upon the eyes. Tearing pain in the eyes, proceeding from the left canthus. A biting in both eyes, with burning and sticking from without inward. Pain in the orbits, as if the eyes were torn out; sometimes, again, as if they would be pressed into the head, with a pressure on the eyes coming from the forehead (458). Burning with itching; desire to rub the eyes and relief thereby.

The secretion is early affected. First, a burning dryness, then involuntary lachrymation, with the pressing in the eyes. It is altered in character; the eyes are stuck togethr by pus in the morning.

Lids. The lids partake of the peculiar aspect of the eye; they are dilated, stand wide open. Various sensations are noted, both nervous and inflammatory. Trembling and twitching; heaviness; they fall shut in the morning with lachrymation. Throbbing pain, with inflammation and lachrymation. Itching and sticking, relieved by rubbing; painful to the touch.

Sight. The sight is specifically affected in a striking manner. Not only in degree but also in kind is the action of the optic nerve influenced.

As to degree, *i.e.*, in sensibility, it is first intensified, photophobia; and second blunted, hence diminished vision with dilated, immovable pupils; can see nothing but the white margin of the book, which appears black. As to kind, there are abnormal action and illusions. As to the former, objects appear double. Objects when near at hand are not seen at all; when distant they appear double. They appear manifold, are seen obscurely and upside down. As to the latter, letters tremble and are parti-colored, gold and blue. Bright red rings are seen around the candle. Flames and clouds appear. A white star is seen on the ceiling and light silver clouds.

Ears. External. Various pains about the

region of the ear involving the zygomatic region, the parotid gland, the maxillary articulation, the cartilage of the ear, and the muscles behind the ear down to the neck.

These pains are, as to the zygomatic process, squeezing pressure on the left zygoma, tearing and drawing and pressure under the right zygoma. In the maxillary joint a violent sticking extending into the ear, induced by chewing and continuing after chewing; fine stickings. In the parotid, stitches extending into the ear; violent stitch extending into the external ear, where it vanishes like a cramp, returning the same day at the same hour. In the cartilage of ear a tearing pain, and pressure in the lower and posterior part. In the muscles behind the ear down the neck, pain as if strongly pressed; the same in muscles of forehead. See below, under internal ear.

Meatus. Stitches in external meatus, unpleasant pressure like boring with finger, as if from pressure.

Internal. Various sensations and pains. A pinching first in right, then in left ear, just after swallowing; unpleasant feeling in right ear as if torn violently out of head. Alternate tearing out and pressing in pain in ears and temples, alternating with similar pains in the orbits. Earache in left ear, sharp shocks, with squeezing; in right ear boring pain, pressing, tearing behind the right ear; a fugitive stitch from ear to chin; stitches also with eructations tasting of food. Drawing from ear to nape. Violent pressure in mastoid process below ear and cutting shocks in it.

Secretion. Discharge of purulent moisture from the ears for twenty days.

Sense of Hearing, Sensibility. Deafness, with stitches in the ear. Increased sensibility (secondary probably, D.). Deafness as if a skin were stretched before the ear.

Various Illusions of Hearing. First, noise of trumpets and rushing in the ears; then a buzzing and humming, worst when sitting, better when standing and lying, still better when walking. Rushing noise, with dizziness and bellyache. Morning, immediately after waking, a rushing and bubbling in front of the ears.

General Complications. 1. Of the ears and temples pains with orbit-pains. 2. Pains in muscles of neck and occiput. 3. Ear-pains with swallowing and eructations.

Nose. In appearance the nose becomes suddenly red at the point, with burning sensation. Various pains and sensations are produced. In the bones of the nose a pressing pain just above the ala, pain as if beaten when touched; above the left half of the nose a painful drawing, a tickling removed by rubbing; in the point of the nose stitches throughout the night and burning with sudden redness.

Eruptions appear on nose as well as lips, ets. At the root of the nose two small red pimples, painful only when touched, as if ulcerated; and on cheeks and nose papules, which quickly fill with pus and cover themselves with a crust.

Sense of Smell. Incresased sensibility; smell of smoke from tobacco and soot is intolerable. Abnormal smells as of rotten eggs (early).

Nostrils, Pains. Left nostril painful, ulcerated together in morning. Painful ulceration of nostrils just on the side where they join the lip. Nostrils and corner of lip ulcerate, but neither itch nor pain. Epistaxis night and morning.

Lips. Majority of the symptoms are those of organic nature, eruptions or other cutaneous affections. On the upper lip, papules near the ala of the nose, covered with a crust, and a corresponding one on the lower lip, with a biting pain as if from salt water. Papules itching when touched. On lower lip burning pain and little vesicles; between lip and chin pustules with burning pain, especially at night. In the corner of the mouth ulcerated spot with tearing pain; rawness as if about to ulcerate. Little pale red papules painless. There are thus eruptions about the external surface of the lips; these are papular, running sometimes into ulcers which cover themselves with a crust. The pains are drawing, tearing biting and burning. In addition the upper lip swells and become red. Functionally the lips are affected, spasmodic motions are observed, also distortions of various degree and foaming at the mouth.

Chin. Eruptions as on the lips, with similar pains.

Jaws. Symptoms referring to motion of the jaws, from sensation of spasm up to absolute lockjaw, resisting violent extraneous force. A large furuncle on the angle of jaw, hard and painless till touched.

Glands of Neck. Drawing and tensive pains in the glands; the glands are swollen and painful at night, but not on swallowing (400-403).

(403-413.) *Muscles of Neck.* Spasmodic tension and cramp-like sensation in the muscles of the neck (without motion). Actual spasm, the head is drawn backward, burying in the pillow, with drawing and pressing pains in the muscles of right side; stiffness of muscless. In the nape of the neck, close to the occiput a pressing pain not affected by motion; and lower down, about the second and third cervical vertebræ, violent frequent stitches by holding head erect. On the side of the neck, arterial pulsation is felt. In the laryngeal region pressing sensation on the left side, increased by touch; fine stickings in throat-pit.

Teeth. As a generality, various symptoms taken from records of poisoning in very high degree, whole muscular system being excited to sepasm. Gnashing of teeth, with foaming at the mouth, smelling like foul eggs (epilepsy) and spasm of right arm.

Gums. Painful swelling on the right side, with fever and chilliness. Vesicle under one of the front teeth, painful as if burnt. The gums are painful to the touch, as if ulcerated; they are hot and throb, with pain in the throat. Gums bleed easily by a decayed tooth, without pain.

Toothache. Various kinds of pain, the symptoms being distinctly marked. The pains are variously characterized, according to their intensity; the majority are drawing; then tearing; jerkings, borings and soreness; digging pains are also mentioned. They occur for the most part in decayed teeth, and if severe, the pain extends to the whole row of teeth in that jaw on that side; the right side is affected by preference. If the pain is severe, or after it has lasted some time, the gums and cheek become swollen, painful and hot to the touch.

The pain gradually rises in severity to a great height, and gradually subsides.

It occurs chiefly at night, or, at least, is much worse at night, preventing sleep; still, it never entirely ceases during the day, to come again at night. It is aggravated by touch, by the open air, and after eating, although often during the act of eating it is relieved (perhaps because nervous system being aflacted attention is withdrawn). The chief complicateions are with pain in the ear. A violent toothache is attended by stickings in the ear; the pains seem to shoot down from the ear to the teeth.

Mouth. Sensation of breadth and depth, as if the tongue were lower down than usual.

Tongue. Various sensations, as if lower down in the mouth than usual, as if asleep, numb or dead, or covered with fur in the morning, and a feeling of coldness or dryness on the anterior half of the tongue. Various pains; painful to the touch; biting pain, as from, a vesicle in the middle of the white-coated tongue; on the tip, a feeling as of a vesicle, burning when touched. Fissured, white-coated (3d Stapf); the papillæ are of a deep red, inflamed and greatly enlarged (3d. Stapf). The tongue trembles and stutters.

Speech. Stammering, weakness of speech, with full consciousness and dilated pupils. Paralytic weakness of speech organs. Difficult speech, dyspnœa and weariness succeeding the anxiety. Speech difficult, the voice is piping. Low speech, attended by headache, as if brain were pressed out close over the orbits in the forehead, which prevents opening the eyes and compels to lie down, with very great contraction of pupils.

Secretion of Mucus and Saliva. Increased, with fissured, white tounge; increased and tenacious hanging and running out of the mouth. Much mucus, especially morning, sometimes with a foul taste; thickened in the throat and like glue on the tongue; he desires to wet the mouth. In the morning, full of mucus; he has to wash it out; disappears after eating. Slimy mouth after waking, with pressive headache. It is also diminished, at least in so far as sensation goes; the mouth feels very dry, with irritable disposition, yet mouth and tongue are moist to appearance; the lips are hot and scaly.

The mucus and saliva are more frequently

altered; thus, the saliva becomes tenacious, yellowish white, coating the tongue, tenacious, thick like glue; he thinks it must smell offensively to others. In connection, it may be observed that the orifice Steno's duct is painful as if abraded.

In the whole mouth and throat dryness, with stickiness and great thirst; the dryness is so great it seems to constrict the larynx and fauces, yet he can swallow liquids, and in most cases the tongue, although feeling as if dry, is really moist.

It is to be remarked that the tenacious foul and foul-smelling slime is found in the mouth chiefly in the morning, removed by eating, etc.

Throat in General. A marked affection. First as to the parts affected.

Fauces in General. Various pains, sensation of dryness and burning in the throat and on the tongue, not relieved by drinking, but diminished for a moment by sugar. Notwithstanding this feeling of dryness the tongue is moist; even food and drink cause a burning as of alcohol in th mouth. (The roof of mouth and palate as of sore and excoriated; painful when touched by tongue and when chewing, as if skin were off; and on swallowing, a scraped feeling as if raw.)

Tearing on the inner surface of corner of left maxilla, in left tonsil and behind it, not affected by touch, worse by swallowing.

Sticking pain in the pharynx, and pain as if from internal swelling, felt only when swallowing and on turning the head and by feeling the side of throat, not during repose or speech; violent sticking on swallowing or breathing. Stickings on left side, equally when swallowing and when not doing so.

Scraping, soreness and constriction, with heat about the throat.

An internal swelling is felt, especially on swallowing and on external touch.

Throat in general is sore, more on the left side;. worse on swallowing and spitting; feeling of internal swelling. (499, 500-503, 512, 515-517.)

Throat feels constricted, violent constriction of throat and œsophagus hindering deglutition; painful narrowing and constriction of the throat, with tension and straining on every motion like swallowing, even if nothing is swallowed; even when really swallowing it is not more painful. (516.) The feeling of constriction is in itself painful. On swallowing, a feeling in the throat as if everything were too narrow and constricted so that nothing would pass down.

Tonsils. Fine tearing in the left tonsil, not affected by touch, worse by swallowing. (492, 507.) Inflammation of the tonsils, going on in four days to suppuration; during these days he could swallow nothing.

Œsophagus. Sensation of constriction, both painful in itself and painful on swallowing and breathing. (513, 517.)

Epiglottis. A scratching pain in the region of the epiglottis, as if it were raw and sore, following immediately after a constriction of the œsophagus (which constriction is excited chiefly by swallowing.)

Second, as to the functions particularly modified :

1. Vegetative.

Deglutition. Increased activity. There is a constant inclination to swallow, a feeling as if he would suffocate if he did not swallow.

Difficult, yet painless. This is observed in one case. Not so frequent, however, as difficult and painful on account of constriction, soreness and internal swelling. Difficult to swallow solid food. He chews food without swallowing it on account of constriction.

Frequent sticking fingers in throat and feeling the neck while unconscious; and hydrophobia. (These symptoms are quoted from allopathic authorities)

When the throat symptoms occur only on one side, they prefer the left.

They occur: 1. Only when swallowing. 2. When turning the head. 3. On external pressure. 4. When breathing deeply.

They are aggravated by : 1. Touch. 2. Swallowing. Ameliorated by : 1. Sugar. 2. Repose.

Taste. The sense of taste may remain natural and be diminished in sensibility, as we find to be the case; or its perceptions may be abnormal; thus there is a flat, a putrid, a nauseous taste in the mouth; the saliva tastes as if spoiled; there is a foul taste after having eaten, like taste of spoiled meat. A foul taste comes out from the pharynx, as well when eating and drinking, although food and drink have their normal taste; a moderately sweet taste; a stickly taste; a saltish sour taste. It is to be noted that in part these abnormal phenomena depend upon the inflammation of the pharynx, tonsils and salivary glands, which Belladonna evidently induces, and which alters their several secretions. This alteration is perceptible to the taste, which itself is normal. Again it is noticed that, in the other case of abnormal taste, the tongue remains clean. Evidently, then, the symptoms do not result from indigestion (*i. e.*, the sense of taste, being normal, does not perceive the abnormal taste of secretions modified by indigestion; no doubt the sense of taste as a nervous function is modified, its perceptions distorted.)

Taste of Food. Food tastes salt; at first it tastes right, then, all at once, it tastes partly salt, partly tasteless and flat, with a feeling in throat as if it did not go down.

Taste of Bread. Smells and tastes sour, very sour; and after eating it, a kind of hart-burn. Taste of coffee repugnant. Camphor nauseates.

Appetite. Many of the phenomena are rather nervous than due to organic derangement.

1. Especial loss. 2. General loss. 3. General increase. 4. Peculiarities.

Repugnance to milk; it has a nauseous small and bitter, sour taste ; lost by continued drinking.

Repugnance to food. Total repugnance to all food and drink, with frequent weak pulse. Repugnance to beer.

Repugnance to acids, and especially to meat ;

loss of appetite, entire and long continued; everything nauseates, especially after smoking. Loss of appetite, with feeling of emptiness and hunger ; if he begins to eat, everything tastes well and he eats as usual. (Again, the loss of appetite is rather a nervous phenomenon.) Appetite only for bread and soup.

Increased appetite (*heilwirkung*).

Thirst. Loss of thirst. Entire thirstlessness. Abnormal. Greediness to drink, without appetite to do so; he brings the vessel to his lips and then sets it down again. Great thirst evening, with watery taste, but all drink nauseates him. Great thirst for cold drinks, while yet there is no heat about the body. Thirst at noon (for several days together).

After Eating. After eating a little, a constricted feeling in the stomach; cough and great thirst; a king of drunkenness; pinching below the umbilicus, close under the abdominal walls; bitter eructations.

After Drinking. After drinking beer, inward heat; after drinking, nausea.

Gastric Eructations. Frequent eructations, bitter and putrid, after eating; these are often incomplete; a half hiccough, often a mere vain endeavor; succeeded often by the raising of a burning, sour acrid fluid and a kind of straining to vomit, with giddiness. (See 526.) The nausea is felt in the throat and not in stomach. A burning on the upper edge of the larynx and a biting at the upper pharynx.

ATROPA BELLADONNA.   233

Nausea. Nausea felt in throat only. Qualmishness after breakfast and on going into open air; nausea in the stomach, with inclination to vomit and great thirst, and with eructations.

Vomiting. As a rule difficult and scanty; rather a great retching, with sweat.

Hiccough. A mixture of eructation and hiccough; hiccough followed by spasm of head and extremities; alternately of right arm and left leg; thirst, redness and heat.

Epigastrium. Painless throbbing; occasional pain, especially a great pressure after eating.

Stomach. Sensation of pressing is the most constant symptom; violent pressure occurring, for the most part, after eating; or else aggravated by eating. It occurs at times only when walking, and compels one to go slowly. Fullness in pit of stomach and under the short ribs, as if gas were pent up there, relieved by flatulent emissions, which increase the nausea; on stopping the fullness is greater, with blackness before the eyes. Distention, with tensive pain evening in bed. The pain are chiefly cramp-like, during every meal; a pain of contraction after a moderate meal; sticking pains in epigastrium, sometimes so violent as to compel him to bend the body backward and hold his breath; and burning felt both in epigastrium and abdomen (these symptoms are doubtful).

Abdomen. Various pains and sensations in the whole abdomen in general (allopathic records);

cutting pain. Tensive, spasmodic pain from thorax down to hypogastrium, not permitting the least motion of the body. Drawing-in pain with pressure, occurring when lying down. Pinching pain, compelling one to sit all crouched up and bent forward, with an unavailing desire for stool and subsequent vomiting; pinching in the intestines; pinching across the upper abdomen, and down the left side, as if in the colon; pinching, with rumbling.

Pressure like a stone, together with pain in the loins; pressing pain, as from a hard burden, only when walking and standing, always relieved by sitting. Pinching, clawing, grasping, as if seized up with talons, in a spot in the abdomen.

Distention and rumbling. (See Flatus.)

Hypochondria. In the hypochondria a pressing outward and pain, whenever pressure is made upon the epigastrium.

Distention. Right. Violent constricting pain in right hypochondrium, with sharp sticking thence through right thorax out to the axilla.

Pinching cutting, so that he cannot rise from his seat. Dull stitches about the last ribs.

Left. A pressing cutting, when lying quietly on the left side, morning, in bed, relieved by lying on the other side.

Umbilical Zone. Various sensations and pains, the greater part of which are referred to a region immediately below the umbilicus.

Sensation as if the intestines were pressing outward, mostly when standing.

A pressing sticking pain in the umbilical region.

Constricting pain under the umbilicus, simultaneously with a feeling of distention in the abdomen; the pains come in jerks and double one up. This pain compels to crouch forward. Drawing up in a knot of the abdomen, as if a coil or lump were forming. A most painful grasping together in the umbilical region; it seems to come from the sides and concentrate about the navel.

Dull stickings.

Right Violent stickings, as with a dull knife between the right hip and the umbilicus.

Cutting sticking over left hip to loins.

Hypogastrium. Sensations attributable not only to intestines but also to genito-urinary organs.

Pressing, like a heavy load, very low in hypogastrium.

Violent cutting pain, now here now there; more violent on left side.

Cramp-like, constricting pain in the intestines, lying very deep in hypogastrium, alternating with dull stitches or jerkings toward perinæum.

Violent tensive, pressing pain in whole hypogastrium, especially in public region, as if hypogastrium were spasmodically constricted, sometimes as if it were distended (not really so); pains which gradually increased and gradually diminish.

Violent pinching deep in hypogastrium, aggravated by drawing in the hypogastrium and by bending the trunk to the left side.

Loins. Pain, with pressure, as of a stone in the abdomen.

A sticking cutting goes from the umbilical region, over the left hip around to the lumbar vertebræ, is if in a single stroke, and is more painful in the back.

Flatus. Distention and rumbling.

External abdomen sensitive. Whole abdomen painful, as if raw and sore.

Heat in abdomen and thorax.

Itching sticking around navel, better by rubbing.

Stool. . Irritation of various intensity, inducing altered secretion and spasmodic action. Sensation in the abdomen as if diarrhœa were about to set in, with heat in the abdomen. The primary effect seems to be the production of a slight diarrhœa; pappy stool mixed with slime; green stool with enuresis and sweat (not inflammatory); several watery stools immediately after a copious sweat. Then the stools become less copious but the irritation is increased. At first soft diarrhœic stools, then more frequent desire for stool, but very scantly evacuations or none at all. Also, desire for stool becomes very frequent and violent, inducing straining, etc.; desire for stool, which is thinner but normal in quantity; frequent thin stool with tenesmus; he must go to stool every quarter of an hour; has to go to stool constantly; as the tenesmus increase the discharge diminishes; tenesums; scanty diarrhœic discharge, followed by increased tenesmus; frequent tenesmus without evacuation; tenesmus without evacuation, followed by by vomiting.

Constant tenesmus, a pressing and urging toward anus and genitals, alternating with painful constriction of anus.

During stool, a shudder; a kind of chill.

After stool, increased tenesmus immediately.

Character of Stool. 1. Consistence, pappy, mixed with slime; diarrhœic, alternating with headache; or with nausea and pressure in the stomach; granular, yellow and somewhat slimy; watery, immediately after copious sweat; at first soft and diarrhœic, then frequent tenesmus but little or no evacuation; sometimes hard. 2. Color: yellow, white, like chalk; green, with enuresis and sweat. 3. Smell, sour.

Rectum. Pressing toward the anus; constrictive pain followed by soreness in the abdomen; quick, slimy diarrhœa and unavailing tenesmus; single stitches.

Itching, and at the same time constriction sensation; itching low in rectum; violent painful itching in rectum and anus; pleasant tingling in lower part.

Anus. Internal itching, violent, sudden and painful.

External itching when walking in open air.

Hæmorrhage several days in succession from hæmorrhoidal veins.

Sphincter relaxation; involuntary discharges (last action in complete intoxication); spasmodic contraction. (See under Stool "constriction and constrictive pains.")

Urinary Organs. I. Pains and sensations. 2. Function. 3. Excretions.

1. *Pains and Sensations.* Twisting and turning in the bladder, as by a great worm, without a desire to urinate. Dull Pressure in region of bladder.

2. *Function.* Discharge suppressed; the first effect seems to be a retention.

The evacuation is difficult; occurs only in drops (secondary). This symptom is attributed to allopathic observers. The most striking noted by a prover, and probably the first, is frequent desire, but evacuation of a very small quantity at a time; the character of the urine is normal, hence the effect of the drug has been merely to produce spasm.

Involuntary discharge during sleep and at other times; this symptom is noted by Hahnemann as well as by allopathists; it is spasm, perhaps, of long fibres:

Complications. During urination, drawing in left seminal cord. After urination, biting in edge of prepuce.

3. *Excretions.* Urine Quantity diminished according to Hahnemann.

Increased, according to allopathic authorities. Character. Turbid and yellow; turbid with red sediment. (Hahnemann.)

Color. Yellow and clear; whitish. White with

white sediment, turbid with red sediment (both Hahnemann).

Genital Organs. 1. Pains and sensations generally. Violent straining and pressing toward genitals as if all would fall out; worse by sitting crooked and walking; better by standing and siting erect. Violent stitches in pubic region as if in internal genitals.

Prepuce. Drawn back, with unpleasant sensation in exposed glans.

Urethra. Stitches, length of it, from bulb to orifice, while walking.

Dull stitches behind the glans, especially during motion.

Seminal Cords. Repeated tearing upward in left cord, evening in bed before sleeping.

Drawing during micturition.

Testes. They are drawn up, with great sticking pains in them.

Semen. 1. Nocturnal discharge, from relaxed penis. 2. Repeated in one night and without lascivious dreams.

Sexual Instinct. Lost entirely.

Menses. Before: lassitude, abdominal pain, anorexia. During: sweat on chest, yawning and crawling chills, anxiety about heart, great thrist, cramp-like tearing here and there in back and arms. Too early and too copious.

Leucorrhœa. White, after pressing as if all would fall out with distention, and then a drawing together in abdomen, with abdominal pain.

Respiratory System. Sneezing. Repeated attacks.

Obstruction of Nose. Nose now obstructed, now discharging water.

Catarrh. With the cough of Belladonna, one-sided catarrh with stinking smell like herring-brine, especially on blowing the nose.

Larynx and *Trachea.* Hoarseness. Voice rough and hoarse.

Cough. The cough is, for the most part, a dry, hacking cough, violent, in repeated attacks at short intervals; the violence of the mechanical action being apparently out of proportion in its intensity to the gravity of the organic affection. Spasmodic cough, as if something had fallen into the bronchia, or dust had lodged in the larynx. A constant inclination to cough. The cough is often accompanied by feeling of dryness and tightness in the chest and in the upper parts of the air-tubes, and is sometimes induced by these sensations. It occurs (at noon, once) in the morning, both early and after rising and at evening after retiring; and on through the night, walking from sleep. It is to be observed that it is the spasmodic cough, violent, which occurs at night, while the morning cough is less violent, and is attended by an expectoration of mucus resembling pus (the accumulation of the night, the affection being in a more advanced stage). The aggravation in the evening, after lying down, is marked.

Expectoration. Tenacious saliva, mucus resembling pus, bloody mucus.

ATROPA BELLADONNA. 241

Exciting Causes. The cough is excited by the slightest irritating cause; even by every inspiration; by sensation as if he had dust in the throat, or something in the bronchia; by a tickling in the back of the larynx (this cough is a violent, dry, irritating cough); by a tightness in the chest; by a feeling as if something lay at the epigastrium.

Complications. During the night-cough he grinds his teeth. Needle-stickings in the left side under the ribs. A violent pressing pain in nape of neck as if it would break in pieces.

Respiration. Difficult and oppressed; the acts of respiration are energetic, small, frequent and anxious; increased difficulty from coffee-drinking; from a pressure in epigastrium.

Chest. Sensations and pains. Pressing upon chest about region of epigastrium, impeding respiration, whereupon nausea rises up into the throat, with faintness; these alternate.

A cramp-like constriction in epigastric region compelling to breathe deeply, walking. Violent constriction as if the chest would be pressed together from both sides. Violent constriction not relieved by voluntary coughing; difficult inspiration as if hindered by mucus in bronchi; at same time a burning in chest.

Burning. Heat rises suddenly from abdomen in chest, quickly passing away.

Sticking pains in various parts of the chest, brought on and aggravated by coughing, yawning, and by motion generally, but not affected by respiration. They occur most frequently on the right side, and on that side under the clavicle from before backward, under the right arm (checking respiration). On left side they occur from sternum to axilla. Sticking pains, too, are felt in the external coverings of the thorax. Pressing pains on the cartilages of the left side; worse on respiration. Pressing in the chest and between the scapulæ, with dyspnœa, when walking and sitting. Oppression in right chest, causing anxiety.

Heart. Pains and sensations. Throbbing pain and pressing unrest and anxiety. Irregular action. A kind of hiccough of the heart on going upstairs.

External Chest. Eruptions. Painful vesicles over the sternum. Small dark-red spots on chest and thighs. On left mamma little scattered papules; itching, relieved by rubbing.

Mammæ. Into the breasts of a woman not *enceinte,* milk enters; it runs out; on left mamma little scattered papules, relieved by rubbing.

Pelvic Region Generally. A dull sensitive drawing in the whole circumference of pelvis; it goes alternately from sacrum to pubes.

The ischia are painful; feel as if without flesh; still they feel better when prover sits hard than when softly (characteristic).

In the crest of ilium over the hips a pain as of a sharp body cutting out, when he rises from seat.

Sacrum and Coccyx. In sacrum and coccynx an extremely painful cramp-pain; he can sit only a short time; becomes by sitting quite stiff, and can then not rise again on account of pain; cannot even lie well, and has to turn to the other side amid great pain; cannot at all lie on his back; most relieved by standing and slowly walking about, but quick walking is impossible.

Loins. Spasmodic sensation in left lumbar region.

Back Generally. Vertebral column; Pains and sensations. Pressing pain on the left side under the false ribs. Sticking and gnawing pain in vertebral column generally; gnawing pain, with cough. Cramp-like, pressing sensation in middle of column, which becomes tense on becoming erect.

Vertebral column and back: Right side, pain as if dislocated or sprained.

Vertebræ. Sticking from without inward, as if with a knife.

Scapulæ. Left: Pressing pain under it, rather toward outside. Right: Fine stitches. Between: Pain as if from a sprain. Repeated stitches, as if electric, from the left to the right scapula. Violent drawing between scapulæ, down the back. Between right and vertebral colum, drawing pain; cramp-pain, almost a pinching.

External Back. Back, and especially the scapulæ, covered with large red papules; whole skin looks red and feels sore to touch, but in the points of the papules are fine sticking pains. Itching eruption on right scapula, tickling on left.

Nape. Painful stiffness between scapulæ and in nape, on turning throat and head either way.

Pressing pain externally in neck and throat on bending head backward and on touch.

Externally. Swelling of the glands in the nape, with confusion of the head. Papules on nape and arm; fill with pus and form a crust.

Upper Extremities. Axilla. Left: Painful swelling of the glands.

Arm Generally. Motion: Stretching, twisting and turning of upper extremities. Motion convulsive. Spasm of right arm, with gnashing of teeth. Jerking in right arm. Drawing down in muscles of right arm, and when down a jerking upward toward shoulder. Convulsive shuddering. Tonic spasm (allopathic observations).

Sensation. Lassitude, ecpecially in hands, which he leaves hanging down. Heaviness and paralysis, especially of left arm. Paralytic pressure and paralytic sensation and weakness in left arm.

Pains. Tearing pain, as if too short; stiffness; tearing pains; drawing pains; pains as if beaten.

Externally. Sensation: Crawling, as of a fly, not relieved by rubbing.

Eruption. Papule under each elbow, dull red, no sensation nor suppuration.

Elbow. Rumbling (*Kollern*) as of water or blood running through the veins. Pains. Cutting pains inwardly, when walking. Sharp stitches externally. Paralytic drawing pains in elbow and in fingers of left hand.

Forearm. Fine stitches in left forearm. Dull sticking in middle of inner forearm, becoming gradually worse and at last very violent. Cutting, tearing pain.

Carpus. Paralytic tearing in the carpal bones.

Metacarpus. Sticking tearing in the bone of left metacarpus.

Hands Generally. Copious cold sweat; swelling; painless stiffness, hindering flexion as if joints were dry.

Fingers. Painful drawing in periosteum. Tearing cutting.

Externally. Little red spots on dorsa, vanishing quickly. Finger, vesicle with painful inflammation. Pustule close to nail.

Lower Extremities Generally. Motion: Stretching, he is obliged to extend the limb. Paralysis with nausea, trembling anxiety (from allopathic authorities).

Sensations. Soreness on inside of limb; sensation as if beaten or rotten in whole limb, with sticking and gnawing in the bones, with great tearing in the joints; this gradually rises from the feet to the hip, relieved by motion and walking, weariness and heaviness of the limbs a marked symptom, with drawing pain, a paralytic sensation.

Iliac Region and Joint. Cramp pain with tension in the glutæi when stooping. In the hip-joint (right) a cold feeling; transient, sticking pain both during rest and motion; paralytic tension when walking, as if luxated. Left: Pain with limping (allopathic), also nervous. Right: Pain when lying on it, relieved by turning to lie on left hip.

Thigh. Excessive heaviness and stiffness when walking; heaviness when sitting; sticking pain, as from a knife in middle of thigh, rather behind (after dinner); sticking cutting in exterior muscles of right thigh, just above the knee, only when sitting; cutting, jerking tearing in posterior muscles of left thigh when sitting; drawing pain outward toward skin at a small spot inside left thigh; throbbing spot inside of left thigh.

Knee. Violent pains; unpleasant sensations, especially in knee and in other joints of lower extremities, as if they would "click" when walking and descending.

Above. Tingling, quivering sensation when sitting.

Patella. Right: Cramp pain near patella, from within outword; sitting, pressing sticking while sitting. Left: Needle stickings under patella, sitting.

Hollow, Motion: Stiffness on motion, as if external (and sometimes the internal) hamstrings were too short; in thigh muscles, jerking upward and pains. Right: Squeezing and pressing pains. Left: Dull sticking.

Leg Generally. Motion: Has to stretch out the foot from horrid pain in leg.

Sensations. Paralytic lassitude in both legs, and especially in calves on going upstairs; trembling heaviness of right leg when it is crossed over the left; a drawing-up sensation, which is externally a mere crawling, but internally is innumerable stitches.

Legs. Pains: Stitches, painful from foot to knee (when stepping with left foot); cutting drawing, first in a little spot on the feet, then through the leg and thigh to the loins and shoulder; compressed and dull tearing, especially at night, relieved by hanging the leg out of bed; a dull burning tearing up the leg through the inner hamstring.

Shin. Tearing in shin-bone; in right shin-bone, with pressing as under sensation. Left: Pressing when standing.

Calf. Left: Sharp sticking from below upward; cramp on bending the leg, evening in bed, relieved by stretching out the thigh; tearing pain inside, not affected by motion or touch.

Feet. Externally. Sweat without warmth; excoriating itching, soles and dorsa; itching, swelling of the feet.

Sensations. Joints. Right: Tension on walking; pain in metatarsus, as if luxated on walking and bending inward the sole; tearing in the great toe joint.

Sole. Cramp, evening in bed on bending up the knee; burning and digging.

Pains. Dorsa. Dull stickings when sitting, not affected by external pressure.

Soles. Heat; boring digging pains.

Heel. Tension in right sole in the region of the heel, becoming a tensive pressure, relieved for a while by pressure.

Tendo Achillis. Boring or tearing sticking.

Generalities. Motion: Constant disposition to stretch, evening; pain prevents it.

Pain advances gradually to a very high pitch; then suddenly vanishes and re-appears in another spot; sudden horrid pain in one side of chest, abdomen, loins or in one elbow, especially during sleep, compelling to crook the part.

Aggravations. All symptoms aggravated afternoon (three and four P. M.); more tolerable forenoon; gnawing pain in affected parts.

Sentitive to touch; parts where sticking pains have been are very sore; crawling, tearing, sticking, itching, here and there, in evening in bed; after rubbing a tearing pain remains.

Glands. Boring pain in the affected glands.

Skin. Ulcers. Burning pain, almost only at night (six P. M. to six A. M.), as if something would be pressed out; the parts as if lame and stiff, violent itching; cutting pain during rest, tearing during motion of the part; soreness around ulcer.

Discharge almost nothing but bloody serum.

Spasm. Spasmodic laughter; convlusive movements of the extremities, *subsultus tendinum,* etc., are attributed to Belladonna by allopathic authorities. Slight vexation induces convulsive paroxysms; he inclines to run up the walls; convulsive movements on waking.

Under title Sleep, frequent mention will be made of convulsive motion on waking and during sleep.

Restlessness. He has constantly to change the position of limbs and body, especially hands and feet; trembling in all his limbs.

Lassitude. Disinclination to work; lassitude generally, and in morning after a sleep, whether long and heavy or interrupted by dreams, forgotten or not; feebleness of hands and feet; uncertain step, the knees give way.

Paralysis. Paralytic weakness of all limbs, especially of the feet. Allopathic authors quote complete paralysis of left side, arm and thigh; stiffness and paralysis of the extremities and whole body.

Syncope. Complete. Allopaths quote an entire apoplectic condition.

Sleep. Sleepiness; stupidity compelling sleep, which lasts about ninety minutes; after it great hunger, with great burning heat in mouth; no thirst; foul breath on coughing; great sleepiness with yawning; afternoon, sleepiness with yawning and stretching, and eyes filled with water; sleepiness at night with inability to sleep, or starting up in a fright at the moment of falling asleep.

Going to Sleep. Starting up in a fright, the feet jerking upward and the head forward; always, on going to sleep, waking and starting with fright. Just at time when he usually goes to sleep he lies long without knowing whether he is awake or is dreaming; in evening it seems as if the bed swims.

Time. Generally late; sometimes early, and, waking early; refreshed for time only.

Sleep. Restless sleep before midnight, tossing and talking in the sleep; restless, being full of dreams about men or about business; restless, the pains become unendurable, with frightful dreams; restless, he wakes frequently, tossing and cannot sleep again; heavy, with anxious dreams which he cannot recall; he even hears himself cry out from fright and yet does not awake; when waked by coughing, he goes to sleep again immediately, yet in the morning is unrefreshed, with lassitude. During sleep, starting continually; singing and loud speaking.

Complication. Whether asleep or awake, interruption of the respiration; the respiratory act lasts only half as long as the pause; expiration follows suddenly and convulsively, and is louder than inspiration; inspiration only a little longer than expiration.

Dreams. Many dreams about men and business; many which are not remembered, they take the refreshment from sleep; not many until toward morning. Character: Lively dreams; fearful, waking him with starting and a cry of murder and robbers; dreams with aggravation of the pains.

Waking during sleep; he awakes full of alarm and fear, as if something under the bed had cried out, with dry heat; waking, with fearful dreams, with sweat on forehead and præcordia.

Waking morning; bad humor, headache and lassitude; headache over the eyes, like a weight in the head, and pain in the eyes when touched; sleepiness.

Sleeplessness. Great sleeplessness for several nights in succession, from anxiety, with drawing pains in the limbs; sleeplessness from phantasies which hold her attention.

Fever. Allopathic authorities mention paroxysms of fever, commencing generally in the night after midnight or in the morning, accompanied by very great thirst, which is greatest after the sweat. The sweat is copious.

(1178-1194) Hahnemann also describes paroxysms: These occur in the afternoon or evening; very severe chill; two hours after, heat and general sweat, without thirst during either chill or heat; the heat is especially great about the head and in the face, and is often attended by dizziness; frequent attacks of fever during the day; chill, followed by general heat and sweat, without thirst during either stage.

Chill. Paleness and coldness; ice-cold hands, dull headache and depression; coldness of the whole body, especially of the feet (with headache *congestio ad caput*), with swollen, red face and hot head, pain in ears, etc.; cold, beginning in the back and epigastrium or in both arms, and going over the whole body.

Shudder in various parts, with heat in others; with heat in ears and head and face and nose; swollen face.

Sweat of feet.

Chill excited by every breath of air, yet air, in other respects, is agreeable.

Heat. Allopathic authors mention violent burning heat, both internal and external; red face; general dry heat of feet and hands, without thirst; pale face.

Internal Heat. Everything taken is too cold.

Internal heat with swollen veins, and especially pulsation of the carotids so great as to make the teeth chatter; heat in head.

Internal heat morning in bed, yet he does not uncover; pain in the parts which he does uncover, as if from cold.

Internal heat and external over whole body, especially the head; pulsation in the temporal arteries, with confusion in the head and subsequent sweat.

Internal heat both sensible and actual, especially in red, sweaty face, with headache and thirst.

Heat. Excited by slight motion.

In Relation to External Surface. Allopathic authors quote: Inflammation of whole body, with quick pulse; heat of the whole body, with violent redness; redness and swelling of whole body; burning hot and red, with pricking, biting sensation; itching of the whole body, with eruption of red petecchiæ.

Eruptive Fevers. Thorax and abdomen covered with little red, elevated, painless spots, which often vanish and suddenly re-appear, with general redness of the skin. Inflamed red spots and spots like scarlatina, of various forms, over the body. Hot erysipelatoid fever, accompanied by swellings inflamed and even gangrenous.

ATROPA BELLADONNA. 253

Allopathic authors in addition give; Blood-red spots on the whole body, especially in the face and chest. Measles-like eruption. Dull, red, scarlet-fever-like spots over the whole body, with small, quick pulse, dyspnœa, violent cough, delirium, increased memory and dilated pupils.

Sweat. Sweat more or less copious after the heat. Fugitive sweats, alternating with coolness; sometimes occurring with heat. The sweat is most apt to occur, or is most copious, on face and forehead, and is often unaccompanied by thirst.

Excited by: Slight motion during sleep; many symptoms refer to night-sweats, very copious; covering one's self in bed, only the parts covered sweat; covering the hands in bed, inducing a general sweat; on uncovering them, a general chill.

Time. Night frequently mentioned. The night-sweat does not debilitate. Immediately after midnight. During sleep. Morning.

Smell. The night-sweat Putrid.

Pulse. Strong and frequent, large, full and slow. Small and frequent. Large, 85.

Anxiety. Crying out on the slightest Provocation, on approach of anybody. During the day, no rest in any place. Great affright. Anxiety in the Præcordial region.

Groaning. Frequent, especially in morning, without knowing why. At every expiration, and during sleep.

Allopathic authors give: Trembling in hands and feet, with sudden cry. Anxiety, followed by sweat, about things formerly hoped for. Anxiety and unrest in præcordia, with headache, red face and bitter taste.

Restlessness. Cannot sit long in one spot, goes about everywhere. Ceaseless motion of the body, especially the arms; pulse not being altered. Constant tossing in bed.

Delirium. Allopathic authors give: Speech without connection. Constant delirium, waking and in dreams. It comes on after eating. Dreams of conflagration at home, of wolves and dogs around him.

Night—delirium, with consciousness during the day. Paroxysms of delirium.

(F. Hahnemann.) She sits idle behind the stove; makes songs and sings them, senseless and incoherent; also she whistles by times; eats and drinks nothing; pale face and sweat on the forehead.

Disposition. Elevated. Shown by disposition to sing and whistle; laughing at she knows not what; frequent laughing and singing, loud and long; laughable gestures, now sitting, now motioning as if washing, counting money, drinking.

Allopathic authors give: Great insane excitement; running half-clad, with wonderful gestures; laughing, singing, dancing, etc.; violent shaking of the head, foaming at the mouth; clapping the hands over the head, saliva running out of the mouth; she distorts her face; her tongue hangs out of her mouth.

Depressed. Anxiety with weeping; she is tired

of life. Fearfulness, with disposition to weep. Whining, sniffling and howling without cause, with fearfulness especially on waking. Indifference. Inactivity of mind and body.

Indifferent to everything; careless of life. Apathetic, unimpressible. Then, after a few days, she is very sensitive and impressible.

Irritable. Irritability about trifles, with pressing headache as from a stone, caused by every noise or visit. She wishes solitude and repose. Quiet irritability, alternating with the natural disposition, with great dryness in the mouth.

Anger. If all be not right, even anger at himself about very trifles.

Irritability and over-sensibility; all the senses are too highly strung.

Rage. Either paroxysmal or constant delirium; first jolly, then raging; howling and crying about trifles, aggravated by kind speeches; with very mobile pupils; violent rage, not to be soothed.

Allopathic authors give: Rage, tossing about in bed, tearing clothes, striking himself in the face with his fist, gnashing of the teeth and convulsions; biting the spoon, barking and howling; great desire to bite the by-standers. This rage is attended by burning heat of the body, open, staring eyes, and spitting at the by-standers.

Mistrust and desire to flee; fear of an imaginary black dog. This is in general a primary and early effect of Belladonna. She seeks to flee; asks her friends to kill her; throws herself into the water.

PRACTICAL APPLICATIONS.

The practical scope of Belladonna in therapeutics may be inferred from a *résumé* of its physiological action. We have seen that it acts upon every part of the nervous system; upon the sensorium, producing confusion, delirium, mania, stupor; that simultaneously it produces heat of the head, redness of the face and eyes, throbbing of the carotids, a full, hard and tolerably frequent pulse, together with perversions of the special senses and spasmodic action of the voluntary muscles.

Now, these symptoms point to the use of Belladonna in diseases which involve not merely the function, but also the tissues, of the nervous center of the cerebro-spinal nervous system. Accordingly, in mania we find Belladonna a prominent remedy, as likewise in inflammation of the brain and its meninges. In these affections, besides the perversion of the sensorial functions and the direct symptoms of cerebritis or meningitis respectively, there will always be present, if Belladonna be indicated, the red face, shining eyes and full, hard pulses, already described. These may not be present along with mania. The face may be of a natural hue or pale; the pulse not fuller, even smaller, than is customary; the expression, far from being anxious, turgid, inflammatory, may be mild or pinched, or again, stupid. In such cases, the true remedy may be Hyoscyamus, Stramonium,

Veratrum, Platina or Natrum muriaticum or some other drug; it cannot be Belladonna.

So of the encephalitis, the face may be pale, the eyes dull or distorted, the patient stupid or nearly so, the pulse slow and soft. The brain or its membranes, or both, may indeed be the seat of inflammation, but Belladonna cannot be the remedy. This may be Helleborus niger or Sulphur or Bryonia or Zincum.

As a generalization, it may be stated that Belladonna seems to be required in cases in which the arterial storm which would have indicated Aconite, having actually burst upon the patient and localized its action in the encephalon, this localization is still in the first stage of engorgement and plastic deposit. When the period of serous effusion arrives, or when the deposit is complete, the case has already passed beyond the province of Belladonna; and now Hellebore, Sulphur and Zinc come into the field.

In affections of the eye, both functional and organic, Belladonna is indicated by the symptoms, and has approved itself in practice. As regards functional disease, cases are numerous in which partial or total blindness has ensued from poisoning with Belladonna. On the other hand, Belladonna has approved itself a frequently indicated and very serviceable remedy in amaurosis, partial or complete.

As to organic affections, while the conjunctiva and the secretions are but moderately affected, the deeper tissues of the eyes seem to be gravely attacked, as is shown by the deep pains in the orbits, the fullness and distention of the eye as though it would burst, the supra-orbital and post-orbital pains and the illusions of vision. It is rarely that Belladonna is indicated, unless the general symptoms characteristic of its action are present, viz., the full, hard pulse, the red and hot face, the frontal weight and heat and the peculiar crescendo character of the pain.

The facial neuralgia produced by Belladonna has been fully described. Many cases of cure are recorded. The pain has the peculiarities already described, and is most likely to be aggravated in the evening. It occurs generally on the right side, and is thus distinguished from the neuralgia for which Spigelia is indicated. From the neuralgia which requires Stannum, and which may also be on the right side, it is distinguished by the fact that the pain which Stannum produces and relieves comes on gently, increases gradually and then as gradually diminishes in severity; while that of Belladonna, after gradually rising to an intolerable acuteness, ceases on a sudden.

Inflammatory affections of the throat can hardly be mentioned in any connection without calling to mind Belladonna as a remedy, so universal is its use and so efficacious. In simple tonsillitis, when the tonsils are swollen and present a bright red appearance with painful and difficult deglutition, at first dryness of the fauces, and then moderate secretion of ropy mucus or saliva, with the characteristic pulse and expression of face, Belladonna suffices to effect a cure in a few hours. It is useful not merely in tonsillitis, but equally so in pharyngitis, in inflammation of the soft palate and uvula, and of the larynx when the mucous membrane and the sub-mucous cellular tissue are both involved. The redness is vivid; the pain is acute, tense and often throbbing; the arterial action very decided. The secretion of the mucous membrane in a typical Belladonna case, though it may be diminished causing dryness, or thickened causing a ropy discharge, is not altered in such wise as to simulate a plastic or a diphtheritic deposit. In such cases the remedy is more likely to be found among Mercury, Bromine, Cantharis, Muriatic acid and Lachesis.

If, again, the affection of the sub-mucous cellular tissue be such as to cause a dropsical effusion into this tissue, so that the soft curtain of the palate, the uvula and the walls of the pharynx become like swollen, translucent water-bags, Belladonna is not indicated. The remedy is Rhus or possible Phosphorus.

Finally, the tonsils may be chronically enlarged. The fissures may be very prominent. In these fissures little white granules are observed, which are very fetid and are oily in their composition.

The swelling of the tonsil is very evident externally, and is painful on external pressure.

Pathologists are not agreed as to the nature and origin of these white granules. I believe them to be the altered secretion of the tonsil. Such a state of things is generally attended by follicular pharyngitis and by cough, loss of voice and accumulations of mucus in the larynx and trachea. In such cases Lachesis is almost always indicated. None of these are Belladonna cases, and the sooner their nature is discoverd and the true remedy given in place of Belladonna, which may have been at first selected, the better for the patient.

Finally, in a case which was, or seemed to be, a Belladonna case, the swelling increases, the difficulty in swallowing becomes very great, the mucous membrane of the fauces grows livid, a sharp sticking pain as from a splinter is felt in the side of the fauces, the external swelling is great and tender the secretion becomes offensive and yellowish, the pulse becomes frequent, but softer and smaller; in fact, it is evident that an abscess is forming in the substance of the tonsil. In such a case Belladonna will do no good. Hepar sulphuris will be more likely to arrest suppuration if that be possible, or else to circumscribe and hasten it, if the case have already gone so far that resolution is impossible.

Of the peculiar throat affection of scarlatina more will be said when we come to speak of that disease.

On the digestive apparatus, on the function of nutrition, as already stated Belladonna exerts but little action. It is rarely indicated in diseases of this apparatus. Nevertheless the general symptoms characteristic of Belladonna may be present in so marked a degree in some disease of these organs as to call for Belladonna. Thus, in acute hepatitis it may possibly be sometimes called for, not so much by the liver symptoms as by the general subjective or objective sympathetic symptoms affecting other organs or systems.

Belladonna may perhaps be indicated in some forms of dysentery, or of inflammation of the rectum, as the symptoms of "constant tenesmus and pressing downward upon both bladder and rectum, with scanty stool and increased tenesmus following the stool," show. Yet the drug does not correspond to the general character of these diseases, and if indicated it will be so rather by virtue of its general characteristics; and although it may be an indispensable remedy at some other stage of a difficult case, it will rarely prove the sole and all-sufficient cure for any case of hysentery.

The urine, as we have seen, is scanty, with frequent tenesmus of the bladder and slight strangury. The urine itself is dark and turbid, and sometimes fiery red.

Belladonna has been frequently used in inflammatory affections of the bladder, attended by the above symptoms and by the general characteristics of Belladonna. Likewise, in the first stage of desquamative nephritis.

Its appropriateness to this frequent feature of scarlatina is an additional item in the indication of Belladonna for that disease.

In its applicability to these affections, Belladonna is associated with Cantharides, Apis, Terebinth, Arsenicum and Mercury.

If we are at all in a position to draw distinctions between the members of this group, I should say that Cantharides corresponds more particularly to affections of the bladder and urethra, and not of the kidney; Belladonna to those of the bladder, especially its neck, and to the first stage of kidney affection, congestion; Terebinth to the kidney and not to the bladder, and to the first stage of the kidney affection, that of congestion and hematuria before albumen is effused; Mercury to the kidney when albumen is being effused, but before dropsy occurs; Apis and Arsenicum to the kidney and to the second stage when albumen in abundance is effused, and when, in addition, the disease has endured so long that dropsical effusions have occurred in the cellular tissue. I cannot give these distinctions authoritatively. They should not influence your prescriptions, unless the other and general symptoms of each case correspond to those of the drug; I believe in most cases they will be found to correspond.

The symptoms of Belladonna which relate to the pelvic organs, and in particular to the uterus, are very graphic. No remedy is more frequently and successfully employed for affections of the genital organs of women.

On the provers, Belladonna produced the symptom: "Constant and violent pressure downward toward the genital organs, as if everything would fall out."

This symptom would suggest the use of Belladonna in cases of prolapsus uteri, whether chronic and constant, or occurring at intervals, or at the menstrual period in case of dysmenorrhœa.

In all of these cases, Belladonna is one of our most valuable remedies. But four other drugs of the "Materia Medica Pura" have the very same symptoms, viz.: Sepia, Nux vomica, Podophyllum and Pulsatilla.

How shall we distinguish the case appropriate for each remedy? Why, by the conditions and the concomitant symptoms.

The above symptom of Belladonna is worse when the patient sits bent over and when she walks, but is better when she sits erect or when she stands. Now, under Sepia, the conditions are just the reverse; the symptom is aggravated by sitting up, still more by standing, and most of all by walking; while it is relieved by lying down; just what you would expect in a case of atonic relaxation of the ligamentous and vaginal supports of the uterus; while the apparent incongruities of the Belladonna conditions accord well with the conditions of an irritable or inflammatory state of the organ.

Nux vomica, again, has the pressing down more in the back, with irritable rectum, frequent ineffectual desire for stool, with scanty evacuations. There is but little leucorrhœa. Pulsatilla, on the other hand, has the same symptom as Belladonna, with aggravation on lying down, but it has also aggravation from heat, and amelioration in the open air, with pressure on the bladder and frequent micturition; but this is copious and not attended by strangury.

Moreover, there is a copious thick leucorrhœa. The general symptoms show a disposition to a hydræmic condition, instead of the hyperæmia of hyperrhinosis of Belladonna.

Podophyllum has not been so carefully proved as to furnish a good idea of its characteristics. But I believe that it is rarely useful in prolapsus, unless there be also prolapsus of the vagina and rectum, or a tendency thereto, and pain in the region of the ovaries.

There is a form of dysmenorrhœa in which Belladonna is capable of effecting a radical cure, even in cases of many years' standing. The pain is often exceedingly severe, driving the patient to the use of anodynes. It is a dragging and pressing downward. There are also cutting pains from behind forward, or *vice versa,* and passing through a horizontal diameter of the pelvis, and not around its circumference (as the pains of Sepia and Platina do). These pains precede the appearance of the menses from six to twenty hours. They are paroxysmal and intolerable. The patient notices that an evacuation of the bowels at this time is painful.

It seems as though the fæces, particularly if the mass be large and tolerably solid, in passing along the rectum, pressed anteriorly upon a sore surface. If the index finger be passed into the rectum, a hot rounded tumor may be perceived about two and one-half inches above the orifice of the rectum. It is extremely painful when gently pressed. A vaginal examination brings the finger in contact with this same body in the posterior *cul de sac* of the vagina. It is the congested or inflamed ovary. In very severe cases of this kind, I have found that Belladonna, persisted in for many consecutive months, given just before each menstrual epoch, would suffice to overcome at least all tendency to a recurrence of these attacks, and would render menstruation normal.

Belladonna has been successfully used in certain cases of uterine hæmorrhage.

While on this subject I may call your attention to a singular affection, the pathology of which I do not understand.

In women apparently healthy, in whom the function of menstruation is in every other respect normal, the flow is sometimes extremely offensive. It has been described to me by the patients and their friends as peculiarly and distressingly offensive. The peculiar character of this odor I could never get intelligibly described. The cases that have come under my observation have been unmarried young women, in good circumstances and of most exemplary habits in every way. I was led to give Belladonna from the symptom (quoted by Hahnemann from Evers' "Berliner Sammlungen," iv.)

"offensive metrorrhagia." The odor ceased to be perceived. No other remedy or treatment had any effect. A similar odor has been observed in the lochial discharge on the fourth or fifth day, and has likewise been removed by Belladonna.

Belladonna has been recommended by allopathic physicians during labor, as a local remedy for rigidity of the os uteri. Cases not infrequently occur during labor, or during the puerperal period, in which the general symptoms characteristic of Belladonna are present, and indicate that remedy.

In affections of the respiratory organs Belladonna is a most important remedy; but especially in irritable and inflammatory conditions of the larynx and trachea, whether isolated or conjoined with the affections of the fauces and the pharynx already described.

The cough is dry, or, if there be any sputa, it is only after long coughing, and they consist often of mucus tinged with blood. It occurs, or is much aggravated, in the evening and early night—more particularly just after lying down.

It comes in paroxysms.

It is accompanied by heat and great redness of the face, sparkling eyes and full, hard pulse. It is provoked by a tickling in the larynx, as if dust were there, in the back part of the larynx, which compels a hard, dry cough.

It is induced by exertion, by lying down and by very deep inspiration.

It is accompanied by a feeling of soreness in

the larynx, as if internally hot and sore; this soreness is felt when pressing the larynx externally. It is also accompanied by oppression of the chest, heat in the chest, dyspnœa, etc.

These symptoms have led to the use of Belladonna in laryngitis of adults, and in the first stages of croup; in certain epidemics, in trachitis, and in pneumonia. The general symptoms must correspond, as always.

It is of the greatest importance to distinguish the cough of Belladonna from those of its cognates, viz., Lachesis, Phosphorus, Causticum, Rumex crispus and Cepa. I will sketch their characteristics now, and repeat them as we take up each remedy, hoping by reiteration to fix them in your minds.

The cough of Lachesis is dry, like that of Belladonna; but there is a sensation as if something were in the trachea which might be raised, and indeed comes partly up, but then goes back again.

It is provoked by tickling in the trachea (below that of Belladonna) induced by touching the trachea or pressing on it, or by pressure of the clothing of the patient, and which he therefore loosens, or by throwing the head back, and also by eating.

It occurs always on awaking from sleep.

It is accompanied by some hoarseness and sore throat, which shoots up into the ear, and by chronic tonsillitis, with oily white granules.

The cough of Phosphorus is dry, or has a scanty, rusty sputum. It occurs night or day. It is provoked by a tickling in the trachea pretty low down, and by feeling of rawness ond soreness in the trachea and bronchi. It is induced by a very deep-inspiration. It is accompanied and characterized by a hoarse, barking sound, by rawness of trachea and whole chest, and by a peculiar and distressing weight across the chest. Hoarseness.

The cough of Causticum is dry. It occurs in the evening. It is provoked by a tickling high in the trachea. It is in long paroxysms. The voice is almost gone. The trachea is sore and raw, but not the chest.

The cough of Rumex crispus is dry and short and paroxysmal, or is a constant hack. It occurs evening and night on going to bed. It is provoked by tickling in the supra-sternal fossa; is induced by pressure in that region; is induced by inhaling a breath of cool air; by a deep inhalation; by any variation of breathing. It is accompanied by great fatigue from coughing, and by stitches through the left lung.

The cough of Cepa is dry, though there are acrid coryza and lachrymation. The cough is induced by tickling in the larynx, and each cough feels as though it would split the larynx in two. The Patient cringes under the pain.

I have traveled out of my record to give these characteristics of the cough of each member of this group and to compare them, because this sharp discrimination it is the business of the practitioner to make whenever he is called upon to prescribe for a patient; and my chief business is to show you what is to be done and how to do it, so that the great object may be best attained, viz., the selection of the right remedy and the cure of the patient.

GENERAL DISEASES.

Passing now from the application of Belladonna to diseases of special organs or apparatus, we come to its use in general diseases of the entire system; and first, in

Fevers. In intermittent fever we should not be likely to select Belladonna. Its proving shows hardly a trace of periodicity, neither is the febrile paroxysm distinctly divided into stages. For this very reason, however, it may be required in some malarious diseases, commonly classed among intermittents, and in which the heat begins early and is nearly continuous, and the head shows signs from the first of being involved; great cerebral congestion or positive inflammation taking place in the encephalon. In such cases, Belladonna may be indicated. The characteristic general symptom will be present. The fever of the Roman Campagna is of this kind.

In typhoid or typhus fever, we should not expect to employ Belladonna save as an intercurrent remedy. Its symptoms give us to picture of blood decomposition. The nervous system, instead of being depressed, unstrung or suspended from its office, is stimulated aroused; and if perverted in its action, perverted through the morbid intensity and energy of trat action.

All this is very unlike the effect of the typhus miasm on the nervous system.

Nor, again, does Belladonna present us the muscular torpor and paralysis peculiar to typhus, and which Rhus toxicodendron and Arsenicum present so clearly.

Belladonna, then, is not suited to a typical case of typhus or typhoid.

Nevertheless, cases may occur that will call for it. Mania, *per se,* or encephalitis, may occur in the course of the disease, and, presenting the characteristic symptoms of Belladonna, may require its use as an intercurrent, but as an intercurrent only.

And let me warn you to beware of intercurrent remedies. Let your aim be to select each drug as a remedy corresponding not merely to the present symptoms, but also to that general character and fabric of the disease which determine its symptoms and their successive productions, course and relations.

Eruptive Fever. While Belladonna may be indicated by the totality of the symptoms at some period during the course of any one of the eruptive fevers, it is particularly to scarlatina that it seems closely to correspond, and in the treatment as well as in the prevention of which it has become a famous remedy.

Prophylaxis. Hahnemann's attention was called to the subject of scarlatina by the prevalence of a severe epidemic of it in Saxony; and which invaded his own family soon after he had began his investigations of the law of cure and his provings of drugs upon the healthy subject. Having become satisfied of the close resemblance existing between the character of the prevailing epidemic and the effects of Belladonna, he went further, and conjectured that Belladonna might prove a prophylactic against the disease. The story of this discovery may best be told in his own words:

"The mother of a large family, at the commencement of July, 1799, when the scarlet fever was most prevalent and fatal, had got a new counterpane made up by a sempstress, who (without the knowledge of the former) had in her small chamber a boy just recovering from scarlet fever. The first-mentioned woman, on receiving it, examined and smelt it, but as she could detect no smell, she placed it beside her on a sofa on which, some hours later, she lay down to sleep. In this way, alone she imbibed the miasm. A week subsequently she was suddenly attacked with qninsy and its characteristic shooting pains in the throat, which were subdued in four days. Several days afterward, her daughter, ten years of age, was attacked in the evening by severe pressive pains in the abdomen, itching of the head and body, rigor over the head and arms and paralytic stiffness of the joints. Her sleep was restless during the night, with frightful dreams and general perspiration, excepting the head.

"I found her in the morning with pressive headache, dimness of vision, slimy tongue, some ptyalism, the sub-maxillary glands hard, swollen and painful to the touch, and shooting pains in the throat when attempting to swallow. She was free from thirst; pulse quick and small; breathing hurried and anxious; very pale though feeling hot; horripilation; leaning forward to lessen the pain; she complained of stiffness with an air of much dejection, and shunned conversation, feeling that she could only speak in a whisper. Her look was dull, yet staring; her eyelids widely stretched, face pale and features sunk.

"Knowing too well the ineffectual nature of the ordinary favourite remedies, I resolved, in this case of incipient scarlet fever, not to act with reference to individual symptoms, but (agreeably to my new synthetical principle) to obtain, if possible, a remedy calculated to produce in a healthy person most of the morbid symptoms I now observed; and my memory and written remarks suggested no remedy so appropriate as Belladonna, which I had observed to produce precisely the above-mentioned symptoms.

"I therefore gave the girl, who was already affected by the first indications of scarlet fever, a dose of Belladonna (432,000 of a grain of the extract, which, according to my subsequent experience, is too large a dose). She remained quietly seated all day, without lying down; the heat of her body diminished, she drank but little; none of her symptoms increased, and no new ones appeared. She slept quietly, and the following morning, twenty hours after taking the medicine, most of the symptoms had disappeared without any crisis; the sore throat only continued, but in a less degree, till the evening, when it went off. The following day she was lively, and ate and played as usual.

"I gave her a second dose, and she remained perfectly well, while two other children of the family fell ill of the scarlet fever without my knowledge, whom I could only treat according to my general plan detailed above. I gave my convalescent a smaller dose of Belladonna every three or four days, and she continued in perfect health.

"I now earnestly desired to preserve the other five chiledrn from infection; their removal being impossible, and I thus reasoned: a remedy capable of quickly checking a disease in its first onset must be its best preventive, and the following occurrence strengthened my opinion. Some weeks previously three children of another family were ill of severe scarlet fever. The eldest daughter alone, who had been taking Belladonna internally for an external affection of the joints of her fingers, to my great astonishment escaped the infection, although in other cases of epidemics she had readily taken them.

"This decided me to administer to the other five children very small doses of this excellent remedy as a preservative, and as its action lasts only three days, I repeated the dose every seventy-two hours, and they all remained in perfect health, though surrounded with infection.

"In the meantime, I was called to attend another family where the eldest son was ill of scarlet fever. I found him in the height of the fever, with the eruption on the chest and arms. He was seriously ill, and it was too late to give the specific prophylactic remedy. But, wishing to preserve the other children of four and two years old and nine months, I directed the parents to give the requisite dose of Belladonna every three days, and had the happiness of seeing them escape the disease in spite of constant intercourse with their sick brother."

By this narrative Hahnemann introduced to the medical world what he thought a discovery of great value. Scarlatina prevailed extensively in Europe at that time and during the first quarter of the present century. Belladonna as a prophylactic was tried in thousands of cases and by hundreds of physicians. The testimony in its favor was not unanimous, but greatly preponderating.

Hufeland, the great protomedicus of Prussia, reported in favor of its prophylactic action. His report was based on observations of his own and the sum of the testimony of others. In consequence of his report the Prussian government, in 1838, decreed that it should be obligatory on physicians to give Belladonna as a prophylactic whenever scarlatina prevailed as an epidemic.

Pareira endeavors to throw doubt on the arguments and evidence in its favor, but Dr. Stillé, of Philadelphia, the most recent writer, speaks as follows (ii. 51):

"On a review of the whole subject we feel bound to express the conviction that the virtues of Belladonna as a protective against scarlatina are so far proven that it becomes the duty of practitioners to invoke their aid whenever the disase breaks out in a locality where there are persons liable to the contagion."

The evidence of the prophylactic power of Belladonna will appear stronger if we consider two facts:

1. As Stillé remarks, the paucity of the cases of some objectors, and the meagerness of the details furnished by others, deprive their evidence of real weight: and

2. It is notorious that epidemics often differ very widely from each other in characteristic symptoms, even though the same name may be applied to them. Now, if Hahnemann's reason for giving Belladonna as a prophylactic be correct, Belladonna would only be a prophylactic against an epidemic miasm, the disease resulting from which closely resembled the symptoms produced on the healthy by Belladonna. In an epidemic which did not resemble the effects of Belladonna, that remedy would not be a sure prophylactic.

Hahnemann himself pointed out this fact in his preface to Belladonna. He says:

"The property I have discovered in Belladonna, given in a small dose every six or seven days, of being a preservative against scarlatina, as Sydenham, Plenciz and others have described it, was for nineteen years brought into contempt by physicians, who, ignorant that the disease belongs only to children, have confounded it with the purple miliary rash introduced from Belgium in 1801, and have applied to the latter my method, which of course failed. I rejoice, however, that of late years other physicians have distinguished the ancient and true scarlatina, establishing the preservative property of Belladonna in that disease, and have thus rendered justice to my labors, so long misunderstood."

Remedies. Little need be added to what has already been said on the subject of Belladonna as a remedy for scarlatina. Its correspondence to the majority of cases in epidemics presenting no peculiar type is very manifest. But epidemics do occur; and we have had several of late years in which the symptoms do not correspond so closely to the symptoms of Belladonna as of some other drug; as, for example, of Stramonium.

It behooves us, therefore, to avoid here as ever the great error of prescribing according to the name which we may have given to the disease; and to study closely the symptoms of each case, and compare with those of various drugs of the Materia Medica, so as to select that which shall best correspond.

If, now, we have thus chosen Belladonna, his remedy may be sufficient to carry the case through to convalescence. Frequently, however, this will not be so. Tendencies to chronic disease hitherto latent may be aroused in the patient by the scarlatisa poison, and may become active. Then we shall require to enter upon a course of treatment of a chronic disease; and it is not probable that Belladonna will be of further service.

This awakening of chronic tendencies often takes place about the third day of the rash. It is of great importance to take it in the beginning. Hence the rule which has been suggested, that on the day above mentioned the careful physician shall carefully examine the patient, with a view of detecting tendencies to chronic disease, and should be prompt to prescribe accordingly. Rhus, Calcarea carbonica, Hepar sulphuris, are remedies likely to be required.

Epilepsy. In this disease Belladonna has been more successful than perhaps any other one remedy. Some brilliant cures of this terrible disease are on record. In all cases which it has favorably affected, the spasms were accompanied by the general symptoms above recited as characteristic of Belladonna.

The same remarks may be made of puerperal convulsions.

Erysipelas. No mention has yet been made of the use of Belladonna in erysipelas. And yet in the smooth, shining affection, specially of the face and head, it has been of greatest value. Mr. Liston, of London, though not a homœopathist, bore testimony to its efficacy in the hands of homœopathists. Its homœopathicity cannot be questioned.

HYOSCYAMUS NIGER

HENBANE.

IS classed along with Belladonna among the narcotics, or among the cerebro-stimulants. It resembles Belladonna in some respects, though lacking its power to act on a number of organs and systems of the body, and acting very differently on others.

It has been used as a medicine from the earliest ages; but was brought into prominent notice by Stoerck.

Swine eat it with impunity. It is peculiarly fatal to fowls. Hence its name.

It acts on dogs as on men.

On men it produces, in large doses, delirium resembling that of drunkenness,—a garrulous delirium, with proneness to altercation and quarrelsomeness. Hence one of its ancient names, *Altercum*. Its power to produce an excited or quarrelsome or fantastic mania is universally conceded. The effects are, moreover, "fullness and heat of the head, flushing of the face, injection of the eyes and cerebral excitement, manifested by indistinct or clouded vision, and sometimes total blindness, giddiness, delirium and hallucinations. Sometimes natural objects assume a grotesque appearance, or the field of vision is filled by luminous figures.

"There is little or no inclination to sound sleep, but a sort of somnolence with incoherent mutterings, like that which is so common in typhoid fever.

"Sometimes the hearing is lost. The pupils are often, but not always, dilated; the muscles of the throat and chest, and of the lower limbs, are affected with tetanic rigidity or clonic spasms; and there is more or less complete loss of power in the same parts, which is apt to continue after the attack. Aphonia is by no means uncommon. General sensibility is in most cases very much impaired, while at the same time there may be severe neuralgic pains in the course of the principal nervous trunks. The skin is apt to be bathed in perspiration, which is sometimes cold when a large dose has been taken. Sometimes the tongue is paralyzed and the pharynx spasmodically contracted." (Stillé, vol. ii., 24.)

The summary taken from Orfila and Stillé shows the homœopathic relation of Hyoscyamus to many cases in which homœopathists have successfully used it, as we shall see.

Our knowledge of its physical action is derived from Hahnemann's proving. (R. A. M. L., iv.)

The whole plant is used in medicine.

The action of Hyoscyamus on the vital power is marked.

1. On the sensorium it produces perversion of perception, so that illusions perplex the patient; he sees things which have no existence; also perversion of intellectual action; he reasons erroneously. A distinct mania of the quarrelsome or obscene character. The patient would escape, or would be undressed and walk about nude, or use offensive and unbecoming language and gestures, or quarrel with by-standers.

2. On the muscular system. It paralyzes and convulses the voluntary muscular system, *e. g.*, the extremities, and paralyzes the involuntary system, produces convulsions and paralysis (with pale face, quiet pulse, nervousness). As, for example, paralysis of the constrictors of the pharynx, and also of the sphincter ani.

The action on the organic substances of the body is so slight that we can hardly define it.

The sphere of action of the drug seems to be confined:

1. To the sensorium, producing the peculiar forms of mania and delirium alluded to.

2. To the muscular system, producing partial or general convulsions, and also paralysis of the sphincters.

3. To the nervous supply of the larynx and trachea, producing a tickling cough.

4. To the sleep: Produces at first, under small doses, an unwonted liveliness and difficulty in get-

ting asleep; sleeplessness and frequent waking, with exaltation of mind and vivid imaginings. Even when it occurs the sleep is very unquiet, the limbs twitch or are contorted into various grotesque shapes, the hands clutch at the bedclothes or grope about here and there; there are convulsive twitches, startings up in affright, grinding of the teeth, groaning and starting in sleep.

The peculiarities of Hyoscyamus may be noted as follows: First the convulsions, the mania, the delirium, the cough, the sleeplessness, all occur almost absolutely without any manifestations of fever. In this respect it presents a marked contrast to Belladonna.

2. The singular and definite character of the mania, which is loquacious and quarrelsome, the subject of it being especially inclined to unseemly and immodest acts, gestures or expressions.

It differs from that of Stramonium in these particulars: The latter produces mania with some degree of fever (though less than Bellodonna), and in it the patients, though loquacious, are good-natured and fully occupied with the observation of the phantoms by which they fancy themselves to be surrounded.

The spasmodic affections may be either *subsultus tendinum* of a single extremity or general epileptic convulsions; the limbs are forcibly curved and the body is thrown up from the bed; the patient then falls with a cry and is generally convulsed. It resembles and is useful in convulsions from intestinal worms, and especially in puerperal convulsions; also spasm of pharynx and œsophagus.

The cough of Hyoscyamus is a dry, nervous, spasmodic cough, which occurs at night, and ceases when the patient sits up; this is a certain characteristic of Hyoscyamus. The Belladonna cough often compels the patient to sit up, but does not thereupon cease.

The symptoms generally are aggravated at night.

The forces sink quickly; the patient gets easily fatigued; syncope is readily produced; the limbs become cold and tremble. These symptoms, with those of the sleep, the paralysis of the sphincters, point to the use of Hyoscyamus in some conditions occurring in the course of continued fevers.

SPECIAL ANALYSIS.

The vertigo of Hyoscyamus is attended by obscuration of vision, and loss of the general sensibility of the external surface of the body.

The head becomes heavy and confused. The pains which, however, are ill defined, are mostly in the forehead. When walking there is a sensation as of a wave within the cranium with pressing in the forehead.

Heat in the head and in the forehead.

The eye presents no evidence of organic affection, whether subjective or objective. On the other hand, vision is eminently affected.

The sight is obscured; illusions are very various;

fiery red objects appear. When reading, the letters move about, small objects appear large; in sweing, the needle goes to the wrong place.

The eyes become short-sighted; they are distorted; they stare and protrude.

Hyoscyamus has proved an excellent remedy for squinting and for double vision.

The face is distorted; the *risus sardonicus* is produced.

There is roaring in the ears.

In the throat, dryness and inability to swallow, but not from swelling or soreness. The affection is purely nervous or spasmodic.

The digestive organs present nothing characteristic.

The stool is inclined to be loose and diarrhœic. It is characteristic that it passes involuntarily.

The secretion of urine is perhaps diminished. The bladder itself is often paralyzed, so that urine accumulates and the patient is unable to expel it or unconscious of its presence.

A number of these symptoms suggest Hyoscyamus as likely to be useful in the puerperal state.

The menses are too copious, and are preceded by labor-like pains.

The symptoms of the extremities have been noted.

The disposition is exceedingly despondent and melancholy (save in the mania). A peculiar feature is the production of a state of mind resembling jealousy. Hence Hyoscyamus acquired some reputation in illness arising from disappointments in love, etc. The physiology of this is a matter of speculation.

PRACTICAL APPLICATIONS.

A few only of the applications of Hyoscyamus which, according to the law *Similia similibus curantur,* would suggest themselves in accordance with the above symptoms, need be specified particularly.

In spasms of various kinds, involving the voluntary muscular system, Hyoscyamus has proved a most valuable remedy.

If general, the convulsion differs from that for which Belladonna is indicated in this particular, that it is neither preceded, accompanied, nor followed by symptoms of cerebral congestion or of great arterial energy of action, as is the case with Belladonna convulsions. Indeed, the absence of all such signs is remarkable under Hyoscyamus. Now, of all convulsive affections that could exist without these symptoms, none are so probable as convulsions from the irritation of intestinal worms, and more particularly the convulsions that sometimes unhappily attend and complicate labor and the puerperal state. Of course some puerperal convulsions are accompained by the cerebral congestion and arterial storm, and these may require Belladonna. But there is a large class which have them not, and of these Hyoscyamus is a conspicuous remedy.

Similar remarks might be made respecting the mania which is curable by Hyoscyamus. The especial adaptation of it to certain non-congestive or non-inflammatory forms of puerperal mania has been fully recognized and established in clinical experience.

The character of the mental affection is one which is prevalent in puerperal mania, or in mania relating to, or in any way depending on, functional or organic maladies of the sexual organs of women.

The tendency to loquacity, to quarreling, to the use of indelicate language and of immodest gestures and actions, all remind one forcibly of the graphic instance of this distressing affection described by Gooch, and which sometimes see.

An example of this kind of mania, occuring, however in an unmarried young woman, in sequence of some menstrual irregularity, and cured by Dr. Guernsey, of Philadelphia, is a remarkable instance of—

1. The efficacy of Hyoscyamus in mania.
2. The efficacy of a single small does of a remedy, if well selected, in the cure of a terrible malady.
3. The value of the homœopathic law as guiding us in selecting the right drug.

A young woman, apparently well, except that she had recently had irregular menstruation, one morning refused to rise from bed and dress herself. She assigned no reason. After a few hours she insisted on rising, but would not wear a single garment of any kind.

Her parents, alarmed, sought advice. Dr. Guernsey called. The patient received him without any apparent consciousness of her singular condition, conversed intelligently, but would not admit that she needed any advice to clothe herself. She refused medicine, and cunningly evaded all stratagems to give it clandestinely.

Several days passed in this way. She escaped from her room, went through the house, and sought to escape into the street. At length, when matters were growing worse, Dr. Guernsey succeeded in getting her to take a dose of Hyoscyamus^{200}. In a few hours she was well, dressed, and behaved as when in good health.

The symptoms which controlled Dr. Guernsey's choice of Hyoscyamus are the following:

(445.) He makes himself naked.

He lies in bed nude and chatters. He walks about insane, naked, wrapped in a skin during the summer heat, etc., and others to the same purport.

In convulsive affections of the pharynx, which interfere with or prevent deglutition, the symptoms would lead us to infer the usefulness of Hyoscyamus; and Hahnemann speaks confidently of its power to cure hydrophobia, the symptoms otherwise corresponding.

In affections of the eye, involving the special sense alone, Hyoscyamus may be a valuable remedy, as the symptoms show.

As regards the digestive apparatus, it will have been observed that Hyoscyamus produces a kind of diarrhœa. This is characterized by involuntary evacuations during the sleep at night, apparently from inertia of the sphincter ani. This must not be confounded with the involuntary defecation which attends the blood dyscrasia in typhus, etc. It is a paralysis of the sphincter.

Dr. Wurmb says : "Hyoscyamus is indicated in those fever cases in which torpor of the entire organism predominates. The patients have a dull, fixed expression of face, delirium is lacking, or if present, it consists of a confused farrago of complex images; the perceptive faculty is almost suspended."

The cough of Hyoscyamus has been described. It is a very useful remedy.

For sleeplessness or dozing with the brain full of figures and bewildering images, Hyoscyamus is a very valuable remedy if other symptoms correspond.

DATURA STRAMONIUM.

THORN APPLE OR JAMESTOWN WEED.

INDIGENOUS in the United States and Europe. So common in our waste places about the cities that cases of poisoning with it are by no means uncommon.

Goats eat the leaves with impunity. Cows, if affected by it, are not easily affected. But after eating it, their milk has proved poisonous to children.

This drug, the action of which resembles very closely in many particulars that of Belladonna, was brought into prominent notice as a remedy by Stoerck, of Vienna, who advised its internal use in mania and epilepsy.

"If," says he, "Stramonium produces symptoms of madness in a healthy person, would it not be desirable to make experiments in order to discover whether this plant, by its effects on the brain, in changing the ideas and the state of the sensorium (*i. e.*, of the part, whatever it be, which is the center of action of the nerves upon the the body), should we not, I say, try whether this plant would not restore to a healthy state those who are suffering from alienation of mind; and if, by the change which Stramonium would cause in those who suffer from convulsions, by putting them in a contrary state to that in which they were, would it not cause their cure?" This was written in 1762.

By allopathic physicians it has been successfully employed against epliepsy in Stockholm, and by both allopathic and homœopathic physicians against mania.

The following general summary of its effects is taken chiefly from Trousseau and Pidoux :

"In moderate doses, Stramonium produces slight vertigo and a disposition to sleep; the muscular energy is lessened; the sensibility is blunted; dilatation of the pupil; slight obscuration of vision ; acceleration of pulse; elevation of the heat of the skin; thirst; a slight burning in the fauces. Generally the bowels are relaxed ; the urine is more abundant than common; there is copious perspiration, provided there be neither diuresis nor diarrhœa.

"But, in larger doses, vertigo, general debility; some degree of stupor; soon the vision becomes obscured; there is enormous dilatation of the pupils, agitation, spasms, furious delirium, continual hallucinations, obstinate insomnia, high fever ; the skin is hot, dry and often covered with an eruption closely resembling that of scarlatina, burning thrist, and very painful dryness and constriction of the pharynx; often impossible to swallow; cardialgia;

vomitings; sometimes diarrhœa; frequent desire to pass water, with but little or no urine.

"When the poisoning is to prove fatal, the extreme agitation is succeeded by collapse, clodness and death. In the more happy and more frequent cases, the hallucinations cease little by little, delirium comes to an end, and of this whole collection of formidable symptoms there remain only the dilatation of the pupils, the obscuration of vision, and sometimes a transient blindness. The delirium and the blindness, however, have been known to persist for several days, and even for weeks.

"The delirium is sometimes gay, sometimes sad, but is always accompanied by singular hallucinations and fantastic visions."

Our more exact knowledge of the effects of Stramonium is derived from Hahnemann's proving of it. ("Materia Medica Pura," vol. iii.)

Upon the vital force Stramonium exerts a very powerful and characteristic action.

1. The sensorium is both exalted in activity, as the vigilance shows; and perverted in its functions, as we gather from the mania, the hallucination and the fantastic visions which universally result from it.

The special sense of vision is perverted, as witness the double vision and the peculiar false vision, as well as the colors seen by the patient; and it is blunted, blindness resulting.

The general sensibility is blunted; the function of voluntary motion is affected; convulsive motions of the extremities ensue, particularly of the arms and of the face. Isolated groups of muscles are convulse.

The function of the secreting surfaces of various organs is suspended. The secretion of urine is suspended, and so is that from the surface of the intestine, by large doses.

2. On the other hand, the organic substance is hardly affected, save in the eruption which covers the skin, and in the greenish diarrhœa which sometimes follows a small dose.

3. There is no marked periodicity of action.

4. The peculiarities of the action of Stramonium are the followinge : The mania and delirium are not attended or followed by high fever; the hallucinations are real as in the second stage of delirium tremens ; the convulsions affect the arms more than the lower extremities; and consist in a trembling and convulsive groping forward with the hands; finally, the peculiar false and double vision in which the patient, looking at an object, sees it repeated a little above and at the left side of the original, or in which only a small part of an object is to be seen at once, as for example the nose on a person's face, etc.

The suppression of urine is a noteworthy symptom.

The convulsions are often provoked by looking at a light, or upon a reflecting surface as a mirror or water, and also by contact.

The limbs feel as if separated joint from joint.

The vertigo of Stramonium resembles that of Belladonna, and makes the gait unsteady.

No special headache is ascribed to it. Considerable congestion of blood to the head is produced, with heat and spasmodic drawing of the head hither and thither.

The face is generally swollen, has at first a pleasant expression, except for the fixed stare of the eyes; subsequently the face becomes distorted.

Vision is much affected, colors are not correctly distinguished. Black objects generally appear gray, everything seems to be tipping over; the letters on a printed page seem to move, or they and other objects appear double. There seems to be a fog before the eyes, or it seems as if one looked through a glass of turbid water. Sometimes absolute blindness ensues. The pupils are enormously dilated. The eyes are sometimes red, and there is involuntary discharge of tears. No organic lesions.

The mouth and throat are very dry, although the tongue is moist. Violent thirst but inability to swallow, because the throat seems to be constricted. The vocal organs seem to be paralyzed, the tongue trembles, the patient stammers and murmurs unintelligibly; or is absolutely dumb, and indicates with signs the objects of his desire; or, if he speaks, his voice is shrill, fine and high-pitched, but he has to make great effort to get out a word.

Notice that this is without fever, without swelling or any pain within or without the throat. There is here, then, no laryngitis, but simply a convulsion of the laryngeal muscles and vocal chords.

The taste is bitter; vomiting of green bile occurs on motion, or, even on sitting up in bed.

Great anxiety in the epigastric region. The abdomen is distended, with rumbling and gurgling in it, and painful to pressure.

As a rule, the evacuations are suppressed, but we find urgency to stool yet no stool. Urine is suppressed; yet there is urgency to pass water.

The menses are increased. The flow occurs in large coagula, with drawing pain in the addomen, in the ilium and other parts.

With regard to the respiratory organs, we find no cough as by Hyoscyamus and Belladonna, but respiration is difficult and constricted, generally with anxious respiration and lividity of the face. A pressing pain in the chest, which is provoked by talking with difficult respiration; it is hardly possible to draw in the breath. These symptoms are of great interest in connection with the empirical use of Stramonium in asthma.

In the trunk and extremities hardly any symptoms are observed, save the convulsive movements, sense of lassitude in the back and drawing pains in the spine, the sacrum and the ilium.

The sleep is either solid and sound and deep. with loud snoring, the patient lying on the back, with the eyes fixed and open; or else it is light, with troublesome dreams and disturbed by startings, cryings and wakings.

The fever is moderate. The chill, if it occur, is general with twitching of single groups of muscles. Heat is chiefly in the face, or, if it be general, it is characteristic that, during it, the patient carefully covers himself up. (Ignatia.) Sweat copious.

The disposition resembles a genuine mania, distinguished by loquacity, hallucinations and ridiculous attitudes and gestures; the hallucinations completely possess the patient.

But sometimes this mania amounts to absolute rage, with disposition to strike and bite, and alternating with convulsions.

PRACTICAL APPLICATIONS.

Remarks on practical applications of Stramonium may best be prefaced by the following remarks from Hahnemann's introduction :

"During its primary action, Stramonium produces no pain, properly so called, though it does cause very unpleasant sensations.

"The primary effect is to increase the activity of the voluntary muscles, and to suppress all the secretions, a state exactly contrary to the secondary effect which paralyzes the muscles and in which the excretions are superabundant. For the same reason, when taken in a proper dose, it soothes spasmodic muscular action, and restores the course of the suppressed excretions in many cases

DATURA STRAMONIUM. 295

where absence of pain predominates; this plant, therefore, can only cure homœopathically when the morbid state corresponds with its own primary effect.

"But, and here I speak from experience, what incomparative curative power has not the homœopathic application of the mental derangement excited specially by Stramonium exerted in analogous mental diseases arising from other causes; and how salutary is this plant in convulsive affections similar to those which it provokes. I have found great benefit from it in certain epidemic fevers having symptoms analogous mentally and physically to its own.

But, as mania shows various modifications, so we cannot always obtain a cure for it by one remedy. In certain cases we must have recourse to Belladonna, in others to Henbane, in others to Stramonium, according as the symptoms correspond homœopathically with one or the other of these three drugs.

"Moderate doses only keep up their action thirty-six to forty-eight hours; weaker doses a still shorter time."

In mania, Stramonium is a most valuable remedy. The form which requires it has less fever than that of Belladonna; more convulsion, and especially convulsion of isolated groups of muscles; more hallucination. It has more fever than that of Hyoscyamus, less loquacity, on quarrelsomeness, but on the contrary, good nature; the hallucinations are real, not, as under Hyoscyamus, half real, bewildering the patient.

Convulsions. Stramonium has been found useful in epliepsy as well as in other forms of spasmodic disease. It is remarkable, however, that the convulsions produced by it are partial, rather than general, affecting the arms rather than the lower extremities; affecting, also, isolated groups of muscles. Thus, we have twitchings of the extremities and of the facial muscles, jerkings of the head, etc.

From these symptoms we should be inclined to draw an indication for the use of Stramonium in chorea; and it has been found the most useful drug in the materia medica in this malady.

It should be noted, however, that chorea being almost always (at least in my experience) associated with, if not based upon, a depraved and vitiated state of the nutrition involving changes of organic substance, no such remedy as Stramonium, which does not modify nutrition nor alter the organic substance, can be relied upon as the sole or even the chief remedy; I have, accordingly, though finding Stramonium very useful to moderate the severity of the purely nervous phenomena, been obliged to trust to such remedies, alterative in their character, as Calcarea carbonica, Natrum muriaticum and Sepia, or Sulphur, for a permanent cure.

In delirium tremens, it is easy to see that Stramonium would be clearly indicated in the second stage too. It has been tried and with admirable success.

The spasmodic affection of the pharynx, and the fact that the various convulsive affections are brought on by the sight of water, etc., suggest the use of Stramonium in hydrophobia. Hahnemann affirms that it has been successfully used in some forms of the disease.

Stramonium has been of greatest service in suppression of the urine, without pain or discomfort, such suppression usually occurring in the course of long fevers, *e. g.*, typhoid or typhus, not a simple retention of urine in the bladder; in such a case Opium would do better.

Likewise in suppression of urine after miscarriage or after labor, where the desire to pass water is great but there is no ability to accomplish it, Stramonium will give speedy relief, provided always the case be not one of retention from a mechanical cause, such as retroversion of the uterus.

In affections of the respiratory organs, Stramonium has acquired a great reputation for the relief of asthma. It was used as follows: The dried leaves were smoked in a pipe, sometimes alone and sometimes with niter; giving often relief but sometimes causing damage.

In scarlatina, Stramonium stands next to Belladonna. The eruption is generally reported as being very like scarlatina. The fever is less than that of Belladonna. The throat affection is less than that of Belladonna. At the same time, from the suppression of urine, we may infer that Stramonium affects the kidneys more than Belladonna. It is thought that Stramonium suits now a larger class than heretofore. (See the article of Dr. Wells on scarlet fever, "American Homœopathic Review," vols. iv., v. and vi.)

The following case of poisoning from the application of Stramonium leaves to an ulcer came under my own observation:

A mechanic, about forty-four years old, whose health had suffered greatly in consequence of a severe bilious remittent fever and the heroic doses of calomel prescribed for its cure, had been under my care several weeks for large irritable ulcers upon both legs. I was called in haste, early one morning, and was informed that my patient was "not right in his mind."

I found him dressed and lying on a lounge. He recognized me and immediately apologized for not rising, stating that his limbs were not under his control; and, in fact, I found afterward that they were paralyzed. His face was covered with patches of an irregular shape, not elevated above the rest of the skin and of a brilliant fiery red color. The conjunctiva was injected, the pupils immensely dilated; the whole expression of the eye was brilliant, restless, suspicious and roving. The brow was corrugated. The appearance of the patient suggested mania and I might have at once pronounced it a case of delirium tremens, had I not well known the temperate habits of my patient.

The tongue was moist, the papillæ enlarged and projecting through a soft white fur. The limbs were motionless. The arms on the contrary were constantly reaching forward and upward with an uncertain tremulous motion, as if the patient were endeavoring to seize some object which he indistinctly perceived in the air. As I sat observing him, he suddenly turned toward the wall, exclaiming, "There are those bugs! help me to catch them!" "What bugs?" I asked. "There," he replied, "a long train of bed-bugs, and after them a procession of beetles, and here comes crawling over me a host of cockroaches." He shrank back in much alarm. Then suddenly he turned to me, saying, "I believe I know they are not really bugs; but, except once in a while, they seem real to me!" This scene was many times repeated. For some time I was at a loss to account for the condition of my patient. At length the peculiar, almost convulsive, motions of his upper extremities while the lower extremities were nearly paralyzed, together with the aspect of the face and the mental condition suggested Stramonium to my mind. His family knew nothing of his having used it, but when he heard me mention the name, be pointed to his legs, where, on examination, I found a quantity of the bruised green leaves which he had applied to the ulcers, it seems, the night before, in the hope of relieving pain.

The poisoning not being very serious, I contented myself with removing the leaves and allowing the effects of the poison to pass away without administering any antidote.

The mental symptoms produced in this case by the Stramonium so closely resembled those of the second stage of delirium tremens, as to point strongly to Stramonium as a valuable remedy in that disease.[1]

---

[1] See a case of poisoning by Stramonium, recorded by Dr. Meigs, in the "North American Medical and Surgical Journal," January, 1827. Also, "Frank's Magazine," vol. ii., p. 230. Case of poisoning from eating Stramonium seeds. Also, poisoning by Stramonium seeds, narrated by Dr. Johnson, "American Medical Times," i., 22, 1860.

OPIUM.

INSPISSATED juice of the *Papaver somniferum*. We derive it from Turkey and from India; it is also made in France. It has been used from early ages. In most countries now, it affords a disreputable but very common means of indulging in intoxication.

No drug is so universally used in the old school of medicine. The great Hufeland affirmed that if he had to choose one remedy from the materia medica for exclusive use it should be Opium. Its extensive use among allopathists follows from these facts. The old school has few specifics, and these are but seldom used. Most diseases being attended with pain, the pain must be either subdued by acting specifically upon the cause of pain, or else the pain must be believed by a palliative anodyne, while the disease is sought to be cured by the use of revulsive agents addressed to other organs of the body than those which are the seat of disease. The latter is the mode almost universally employed. Hence the constant use of anodynes. For examples, in severe sclerotitis, the old school would use revulsive agents addressed to the bowels (purges) and to the skin (blisters); but, at the same time, to subdue the pain in the eye, a dose of Opium would be given.

Homœopathy does not do so. It gives a drug that acts specifically on the cause of disease and upon the organ diseased, and no other, and there is no need of an anodyne. These are the reason why Opium is so much used by allopaths and so little by homœopathicians.

Hahnemann's observations, though requiring some modifications perhaps in consequence of the wider experience of later years, are most instructive. "The primary result of weak and moderate doses, during whose action the organism is affected in a passive manner, appears to be to excite for a short time the irritability and activity of the muscles subject to its action, but also to diminish for a longer time that of the muscles which are not subjected to its influence; to excite the imagination and the courage, but also to deaden and stupefy the feelings, the sensibility and presence of mind. Under a longer continuance of its action the organism, by its power of reaction, produces a condition exactly the reverse,—a want of excitability and activity in the involuntary muscles, an absence of ideas, languor of imagination with timidity and over-sensibility of the general feeling. Certain symptoms are more palpable in some individuals than in others. No medicine relieves suffering sooner than Opium. It is this property that has induced physicians to employ it so largely—a source of innumerable evils. If the use of Opium in disease were as beneficial as it is frequent, no other medicine would make so many cures; but exactly the reverse takes place.

"The power of this medicine and its rapid action indicate that its effects should be thoroughly studied before using it.

"Now, as Opium has hitherto been but little used, excepting as an antipathic and a palliative, and its primary effects only have been opposed to diseases, no medicine has appeared so soothing or has so apparently suppressed morbid symptoms, although soon followed by results more distressing than the original disease. In short, nothing has caused more positive evil after apparent good.

"In all kinds of coughs, diarrhœas, vomiting, sleeplessness, melancholy, spasms, nervous affections, and, above all, in severe pain, Opium is indiscriminately given, on the ground that it is the best remedy in such cases. But its innumerable evil results do not appear among the primitive effects of Opium, which are precisely the reverse.

"Therefore, we may easily imagine how few salutary and enduring effects can be obtained in the greater number of morbid and physical affections; and this is proved by daily experience.

"If Opium has been found to cure cough, diarrhœa, sickness, spasms, etc., etc., in a few cases, it is only when these symptoms first show themselves in persons previously in good health and are but slight. Opium will sometimes restore the patient quickly to health, because, if these symptoms are at once destroyed, the body is restored to its former condition, and the tendency to their return is suppressed.

"But, because this palliative action on slight and recent cases succeeds in a few instances, it does not follow that Opium really possesses the power of curing them permanently in all cases.

"It cannot convert them into sound health because they are symptoms of other diseases with which Opium does not coincide homœopathically. For this reason it has seldom been used without injury to the patient in long-standing coughs, continued diarrhœas, habitual wakefulness, chronic sickness, spasms, anxiety and tremors, when they have been for some time establishd.

"In administering Opium for these complains, we see that it is on the principle of soothing, procuring a temporary suspension of suffering; that subsequently it will relieve only by increasing the dose, which even then becomes less effective and at the same time creates new disease,—an artificial malady, still more serious and distressing than the first.

"But it is yet more striking to observe that up to the present time the use of Opium has been abused by giving it in all kinds of pains, however deep seated and of however long standing. It shocks our understanding and seems like returning to the absurd idea of a universal medicine, to expect from it the cure of diseases totally different to each other.

"All pains soothed for the moment by Opium return after a short time, when the stupefying effect is past, and very often are still more intense than before; so that at last they will only yield to stronger and larger doses, which create in return other serious diseases new to the sufferer. The use of Opium in confirmed pain is therefore empirical and deceptive to the patient, leading him to attribute to other diseases the mischievous consequences that are due to it alone.

"By treating all pains antipathically by Opium, we have seen the use of this drug bring on a train of evil consequences,—stupor, constipation, and other serious symptoms which appertain to Opium, and without which it would not be what it is. But persons have deceived themselves as to the character of these inevitable effects. Instead of perceiving in them results inherent in the nature of Opium, they have considered them as derived from some accessory properties which they have taken unwearied pains to separate from it. Hence the various correctives that have been tried for two thousand years, in the hope of soothing spasms and pains, without bringing on delirium or constipation; of suppressing vomiting or diarrhœa without causing stupor; of procuring sleep without heat, headache, tremors, languor, depression, and extreme sensitiveness to cold.

"But all this is fallacious. By all these means Opium is only rendered less active, without changing its nature."

By a series of arguments and illustrations of this character, Hahnemann shows that the almost universal use of Opium is a resort to a temporary palliative of suffering, not to a specific for the cause of that suffering, whatever that cause may be. Whereas Opium can only be used with propriety in those diseases for which the correspondence of its symptoms shows it may be a specific remedy. These are very few in number. Hence homœopathists make infrequent use of Opium.

Instead of an elaborate analysis of the Opium symptoms, I shall call attention only to a few of the infrequent applications of Opium, viz.:

In apoplexy; constipation; lead colic; wakefulness.

Apoplexy. The following description of the effect of a large dose of Opium is taken from Stillé and Beck:

"The head feels full and hot and sometimes light, there are buzzing noises in the ears, the face and eyes are injected, while the pupil is more or less contracted. Flashes of light are apt to appear before the eyes; the ideas are confused and extravagant, and sometimes there is delirium; the pulse is fuller and more frequent; the skin is hot, the mouth and fauces dry; generally there is nausea and, in some cases, vomiting. To these symptoms depression succeeds. The pulse beats more slowly and often irregularly; the head feels heavy and full, and all the senses lose their acuteness; the countenance assumes a stolid, stupid, besotted expression, produced by the turgidness of the features, the dullness of the eyes and the drooping of their lids; there is a strong indisposition to think or move, or, more properly, an inability to make any exertion, either of mind or body; the speech is thick and hesitating; the muscles of the limbs are affected with spasmodic movements, and, if the patient attempt to walk, he feels dizzy and oppressed, and staggers like a drunken man.

"An irresistible propensity to sleep follows these symptoms, and when yielded to, the breathing becomes laborious and often stertorous, while the general surface of the body grows pale and damp, and the hands and feet cold. The effects of still larger doses are similar, though more decided and not preceded by a period of excitement. They are giddiness, insensibility and immobility, respiration hardly perceptible, and a small, feeble pulse, which sometimes becomes full and slow. The eyes are shut, the pupils contracted, and the whole expression of the countenance is usually that of deep and perfect repose. As the effects increase, the lethargic state becomes more profound, deglutition is suspended, the breathing is occasionally stertorous, the pupils are insensible to light, the countenance is pale and cadaverous, and the muscles of the limbs and trunk are relaxed."

These same words might be used to describe one form of cerebral apoplexy.

"After death from Opium poisoning, the convolutions of the brain are found to be flattened, the vessels of the cerebro-spinal axis and its investing membranes are gorged with black blood, and the capillaries of the brain give out on incision minute drops of the same fluid. A serous liquid is usually met with in the ventricles of the brain and under the cerebral face of the arachnoid membrane."

Thus both the symptoms and the post-mortem appearances resemble those of one form of apoplexy, and it is not, therefore, surprising that Opium has been found a most valuable remedy in even apparently hopeless cases of this affection.

It would seem that we should hope more from it when the apoplexy had not been preceded by chronic symptoms of lesion in the substance of the encephalon, such as would indicate a destructive process (softening, for example) as going on for some time prior to the apoplectic stroke. In such cases we have undoubtedly a considerably coagulum in the brain substance, and the case would naturally be almost hopeless.

In several severe cases of cerebral apoplexy, with very profound coma, where Opium had entirely failed, Dr. J. Barker, of Brooklyn, has succeeded in effecting a cure with Apis. In his opinion, which is based on much experience with this remedy, Apis is a medicine of great importance in cerebral and spinal affections, whether they manifest themselves chiefly by coma or by spasms.

Constipation. Opium produces a suspension of the secretion from the mucous surfaces of the digestive canal, *e. g.,* the dry mouth and fauces. It probably, therefore, lessens the amount of excrement. It also paralyzes the intestine. These two actions combine to produce an obstinate constipation, an effect of Opium which is universally admitted, recognized, and, by allopaths, regretted. We are, however, enabled by it to cure certain analogous forms of severe constipation.

Most prominent among these is the constipation from paralysis of the intestine caused by lead, and known as a concomitant of "painter's colic."

Retention of Urine. It is doubtful whether Opium diminishes the secretion of urine, but it certainly does cause its retention in the bladder. This it does, perhaps, chiefly by blunting the sensibility of the lining membrane of the neck of the bladder, so that the fullness of the bladder is not recognized by the patient. It may also paralyze the longitudinal and circular muscular fibers of the bladder. Though the mass of the urine is retained and the bladder full, yet some urien may dribble away unknown to the patient.

This whole condition is very different from that produced by Stramonium, which produces suppression of urine, causing the kidneys to suspend their function.

In retention of urine, Opium is our best remedy.

It may occur in fever, in acute illness, or, frequently, after child-birth.

Do we never use Opium as a palliative in acute and very painful affections for which we have not found a specific remedy? I have twice thought it necessary to do so. On each occasion I regretted it. It did mischief. The patients, after a temporary relief, got worse, and then, after all, I found, by hard study, the proper remedy (as I ought to have done at first), and cured the cases, as I might and ought to have done in the beginning, without Opium, had I known enough.

In evidently incurable diseases when the patient is moribund, as in cancer, etc., Opium may perhaps be given, but even in such cases, though there be no hope of recovery, it should be sparingly used.

HELLEBORUS NIGER.

BLACK HELLEBORE—CHRISTMAS ROSE.

BEFORE passing from this group, I desire to say a few words upon this drug, of which we know but little,—that little being, however, very precious. It was used by the ancients in the treatment of insanity, of epilepsy and of dropsy. It is rarely used now by allopathists.

1. Its action on the vital force is well described by Hahnemann in a foot-note to the proving:

"I conclude, from various observations, that stupor, blunting of the general sensibility, a condition in which, with unimpaired vision, the patient, nevertheless, sees imperfectly and does not regard the objects he sees; with the apparatus of hearing intact yet hears nothing distinctly nor comprehends, with his organs of taste in working order, yet finds not the proper taste in anything; is always or often distraught, hardly remembers, if at all, the past or what has but just happened; has no pleasure in anything; slumbers but lightly, without a sound or refreshing sleep; undertakes to work without having power or strength to attend to his work,—these are characteristic primary effects of Hellebore."

2. On the organic substance it acts as a producer of watery accumulations in various parts of the body and general anasarca. The peculiarities of its action have been described. In addition, it produces a severe headache, similar to that of Belladonna, and of Silicea as follows:

Headache in occiput; dull pain; worse on stooping, from the nape of neck to the vertex, aggravated and changed to burning on rising to the erect posture.

The pain is so violent he knows not where or how to rest the head; he lays it every moment in a different position, at last finds it most tolerable when he compels himself to lie quiet and with closed eyes to half doze, and so forget his pain. Heat in the head, stupidity and heaviness, internal heat in the head, with coldness of the hands, etc.

The eyelids tremble and quiver; a sensation as if the eye were pressed shut or out from the eye and yet the vision is normal.

A bitter taste in the throat, increased after eating; nausea from the epigastrium, without ability to vomit, sometimes a feeling of nausea in the stomach, as if from hunger, but food is repulsive; pain in the epigastrium and in the region of the pylorus; every step is painful, increased by talking and by pressure, a sensation as if the epigastrium were drawn inward.

Heaviness in the abdomen; flatulence.

Stool. The stool is mostly diarrhœic, being slimy and jelly-like, and yet the evacuation requires some urging. A hard and scanty stool is attended by violent cutting pain in the rectum from below upward, as if it constricted over a cutting substance.

Frequent urgency to pass water and very scanty evacuation; or, as a secondary action, copious and easy discharge.

Respiratory Organs. Spasmodic sneezing from tickling in the nose; also a similar cough, with dyspnœa.

Back. A contracting pain in the loins, and a pain in the dorsal and cervical regions, as if beaten, and a stiffness.

Exterior. Tearing in the medulla of the bones and in the dorsa of the fingers, where it is combined with a kind of paralytic sensation; various drawing and pressing pains.

In the skin we see a general anasarca.

Sticking boring pains in the periosteum and other parts of the body, aggravated by cool air and by physical exertion.

The sleep is restless and full of confused dreams and of fantasies.

The fever is made up chiefly of chill, without thirst, and with painful sensibility of the head to touch and motion; with drawing tearing in the limbs and stitches in the joints.

The heat is chiefly in the head.

PRACTICAL APPLICATIONS.

Hellebore has been useful in general dropsy when accompanied by the stupor and general paralysis of sensibility, of which Hahnemann's description has been quoted.

Its most frequent use, however, has been in typhoid and nervous fevers characterized by a similar stupor, and in the second stage of acute meningitis or acute hydrocephalus, when the effusion has already taken place. Its use in these cases was first demonstrated by Dr. Wahle, of Rome.

Dr. Bähr, of Hanover, thus speaks of it: "In acute meningitis, Helleborus niger is one of our most important remedies when the exudation is regarded as accomplished. The exact time for its administration is when the reaction has become almost nothing, and the phenomena of paralysis have become more or less complete."

This indication again throws us back to Hahnemann's very comprehensive and terse characterization of the chief action of Hellebore, which comprises all that can be said of the remedy.

The fact that Hellebore produces anasarca, would suggest its use in post-scarlatinal dropsy; and Altschul speaks very highly of it in such cases, particularly when the general symptoms are those of stupor, etc., as they often are. If, on the country, the patient be restless, excited eand erethistic, although weak, Arsenic will be better indicated. Apis, also, has been found of great value.

In mania of a melancholy type, with fixed ideas, or in mania dæmonica, in which evil spirits are seen at night, Hellebore has been an approved remedy from the earliest ages.

SILICEA.

SYNONYMS: KIESELERDE, TERRA-SILICEA, ACIDUM SILICIUM.

THE proving of Silicea upon the healthy subject was published by Hahnemann in vol. iii. of the "Chronic Diseases," 1828. Additional symptoms are found in the "Materia Medica" of Hartlaub and Trinks, vol. iii., and a fragment by Wahle, in the "Archiv fur Homœopathische Heilkunst," xv., 2, 87. These are all incorporated in Hahnemann's essay in the second edition of "Chronic Diseases." A proving by Ruoff was published in "Hygea," viii. (1838), and one by Hencke in "Allg. Hom. Zeitung," 55, 17 (1857). A proving of Aqua Silicata, by Becker, was published in "Hygea," xxii. (1847), and a paper by Dr. Colby in "New England Medical Gazette" (1871).

In our study of Silicea we shall follow Hahnemann's essay in the second edition of "Chronic Diseases."

SPECIAL ANALYSIS.

1. *Head.* (*a.*) *Sensorium.* Confusion in the head; mental exertion is very difficulty; confusion in speaking; it is difficult to seize the right expres-

SILICEA. 317

sion; a brief conversation causes confusion of the head and general lassitude; memory is enfeebled; dullness in the head without pain, as if it were too full of blood.

Vertigo is a very prominent symptom. It occurs when the prover rises from the recumbent position or from stopping, or when sitting or walking. Also when looking upward. It seems to come from the dorsal region up through the nape of the neck into the head (as does the headache of Silicea). The vertigo makes the prover incline to fall forward or to the left, and is so severe that he fears he shall fall. It is aggravated by motion, and by looking upward and is accompanied by nausea.

(*b.*) *Headache.* The headache of Silicea is characteristic. Its location is for the most part in the forehead, extending often to the temples and involving the eyes, especially the right eye and temple. There is also a characteristic aching and pain, extending as if from the back up the nape of the neck through the occiput to the vertex. Many of the pains, especially the pressing, eaching pain, are described as affecting the whole head.

The pains are chiefly aching, pressing; also tearing and borineg; and heaviness and fullness, as though there were too much blood in the head.

The headache occurs after mental exertion or annoyance. It is decidedly aggravated by mental or bodily exertion, by quick movements of the head or body, which convert the dull aching pain into acute stabs; by noise and by light. It is relieved by quiet, darkness, lying down, and, which is characteristic of Silicea, by wrapping the head up warmly. This condition, relieved by warmth, we shall meet in other Silicea symptoms. It is to be remarked that the relief is not afforded by simple pressure, as with Menyanthes, but by warmth, *e.g.* by warm-water compresses. Indeed, the pressure of the hat increases the occipital headache.

The concomitants are pain in the eyes when the globes are revolved laterally in the orbits, chilliness and nausea and vomiting.

The similarity of this headache to that of Spigelia, Paris quadrifolia, Cocculus and Gelseminum, should be noted.

The Silicea headache is mostly on the right side. The scalp is sensitive to touch ; the hair falls out when combed; upon the scalp are itching pustules.

2. *Eyes.* In the orbits, pressure and soreness ; the eyes pain in the morning, as if they were full of sand and too dry; the lids quiver; they are agglutinated; they are spasmodically constricted, and can hardly be opened; there are symptoms of conjunctivities, with moderate lachrymation and muco-purulent discharge.

Itching in the eyes ; aching of the globe, with redness of the sclerotica.

Considerable photophobia in paroxysms; muscæ volitantes; objects confused before the eyes; throbbing in the ears; shakes the eyes so that objects move up and down.

SILICEA. 319

From the paroxysmal character of some of these symptoms, it would seem probable that most of the eye affections of Silicea are sympathetic.

3. *Ears.* Itching, aching, drawing, pinching pains in the external meatus. These pains sometimes occur, and often are aggravated, when blowing the nose or swallowing. The external ear is swollen, with discharge of fluid from the meatus, with hissing noise and deafness ; deafness ; noises of various kinds in the ears; hard and painful swelling of the parotid gland.

It would appear from these symptoms (as well as from clinical results) that Silicea corresponds to a catarrhal affection of the ear, both external and middle and of the Eustachian tube, producing deafness. There is also exalted sense of hearing, probably sympathetic, with headache.

4. *Nose.* Tenderness of the septum marium and of the end of the nose. Pressure and aching at root of nose. Drawing pain in root of nose, and zygoma. Throbbing in nostrils, extending into the brain, with throbbing headache in the forehead. Fluent coryza, acrid watery discharge. Discharge of bloody mucus. Epistaxis. Dryness in the choanæ. Morsels of food lodge in the choanæ on swallowing. The sense of smell is unnaturally keen.

5. *Face.* The cheeks, lips and chin are affected. The complexion is pale, as after a long sickness. From time to time white spots appear upon the cheek. In the malar bones and behind the ears

and in the temporo-maxillary articulation, pairs of a drawing, tearing character, aggravated by motion and by touch. Painful constricting spasms in temporo-maxillary articulation, and then in the temple. Itching and papular eruption on the forehead and nose, cheeks and lips, painful when touched.

6. *Lips.* Vesicular eruption on the margin of the lips, smarting when touched, and very painful. The corners of the mouth are ulcerated. The submaxillary glands are swollen and painful to touch and on swallowing.

7. *Gums and Teeth.* Gums swollen, sensitive and ulcerated. Vesicles on the gums. Dental ulcers, painful from contact of cold water. Toothache, shooting and soreness, chiefly in carious teeth, worse at night, aggravated always by cold air and water, sometimes also by very hot food, as well as by cold, accompanied by sore gums, heat in head and bruning cheeks.

8. *Mouth.* The mouth and lips are dry (primary, 30 hours); much saliva (secondary, 8 days).

9. *Taste.* Bitter, foul bloody, sour.

10. *Tongue.* Sensations as if a hair lay on the tongue. Tongue sore at the tip, coated and numb. The right half is swollen.

11. *Throat.* In the hard palate and in the velum, itching and stitches, Uvula swollen and elongated.

Itching at orifice of Eustachian tube, with hoarseness and dry throat. Sticking pain in the throat, only when swallowing the throat being painful when touched; sore throat as though a lump were on the left side of the throat.

12. *Œsophagus.* Difficult deglutition; the food passes slowly into the stomach.

13. *Stomach.* Sensations of weight and pressure in the stomach. Pinching and griping pains. Gnawing sensation, relieved by lying with the limbs drawn up. Most of these sensations and many other symptoms come on or are worse after eating, are increased by walking, and are accompanied by flatulence.

(*a*) *Appetite.* Unnatural hunger, especially toward evening, but no real appetite; the food will not go down; after eating a small quantity, nausea; also a sensation of weakness in the stomach. After eating, eructations, tasteless, also acid; feeling as of a stone in the stomach; also vertigo without nausea; also deafness, chilliness, palpitation, sweat of the face, sleepiness, heartburn, hiccough. Aversion to meat.

(*b.*) *Thirst.* Increased.

14. *Hypochondria.* Across the stomach and hypochondria griping and pinching pain in paroxysms for weeks. Drawing and pinching pain extending to hip-joints. Drawing and pinching pain extending from the hypochondria to the spinal column.

(*a.*) *Right Hypochondrium.* Continued pressure, stitches, pain posteriorly (near the region).

(*b.*) *Left Hypochondrium.* Pain as if something would tear away.

15. *Abdomen.* Abdomen distended and hard; not much flatulence. Tearing griping and cutting pains, affecting chiefly the umbilical region, occurring or worse when walking, relieved by applying Warm cloths. Pain in the inguinal region, as though a hernia would protrude. The inguinal glands are swollen and painful. Much offensive flatus.

16. *Stool.* Constipation, will desire for stool. Sensation as though fæces remained in the rectum, which has not power to expel them. When, after much violent effort of the abdominal muscles, fæces have been nearly expelled, they suddenly recede into the rectum. This symptom has often been varified in practice. Silicea produces likewise diarrhœa. Stools are pappy with mucus, like particles of membrane; or are fluid, scanty and putrid-smelling, and are attended by a biting, burning sensation in the anus; or they cansist only of bloody mucus, with burning and biting at the anus. Frequent desire for stool, with chilliness and nausea.

After stool, burning in anus; pressure in head; constriction of chest; relief of colic, and great exhaustion; he falls into a slumber from which colic wakes him.

17. *Anus and Rectum.* Stitching, cutting and burning in rectum and anus. Stitches towards the genital organs. Moisture of the anus. Hæmorrhoidal tumors protrude with stool, return with difficulty, and discharge bloody mucus. They are

very painful (sticking) and tender. Spasmodic, boring pain from anus up into the rectum and to the testes.

18. *Urinary Organs.* (*a.*) *Bladder.* Pressure upon the bladder while urinating; burning after it.

(*b.*) *Urethra.* Smarting and burning while urinating. Fine stitches continually in anterior part.

(*c.*) *Urine.* Scanty, with yellow or red sandy deposit.

(*d.*) *Micturition.* Frequent desire; constant desire, with discharge by drops and burning in the urethra; need to urinate frequently, every quarter of an hour; must get up almost every night to urinate.

Accompanied by burning and smarting in urethra; accompanied by itching in the pudenda.

19. *Genital Organs.* Male. (*a.*) *Pains.* Pressure from the prostate forward prepuce swollen, with itching and moist eruption externally; redness near the corona, as if abraded, with itching.

(*b.*) *Testes.* Pain in the right, as if indurated; pain at night, but only when lying.

Hydrocele (reported by Wahle). Sweat and itching of scrotum; itching and moist eruption on scrotum; aching in spermatic cord, the testes hanging lax.

(*c.*) *Special Function.* Frequent erections; sexual desire enfeebled ; frequent nocturnal emissions; great prostration after coitus.

Discharge of prostatic fluid, with a difficult stool, or at every stools.

20. *Genital Organs. Female.* (*a.*) *Vulva* Itching, with watery leucorrhœa.

(*b.*) *Vagina.* Sensation like labour pains; leucorrhea copious, watery, with violent itching of the vulva, or following a pinching pain around umbilicus on micturition; bloody mucus immediately after menstruation.

(*c.*) Menses first anticipate, then are increased in quantity. The secretion has a strong odor, preceded by a strong pressure and a compressed feeling over the eyes as of a weight, and by constipation.

At the commencement of menstruation, paroxysms of icy coldness of the whole body. During the menses cold feet, melancholy, anguish in epigastrium; drawing between scapulæ, only at night, relieved by bending backward; strong burning and soreness of the pudenda, with eruptions on the inside of the things.

After the menses, immediately a discharge of bloody mucus from the vagina.

21. *Respiratory Organs.* (*a.*) *Nasal Mucous Membrane.* Frequent sneezing, which causes bursting pain in chest; nose obstructed, cannot speak or breathe through it; fluent coryzx; coryza sometimes dry, sometimes fluent, but persistent. This and the cough are accompanied by swelling of the sub-maxillary gland, sore throat on swallowing, great chilliness, compelling to lie down; then, after an hour in bed, great burning heat.

(*b*) *Larynx and Trachea.* Hoarseness; roughness and dryness in the throat, with irritation, inducing cough after lunch.

Sore feeling in top of larynx.

Tickling itching in the region of the supra-sternal fossa, which threatens suffocation, until a deep shattering cough comes on, which lasts several hours, and produces pain in abdomen and throat.

(c.) *Cough.* Deep, exhausting; at first dry, then loose, with abundant purulent expectoration, provoked by tickling in the throat and supra-sternal fossa; by a sensation as if a hair lay from tip of tongue to the trachea and produced a tickling, compelling to cough, hack and scrape; by tickling in larynx at night; excited by cold drinks (Rhus), by every act of speaking; by lying down at night; occurring chiefly at evening, and at night when lying.

Accompanied by pain in thorax and sternum; rawness of chest and throat; vomiting of mucus; pain in epigastrium.

(d.) *Sputa.* Abundant transparent mucus; matter which sinks in water; yellowish green, offensive masses; thick masses of pus; bloody mucus or pure blood.

(e.) *Thorax.* Pressing pain, stitches; general sensation of weakness in chest; weakness when speaking; has to use the whole chest to utter his words.

Induration in left mamma.

(f.) *Respiration.* Deep sighing; dyspnœa; better after eating,

2. *Heart.* Palpitation when sitting quietly.

23. *Back.* Coccyx pains, as after long riding in a wagon; sacral pain on standing up; aching and tension and violent stitch.

Stiffness and pain in the dorsal region; tearing or aching with chill, finally passing into a dull headache; rending pain between scapulæ; drawing pain in scapulæ in paroxysms. Then it goes into nape of neck and head, where it becomes a vertigo, so that he feels as if he should fall.

Pain and burning in scapulæ.

In nape of neck, stiffness, causing headache; stiffness of one side of neck, preventing turning the head; swelling of cervical glands; eruption, like nettle-rash, in the nape of the neck.

Swelling of thyroid body.

24. *Extremities. Upper.* Pressing pain in the shoulder, extending to the hand, with the feeling as if one could not lift a heavy weight; also at night in the shoulder, extending to the elbow, aggravated by uncovering, relieved by warm wrappings; drawing soreness in the axillary glands, in the hands and fingers; jerking pains in shoulders and arms; sticking in the fingers, as if from splinters of wood; the arms and hands are heavy, and feel paralyzed; tonic spasm of the hand when writing.

25. *Lower.* Similar sensations to those described in the upper extremities. Pains and stitches under the great toe-nails, very severe; sweat of the feet, especially of the soles and between the toes, which become abraded and sore from walking; very offensive smell of the feet, without sweat;

the limbs and feet feel very tired, and as if paralyzed; painful tonic spasm in the feet and toes during a long walk.

26. *Sleep.* The prover is wakeful in the evening, by reason of thronging thoughts; the sleep is either frequently interrupted by frightened waking, or disturbed by dreams and fantasies; at night the circulation is excited, with throbbing in all the vessels and a jerking of the whole body; burning in the stomach, with nausea and vomiting of food, and flatulence; anguish and restlessness; sleep-walking; nightmare.

27. Fever in a definite form is not produced by Silicea. Some chilliness, especially after lying down at night, and heat during the night, with thirst; copious sweat at night, especially toward morning.

28. *Skin.* In many places itching or burning itching. Itching eruption, papular or vesicular, upon the chest, thighs and back. The skin is sensitive and irritable, and the whole body is painful as if beaten. Abrasions readily take on the suppurative process.

In ulcers already existing there are boring or aching, stitching pains, with abundant formation of pus.

29. *Mind.* The faculties are depressed, and memory weakened.

30. *Disposition.* Anxiety and restlessness, such as follow fright; preevishness and angry irritation; ill humor and contrariety, with disgust of life.

GENERAL ANALYSIS.

1. *Vital Power.* Silicea manifests but little distinct action upon the vital powers. The sensorium is somewhat depressed in its activity. The special senses of sight, hearing and smell are exalted in connection with the headache hereafter to be described, but no perversions of sense are recorded. The peculiar pains affecting the head, nape of neck and the eyes, show a definite field of action. The muscular system exhibits only a moderate degree of depression. The sphincters are not affected.

2. *Organic Substance.* On the other hand, the organic substance of the body is profoundly and variously affected. The mucous membrane of the large intestine and of the nares, pharynx and respiratory tract generally is affected, secretions being increased, and so modified in respect of, at least, the respiratory tract, as to resemble pus. Pustular eruptions appear on the skin, abrasions readily take on suppurative action, and ulcers already existing increase in size and activity, and become the seat of stitching, borning pains. Clinical experience abundantly confirms these deductions.

3. *Sphere of Action.* The head, orbit, eyes, and at least the upper part of the spinal cord; the nasal and pharyngeal mucous membrane, including the Eustachian tube and the middle ear; the large intestine, the bronchial mucous membrane and the genital organs, the skin and the lymphatic glands.

appear to comprise the sphere of action of this remedy.

4. The sensations which it produces are in the head and eyes, pressing, shooting and tearing; in the limbs, a paralytic weakness; in the skin, itching and burning itching; and in ulcers, a sticking and burning pain.

5. *Periodicity.* Not marked.

6. *Peculiarities.* It at once appears on reading the pathogenesis of Silicea that the symptoms, with hardly an exception, are aggravated by cold and decidedly ameliorated by warmth. This is noticed of the headache, which is relieved by wrapping the head eup warmly, not by the pressure of envelopes, as is the case with Menyanthes, Veratrum and some other drugs, but by the warmth. It is true, also, of the abdominal pains, which are relieved by warmth; of the cough, which (like that of Rhus) is provoked by cold drinks and relieved by warm ones; and of the shoulder pains, which come on at night when the shoulders are uncovered, and are relieved by covering (in contradistinction to Ledum, the pains of which, at night, compel the throwing off of the bed covering). The only apparent exception to this statement is found in the aversion to warm food; the prover can tolerate only cold food.

7. *Characteristic.* The characteristics of Silicea are summed up as follows by Bœnninghausen:

"Profuse sweat of the head, the body being dry, or nearly so. (Rhus toxicodendron has sweat of the body, except the head.) Desponding disposition, sensibility of the pericranium; headache, relieved by warmth; pale, earthy complexion; disgust for meat and for warm food; abdominal pains, relieved by warmth; much sneezing, with acrid coryza; going to sleep of that part of the body on which one lies; unhealthy state of skin; many ulcers form; sleeplessness, on account of orgasm of blood; quickened pulse; chilliness, even by every movement."

PRACTICAL APPLICATIONS.

From the very year that its proving was published, Silicea has taken high rank as a remedy for cases involving profuse suppuration, causing abscesses to come speedily to maturity and moderating the secretion of pus. In this regard, and as a remedy for "simple ulcer," ·it has a brilliant clinical record. It seems to be equally applicable whether the suppurative process be set up in the cellular or muscular tissue, in a gland or in a joint. In fistula lachrymalis, Silicea has not infrequently been beneficial, sometimes completely curing. It compares with Natrum muriaticum and Petroleum in this respect. It has gained a high reputation for the arrest and cure of withlow, as well as for the affection of the matrix of the nail, popularly called "ingrowing toe-nail," and to cure which the toe-nail is so often unnecessarily torn out. When Silicea fails in these cases, Graphites often succeeds.

Silicea is a most valuable and efficient remedy

in caries in and periostitis. It is related in these respects to Asafœtida, Graphites and Conium maculatum, and to Platinic chloride, which I have used successfully in two cases of caries of the tarsus, and for a knowledge of which I am indebted to Dr. Wm. S. Searle, of Brooklyn, N. Y. Its value in affections of the bones would naturally suggest its use in rachitis in children, in which the symptoms of "sweating in the head only," and tenderness of the surface of the body, indicate its homœopathicity. (Hughes.) It has been recommended from experience as a valuable remedy in *tabes dorsalis,* though not so well indicated, I should think, as Alumina or Ruta. Where a remedy is so decidedly indicated, and has proved so successful in certain defined morbid processes of a chronic nature, such as suppuration and rachitic dyscrasia, there is danger of our overlooking its applicability to more acute and transitory functional diseases; we are likely to have a too limited estimate of its powers to help the sick.

The headache produced by Silicea is so characteristic and well defined, and, withal, corresponds to a form so frequently met with, that it is one of the remedies most frequently employed by me for headache. The pain involves the occiput, nape of the neck, vertex and the eyes, or generally the right eye. It is a sticking or a tearing pressing pain, generally beginning in the neck and shoulders and going upward to the occiput and vertex, and extending through the head to the right eye.

Its conditions are characteristic, for it is much aggravated by motion, noise or light, the senses of sight and hearing being unnaturally acute. The patient prefers to lie down in a dark, quiet room. It is relieved by warm applications to the head. When most violent, it is accompanied by nausea and vomiting, and it passes away during sleep. The face is pale. In its conditions of aggravation this headache resembles that of Spigelia, but the latter affects the left eye and temple rather than the right, and is not relieved by warmth; but it is mitigated by pressure, and the pain does not come from the neck and shoulders.

The headache of Paris quadrifolia (a valuable remedy in headache) has some resemblance to that of Silicea. The sensation is, however, a kind of tightness, as if the cerebral membranes were on the stretch, with pressure on the temples and a very painful feeling, as though a cord were stretched tightly from the back of the eyeballs to the center of the brain. This headache is aggravated by thinking and relieved by pressure. The eyeballs feel too large for the orbits.

The headache of Menyanthes is a pressure from above downward; or, in the forehead, from without inward; or, in the temples, a lateral inward pressure, with pressure in the eyeballs. It is relieved by compression of the head, but neither this nor the other remedies except Silicea has mitigation by warmth. I mention these remedies (Paris quadrifolia and Menyanthes) because, like Silicea, I

SILICEA. 333

believe they are not so frequently used in treating headache as they might be with advantage.

In chronic bronchial affections also, Silicea is of value. The cough and sputa furnish characteristic indications, prominent among which is, that the cough is "provoked by cold drinks." I may add, from observation, that the pains, soreness and weakness of the chest, are relieved by inhaling moist warm air.

In uterine or vaginal catarrh, Silicea has proved a valuable remedy, the occurence and character of the leucorrhœa furnishing an indication.

GENERAL VIEW OF ITS ACTION.

In the pathogenesis of Silicea the action of this substance is shown to be marked, first, upon the nutrition, the vegetative sphere; emaciation, loss of appetite, retarded digestion, constipation, sweat confined to the head, but profuse on that part of the body; offensive sweat of the feet, swelling and suppuration of the lymphatic may be cited in evidence. The sweat confined to the head is a pathognomonic symptom of rachitis, and the inference from it that Silicea might be of service in this disease is confirmed by clinical experience. Experience has likewise confirmed Hahnemann's declaration that Silicea has a wonderful control over the suppurative process, whether in the soft tissues, the periosteum, or the bone itself.

Second. Upon the nervous system Silicea exerts a peculiar action. With evidence of exhaustion, furnished by sensation of weakness, paralysis, etc., there is an exalted condition of susceptibility to nervous stimuli; the special senses are morbidly keen, the brain cannot bear even moderate concussion, nor the spine concussion or pressure, and the whole surface is unnaturally tender and sensitive, cold aggravates and warmth relieves. There is, then, an erethism conjoined with exhaustion.

Nor is this all. This erethism, which is not evanescent, but endures for some time, is of such a nature that, while it lasts, spasm is easily induced—indeed, spasm often occurs without any evident provocation, or with only the provocation of muscular exertion and fatigue. Thus, for example, the sensation of weakness and the cramp in the feet at night and when walking, the sensation of weakness and the spasm of the thumb and hand when writing, the sensation of paralysis in the rectum and the spasm of the sphincter ani when making an effort to pass fæces, a spasm which characterizes the peculiar form of constipation observed under Silicea, and so often cured by it.

Clinical experience has taught us that general spasms occur on slight provocation in case of this Silicea erethism.

As an instance of this condition of the nervous system, we may cite the headache of Silicea. It comes on after much exertion, which has exhausted or worried the patient. Its seat is the supra-orbital region, generally the right, or the eye itself, and the pain extends along the base of the brain to the occiput, and down the nape. Noise, motion, light and concussion are intolerable. Repose, quiet, darkness and external warmth give relief.

In subjects whose nutrition is at fault, aching and sharp pains in the nape of the neck frequently occur on the occasion of any nervous strain or exhaustion, and when they exist are aggravated by exertion or excitement. Silicea presents an analogous symptom, with similar conditions.

For patients, on the other hand, in whom fatigue and impaired nutrition produce sluggishness and inaction of the nervous system, Silicea is not at all indicated. It is, for example, very different from Lycopodium in this regard.

The following clinical case illustrates the action of Silicea, as above described:

August 19th, 1869, I was consulted in regard to A. G. W., resident in Boston; a well-grown, bright-looking lad, twelve years old, of dark complexion and hair. His health had been good until the injurey soon to be described. There was no inheritance of spasmadic disease. When he was brought to me he was suffering from epileptiform spasms, of which he had for three months had one or more every day. The history of his injury and its results may best be given from his mother's manuscript as follows (dated March 4th, 1870):

"On the 5th February, 1869, Albert fell upon the ice, making a very severe bruise directly over the right eye. He said, when he got up from the fall, he was a littele dizzy, but it did not hurt him any. That night he complained of being very chilly; the next morning on rising, seemed as bright and well as usual, but late in the afternoon complained of feeling tired, and wanted to retire that night earlier than usual. The following morning he rose with the same tired feeling, accompanied by chilliness, was very quiet, and said he did not feel well enough to go to school. During the week commencing February 7th he was very quiet and not well, the chilliness continuing, and he complained a great deal of his eyes, which were weak; and he could not look at print or anything that required close observation; and at times said everything looked dark as if it was night. He also complained of dizziness, and felt as if his limbs would give out and he should fall down while walking.

"After that week I do not think he complained of objects appearing dark, but all the other symptoms continued, with pain and swelling of his bowels. This last symptom he did not complain of so much the first two or three weeks, but it increased very much, the bowels being swollen, full and hard a great part of the time, particularly late in the afternoon and at night.

I think I may safely say it was in the early part of March he began to be very restless and uneasy, seldom getting to sleep before ten o'clock or eleven, or even later. The only way he could be induced to be quiet or lie still, was by reading to him. As time advanced, that would quiet him but a very short time; he would start up suddenly, running through the rooms, up and down stairs, as fast as he could, and finally throwing himself on the lounge, would sink into unconsciousness. These turns gradually become more severe. I could hardly detect any change from day to day; only by looking back a week or a fortnight could I tell that he grew worse. The attacks grew more frequent and more severe until he was rigid (every limb and every part of his body), his eyes became set, and sometimes one side of him would be convulsed, jerking and twitching. These spasms would vary, lasting from five to twenty minutes usually; but the most severe ones were thirty minutes. From these he would gradually relax, his eyes would close gently and he seemed to sink into an unconscious sleep. At first he would sleep a short time, rouse up suddenly, and always ask where he had been and what time it was.

"After a time, he would not wake from these unconscious turns, but would seem to pass into a natural sleep for the night. These spasms he had every night with but few exceptions after May 1st Commencing about six, P. M., or shortly after, and having from four to six spasms, and sometimes more, until near ten o'clock, and during the intervals between the spasms, he would listen to reading, or be crawling over the bed, pulling the pillows round his neck, tossing them up, and doing such unnatural things, apparently not conscious. The latter part of July, and after, he would at times have these attacks in the day; then they seemed to be brought on by over-excitement, extreme fatigue, or disappointment. On one or two occasions, while walking in the fields with his father, he fell down, lying a few moments, then recovering.

"His appetite was very changeable all through his trouble; sometimes he wanted to eat too much, then for a long time would have but little appetite.

"He was very nervous, and could hardly be induced to sit down to take his meals; was constantly in motion, wanting some amusement all the time. When going into his room to prepare for the night (during July and after), he would, before removing and of his clothing, go into these spasms. His mind always seemed active, bright and quick, except when in these spasms, and I have not had occasion for a moment to think it was at all disturbed; in fact, he seemed more keen and quick than before his injury. His disposition was very much changed. Being naturally pleasant, cheerful and happy, and quite persevering and firm, he became peevish and irritable, very persistent in his own way and wishes; always unhappy if opposed, and seemed in this respect altogether unlike himself.

"He continued as I have described him, apparently growing worse, until he consulted you in August. In about one month from that time, we began to hope (through fears) that he was a very little better; the attacks seemed lighter, more severe ones once in a few days, then less severe again, the severe turns growing less frequent, with longer intervals between. In this way he showed improvement for a time, then would pass a night or two without a spasm; then three or four nights, more or less; the spasms diminishing in this way, until the last spasm he had was October 23, 1869. Since that time, he has been extremely nervous at times, and showed strong symptoms of spasms; but these passed off without further trouble. Twice since you discharged him he has been very nervous and excitable, and on these occasions, following your advice, I resorted to the powders for nervousness (Silicea^{200}), which seemed to have the desired effect. Act times, when tired, he seems more nervous and irritable than is natural; but this wears off by degrees. It might be well for me to mention that a bath does not always affect him pleasantly, and quite recently he complained of feeling badly after getting into it, and appeared stupid and inactive; not because he remained in the bath too long; it seemed more the result of the shock when he first got into the water. Twice within the last two months it has affected him in this way. Aside from this and the nervousness, I am happy to say he seems quite well. In regard to medical treatment, there was no medicine advised by any physician consulted, before yourself, but the bromide of potassium, with great care to be taken respecting his diet, and the quantity, quality and regularity of his meals. Our family physician felt that unless an operation were performed, his trouble would result in loss of intellect, and that was the only treatment that could save him from such an affliction. We consulted one of the first surgeons in Boston regarding it; his opinion was, that it would not be a safe operation, and he did not think favorably of it. With the bromides and plenty of exercise in the open air on a farm, he might ultimately be better."

The above account was written by the patient's mother, March 4th, 1870, and I have quoted in *in extenso,* because of its clear description and history of the origin, progress and decline of the disease. I purpose now to supplement it from my clinical record, made while the case was under treatment, and which does not, in every particular, agree with the mother's narrative, made from recollection, four months after the last spasm occurred. I saw the patient at my office, for the first and only time (the treatment was conducted by correspondence), August 19, 1869. He appeared very bright and intelligent, responding promptly and clearly when questioned. His mother described the case as already detailed, stating, however, that on the steamer, the preceding evening, he had had a worse attack than ever, in consequence, probably, of the excitement produced by traveling. She described the attack as follows, saying it was like those he had had for a fortnight previous, though more severe and lasting longer:

"When in the bedroom, and about to prepare for bed, he, would fall or throw himself upon the bed, then he would plunge head foremost on hands and knees and thrust his head against the bolster or the wall, seemingly unconscious of what he was doing. His friends were obliged to be ready to put cushions between his head and the wall or object against which he seemed about to plunge, in order to guard him from injury. If touched, checked, or resisted while in this condition, he would bite or violently resist. After a time, from five to twenty minute, he would sink upon the bed, become convulsed, and then generally sink into a deep sleep. The bowels were regular. Urine appeared normal. Appetite capricious. The seat of the injury appeared swollen and irregular to the touch, as though there had been a fracture of the outer table of the cranium and some displacement of the fragment. He said that stooping for any length of time produced a sharp pain in the right side of the forehead and heaviness over the eyes, so that he could not keep them open. I noticed a symptom which had never before been observed, viz.: That pressure upon the spine, in the lower part of the dorsal region, as from the fifth to the ninth dorsal vertebra, produced sharp pain in the right forehead, in the seat of the injury.

His mother's attention being quietly called to this fact, she reported from time to time that it was a constant symptom so long as the spasms continued, and that it gradually disappeared, *pari passu*, with the nervousness, which remained for some months after the last spasm. Pathologically this symptom is one of great interest. The lad was much excited during my examination of his case and was quite loquacious, and on this account, and because of the peculiar combative disposition evinced in the attack of the previous night, I gave Hyoscyamus^{200}, ordering that all other medication should be discontinued.

August 26. His mother reports that his condition is as before. She notices, however, that the spine is sensitive at the nape and throughout the cervical and upper dorsal regions, even more than below. Pressure upon the spine Produces pain in the head. She had not noticed these symptoms before, but cannot say that they have not existed. Her attention was never directed to them. Appetite sometimes ravenous, sometimes very poor. Tenderness in the epigastrium is a constant symptom. The abdomen always large and protuberant. Calcarea carbonica^{200}.

Sept. 10th. His mother reports that on the 8th he fell and struck his head in the same place, producing swelling and pain. He was unconscious for some time after the fall. Prior to this his spasms had seemed to be lighter, and his appetite had been more regular, but his excitement and and irritability greater. Belladonna^{200}.

Sept. 22d. He has occasionally passed to day without any spasm, but every few days has had a severe one. He is less irritable, and seems more like himself than since his injury. When excited he moves his eyeballs continually, and snaps his eyelids together spasmodically for a short time. Belladonna^{200} again.

Sept 28th. He took three doses of Belladonna. Had severe headache with spasms in the evening, and unconsciousness. His mother thought the medicine did not agree with him,—aggravated his nervousness and inclined him to spasms. She discontinued it. Calcarea carbonica^{200}.

Oct. 9th. He improved for a few days. Then had more headache, and at night nervousness and spasms. He says it is pain in his head which makes him nervous, and he cannot keep still. The pain is sometimes in the forehead and sometimes in the side of the head. When the pain becomes very acute he passes into unconsciousness. This pain is in and around the seat of injury, and extends thence to the occiput. It is aggravated by motion and noise and relieved by warmth. Silicea^{200}, to be dissolved in water, a tea-spoonful every six hours until some effect appears.

Oct. 19th. He has been freer from headache since the last report, and has not complained of the pain at all.

Oct 28th. Was quite well and free from spasms till 23rd, on which day, having struck his foot while at play, and suffered a good deal of pain and some excitement therefore, he had a hard spasm, passing off in unconsciousness. His eyes have been much better Silicea^{200}, as before.

Nov. 9th. No spasms nor unconscious turns since Oct. 23rd. No complaint of pain or headache. There is no longer any tenderness of the spine, nor pain produced in the head by pressure on the spine. The nervous movement of the eyes is slight. He continued to improve steadily, except for a few days toward the end of November, when disordered digestion seemed to produce an increase of irritability, which, with the indigestion, was speedily relieved by a dose of Nux vomica^{200}, until Dec. 5th, when he complained, while taking a bath, that when the water touched his shoulders it caused pain in the forehead, in the seat of the injury. This aggravation was ascribed to the effect of a blow on the head from a falling door the preceding day. No other bad effect resulted. After Dec. 4th he had only Saccharum lactis.

Jan. 7th, 1870. Continues quite free from spasms, and grows steadily less irritable. No headache, pain or tenderness of the spine. Appetite regular and normal. Digestion and sleep good. Likes to read, and can take a lesson of an hour in length without fatigue.

Discharged, with instructions to take a dose of Silicea^{200} in case of any unusual amount of excitement or return of pain. The lad continued to improve without interruption, and in October, 1870, appeared perfectly well and resumed attendance at school. No symptoms of illness of any kind had appeared up to Jan. 15th, 1871, nor to December, 1871.

On a review of this case, it appears that disturbance of the circulation was apparent, in a slight degree, within a week after the blow upon the head; that the disturbance gradually increased, and was then replaced by nervous irritability, conjoined with a sense of physical prostration and with disturbances of nutrition, until, nearly two months after the injury, the first paroxysm occurred. The spasms increased in frequency and severity until he had been a month under homœopathic treatment. At what period the tenderness of the spine first existed we have no means of ascertaining. It continued until some time after the spasms ceased, declining in intensity as they became less severe. It is noteworthy that with all this disturbance, the intellect and the special senses were not blunted, but came into a condition of erethism or exalted activity. And, moreover, that excitement from unusual stimulus, or from opposition, or from physical injury, caused an increase of nervous excitement, of tenderness of the spine, of headache, and of disposition to spasm. These features of the case are in marked correspondence with the pathogenetic action of Silicea.

Reviewing the result of treatment, it appears that the bromides, though steadily given under skillful direction, had no effect to diminish irritability or control spasm. The effect of exercise in the open air on a farm, as recommended, was faithfully tried from May 1st to August 19th; but the lad grew steadily worse, and the more he exercised, even in moderation, the worse he was. Of the homœopathic remedies, Hyoscyamus probably did no good, and was not a wise prescription, being based on too partial a view of the case. Belladonna appeared to allay the violence of the spasms to some extent, and to moderate the nervous irritability. Under Calcarea carbonica the digestion and assimilation, which had been much impaired and perverted, were nearly restored to the normal state. It must be noted, however, that although in these respects improvement followed the use of these remedies, nevertheless, while they were being taken, the headach and tenderness of head and spine steadily increased, the spasmodic action of the eyes and lids set in and increased, and the spasms, though less frequent, increased in severity. The irritation of the nervous centers was evidently not controlled, and the case assumed more and more the aspect of a well-established centric epilepsy. While, therefore, the remedies produced beneficial results and undeniably contributed to the cure, they did not cover the entire case, and it is a question whether the ultimate favorable result would not have been more speedily attained had the Silicea been administered at an earlier date. This remedy I regard as the chief instrument in the cure. For, so soon as the patient came under its influence there was evident that mitigation of all the symptoms and their disappearance, one by one, which the homœopathist is wont to recognize as evidence that he has found in his remedy a similimum to the case. The amelioration began at once in the symptoms immediately referable to lesions of the nervous centers. The headache ceased; the spine became less tender; pressure upon it no longer caused pain in the seat of the injury. The susceptibility which had, under other remedies, persisted coincidently with improvement in other respects, rapidly decreased. In a word, from the time Silicea was given, universal improvement began; and it was scarcely interrupted until the child appeared perfectly well again.

Happily for the patient and his parents, no opportunity was afforded for obtaining by inspection a certain knowledge of the organic lesions existing in this case. Whether, as was supposed by the attending physician, a depression of the inner table of the cranium or a spicula of bone protruding therefrom, produced pressure upon the brain, and consequent irritation, or whether a low grade of inflammation resulted in tissue degeneration in some part of the encephalon, must be matter of conjecture; other hypotheses may be formed. If the former, the recovery could hardly have been expected, and can hardly be explained. If the latter, then under the action of remedies a retrograde metamorphosis must have occurred, and the normal tissues must have gradually replaced again the degenerate substitutes. In any view, this was not a case in which we could reasonably anticipate a spontaneous complete restoration to health. The recovery, therefore, under the administration of homœopathic remedies is an interesting phenomenon; nor is the interest of the case the less that these remedies were all given singly and in the 200th potency.

STRYCHNOS NUX VOMICA.

THE seed of the fruit of a large tree found in the East Indies. Whether this very powerful and most useful drug was known to the ancients is a disputed question. It is only within the last 150 years that its value in medicine has begun to be recognized.

Nux vomica is supposed to owe its activity to two alkaloids, Strychnia and Brucea; but it is found in practice that the action of Nux Vomica on the organism is not identical with that of either of these substances.

Nux vomica is very bitter, and Strychnia is so intensely bitter that a solution of one grain of it in 666,700 grains of cold water still retains a decided and strong bitter taste.

Nux vomica is classed among the spinants or tetanica, the current physiological theory of its action restricting it to the spinal marrow.

When taken in very small doses, Nux vomica is said by Stillé ("System of Materia Medica and Therapeutics," Phila., 1864) to "derange the digestion; to augment the secretion of stomach and mouth and of liver and pancreas. It disposes to frequent urination, and, when given in larger doses, causes retention of urine; first, by producing spasm of the neck of the bladder, and ultimately loss of power in the muscular coat of the bladder. It excites uterine contraction and promotes the menstrual flow.

"It acts more quickly on paralyzed muscles than on others (perhaps because these are withdrawn from the realm of volition and are affected through reflexion alone), and produces formication in the limbs, and a slight right rigidity of the lower jaw and limbs; a sense of heaviness and debility, with general stiffness of the muscles and clonic spasms.

"In larger, poisonous doses, after general uneasiness, soreness, stiffness and heaviness of the limbs and joints, spasmodic symptoms set in, clonic spasms or violent muscular twitches, seeming like an electric shock.

"Then come tetanic spasms of all the muscles, during which the limbs are rigidly flexed or extended, the lower jaw firmly set against the upper, and the body arched as in opisthotonos. The rigid contraction of the respiratory muscles renders breathing laborious, or even suspends it for a time, and the skin becomes livid from stasis of the blood. The corners of the mouth are contracted, showing the set teeth, with foam issuing from between them; the eyes stare and the brow is contracted.

"Amid all this horrible array of symptoms the

mind is not at all affected, and it is probable that but little pain is felt.

"The convulsions are generally interrupted by periods of calm, from which, however, the least noise, a breath of air, or the lightest touch may act with the suddenness of lightning to renew the scene. (Stramonium.)

"Death at last occurs either from asthenia or asphyxia."

The smallest fatal dose of Nux vomica is three grains; of Strychnia, one grain.

"The anatomical lesions are not uniform. The muscles are rigid, all the internal organs are gorged with blood;" and this is all.

These are the effects ascribed by the most recent authorities to Nux vomica. They may be reduced by analysis into the following :

Nux vomica acts chiefly upon the spinal marrow. It affects that portion which presides over the reflex function of the muscular system. The variety of effect produced by it is this : it excites muscular action, causing incoherent contractions to take place; deranges the normal order in which muscular motions succeed each other; finally it puts an end to these motions altogether, producing a kind of paralysis.

Our much more exact and available knowledge of Nux vomica is derived from a proving by Hahnemann and his pupils; a most excellent proving from which we make the following analysis of the action of Nux vomica on the healthy organism :

SPECIAL ANALYSIS.

The effects on the sensorium are as follows: There is indisposition to mental exertion, and particularly to that form which involves the elaboration and connections of subjective ideas independently of external objects (subjective ratiocination). The prover easily errs in speaking or writing. This corresponds with a certain manual clumsiness.

Vertigo is produced, with momentary loss of consciousness, obscuration of vision and staggering. It occurs more particularly while eating and immediately after eating; when walking and even when lying down in bed. It resembles vertigo produced by alcohol; for which, indeed, Nux is a specific remedy.

Head. Nux produces, moreover, confusion and dullness in the head, especially in the morning and after meals. Also great and bewildering heaviness, especially on stooping.

The headache is pressing, tensive and drawing. It affects chiefly the forehead and the supra-orbital region; sometimes extending through the base of the brain to the occiput.

It is sometimes described as a feeling of internal soreness, as though one had received a blow with an ax. With the acute headache is conjoined, almost always qualmishness, nausea, and even vomiting.

When the prover walks, the brain feels shattered. Externally the scalp is sensitive and sore.

Rhus toxicodendron has the sensation when the patient walks, and especially when he goes upstairs, as if at every step or rising the brain were loose and struck against the skull; hence worse from motion. China has, along with a sensation of great fullness in the head and outward pressure in the temples, a feeling as if the brain were balancing to and fro within the cranium and were striking against the skull, occasioning great pain and obliging one to move the head (hence better from motion).

Face. The chief symptoms noted on the face are small papules,—some of which even contain pus,—isolated, occurring on the forehead, cheeks and scalp, a kind of acne. Nux is a remedy for the acne which is aggravated by eating cheese, although the great constipation sometimes produced by cheese is relieved by Colocynth.

Eyes. Drawing and pressing pains in the eyelids, the margins of which become thickened and sore. The lids are agglutinated in the morning.

In the eyes themselves biting, burning and itching, relieved by rubbing.

The conjunctiva sometimes becomes very red, and there is great photophobia.

Clinical experience has led me to regard morning and forenoon photophobia as especially indicating Nux vomica. (See Euphrasia.) The patient covers the eyes or buries the head in a pillow in the forenoon, and looks around without suffering in the afternoon.

As regards the special sense, there have been observed a glittering appearance just outside the field of distinct vision, and also black and gray points floating before the eyes.

Ears. In the course of the Eustachian tube, an itching and tickling, inducing a desire to swallow. (Gelseminum has produced and cured a similar tickling compelling the prover to cough.)

Stitches, pressure and shocks in the ear, often violent. Hissing and whistling in the ears, and sometimes a whirring and noise like that of a mill.

The cuticle peels off from the lips; on the inner part of the lips and on the vermilion border ulcers form, which burn and stick.

The gums swell and pain like ulcers; indeed ulcers actually form upon them, having a drawing and burning pain.

The stomatitis indicating Nux vomica must be distinguished from that which requires Alumina, Borax, Carbo vegetabilis, etc., chiefly by the symptoms of stomach and bowels and sleep.

In the teeth various pains occur; soreness increased (as all the Nux vomica pains are) by mental exertion, and by going into the open air. The pain may be throbbing, boring, drawing; extending into the gum, which is swollen, and into the bones of the face. It is worse after eating, and from cold water or cold air, and from exertion of mind or body.

The tongue becomes heavy as if half paralyzed. Papules and vesicles appear on it.

The mouth is dry, even without thirst, as after alcoholic drinks. In the morning the mouth and fauces are full of thick and unpleasant mucus.

The fauces are sore as if raw; felt on swallowing and on contact with cool air. The mucous membrane covering the hard palate, and the velum and uvula become swollen with a pressive pain felt particularly on swallowing saliva. There is a sensation as if there were a plug in the throat, felt no more when swallowing than at other times. Probably a gastric symptom. Pulsatilla and Lachesis have a similar sensation; as if a mass of food had remained in the throat.

A kind of burning in the throat and a scraped, raw sensation in the pharynx, as after waterbrash.

It is apparent that Nux does not correspond to angina tonsillaris or submucosa, but rather to a subacute affection confined to the mucous membrane of the palate, uvula, and pharynx.

The taste is much altered, especially early in the morning. It is sour, hereby or metallic, or all three combined; sometimes putrid, especially after eructation.

Sometimes it is bitter, especially just after ejecting mucus from the mouth and fauces. As a general thing, food and drink have their normal taste.

Under Pulsatilla, food and drink very often do not have their natural taste. Under Natrum muriaticum they have no taste whatever.

The appetite is generally impaired, and there is a general repugnance to food and to the accustomed stimuli, wine and tobacco.

On the other hand, there is sometimes an abnormally great hunger.

I have often observed that persons subject to frequent attacks of gastric disorder requiring Nux vomica have, for twenty-four or thirty-six hours before an attack, a wonderfully good appetite, especially for meat and fat. If, as soon as this unnatural hunger is noticed, they cut down their bill of fare to bread and water for one day, they avert the attack.

After the midday meal, a host of symptoms of all kinds appears, relating to the stomach and also to the head and entire organism,—a general aggravation after dinner (different from Pulsatilla).

The eructations are generally painful, as if from spasm of the œsophagus. In taste they are bitter and sour.

Hiccough is a frequent and distressing symptom. There is a good deal of thirst, but water burdens and distresses the stomach.

Nausea is a constant symptom. It occurs especially early in the morning and just after a meal, and is conjoined with a kind of faintness and feeling of illness, such as is produced by a strong purgative.

The vomiting is generally of sour mucus and food, sometimes of blood.

The region of the stomach is very sensitive to

external pressure, and so indeed is the abdomen generally. Tight pressure from clothing is unpleasant. There is a pressing pain as from a load in the stomach, and this even though the amount of food or drink taken has been very small.

Several remedies resemble Nux vomica in these symptoms. Mercurius has a peculiarly deadly faintness produced by pressure in the pit of the stomach. Calcarea carbonica has tenderness of the pit of the stomach.

Lycopodium has pain in the pit of the stomach when the hypochondria are pressed, and pain in the hypochondria when the pit of the stomach is pressed. Lycopodium has also a sensation of fullness in the gastric region as soon as one has eaten but little, although one sat down with a good appetite. Lycopodium has also much flatus incarcerated here and there, but it lacks the irritability of the large intestine so characteristic of Nux vomica.

Sepia and Murex have an all-gone sensation in the pit of the stomach, worse about eleven A. M., and relieved by eating and lying down.

The abdomen feels greatly distended and is moderately so; respiration is embarrassed. These symptoms are all worse from walking in the cool air.

There is much flatus in the bowels. Sudden attacks of spasmodic pain in the region of the stomach.

Burning in the cardiac and pyloric region.

Nux produces sticking pains, and soreness and swelling in the region of the liver, which are aggravated by motion and by deep inspiration, as well as by pressure.

All varieties of flatulent colic are simulated; griping pains, pains as if the intestines were squeezed; between stones, etc.

Great distention immediately after eating or drinking. Frequent sharp pain with desire for stool, ineffectual.

Nux vomica is often a better remedy than Chamomilla for the colic of infants, that is, when it is better indicated; as by the large amount of flatus and by the constipation with apparent frequent desire and effort to evacuate the bowels; Chamomilla having, rather, a diarrhœa.

All symptoms relieved by repose, when sitting or lying down.

In the abdomen a sensation as from a load or burden,—a pressure or dragging toward the genital organs, as from a constrictive cramp; the abdomen is sore and sensitive.

The following symptoms is very important: a sensation of weakness in the region of the abdominal ring, as if a hernia would occur or were getting strangulated. Hernia actually appears. This symptom has led to the successful use of Nux vomica for incarcerated and other hernia.

As regards the stool, Hahnemann remarks that copious diarrhœic stools are never produced by Nux vomica; but that what is called diarrhœa from Nux are rather small evacuations mixed with muscus, and attended by tenesmus and straining. This tenesmus is attended by a smarting burning in the rectum.

The most frequent primary (?) action of Nux is the production of constipation, as if from constriction or inactivity of the intestines, or rather, it produces an ineffectual urging to stool, and whenever at last the stool takes place, it seems to be incomplete and unsatisfactory, and as if a part of the fæces failed to be expelled; or the stool is very hard, and its evacuation requires great effort, and leaves a stitching and aching pain in the rectum. But, after the evacuation, there is no desire to sit and continue to strain, as with Mercurius.

Often, the stool is soft, mixed with mucus and streaked with blood; or there is clear blood along with the fæces. (Dysentery and hæmorrhoids.)

In the rectum and anus, sharp, pressing pain, especially after mental exertion. Painful constriction of the rectum after mental effort and after eating.

As regards the urinary organs; painful, ineffectual effort to pass water, with scantly discharge. Often, with the urine is mixed a tenacious mucus. Burning pain during micturition.

The menses occur too soon and continue longer than they should. The inter-menstrual interval is too brief.

They are accompanied by nausea, chills, and faintness, after previous spasmodic movements in the abdomen. Sometimes great prostration and severe headaches and pains in the limbs. (Useful in anticipating menorrhagia and in menstrual colic.)

In the respiratory tract Nux produces a variety of catarrhal symptoms, but none of sub-mucous or parenchymatous inflammation.

The nares become sore and ulcerated, the smell perverted; there seems before the nose a smell of sulphur, or of bad cheese or of candle-snuff. Frequent discharge of thin, acrid fluid from the nose, and yet the nares are obstructed.

Much sneezing. The coryza is fluent early and by day; and in the evening it is dry and so is the mouth.

Coryza fluent during the day; dry evening and night.

The voice is hoarse and raw; the larynx pale, rough and scraped; the prover hems and clears the throat constantly. There is a moderate amount of mucus in the throat and chest. (Coryza and influenza.)

The cough of Nux is induced by motion of the body or exertions of the mind; by forced expiration, reading, etc:; is worse every other day; appears in the evening or at night after lying down, and prevents going to sleep. It is short and dry but fatiguing; lasts often from midnight to day-break, and is accompanied by severe headache and pain and soreness in the epigastric zone.

It is not a deep, chest cough, but seems to

come from the larynx. A more important remedy in coughs than has been supposed.

Respiration is embarrassed; a kind of asthma worse at night and after a meal; worse from having the clothing tight on the thorax, relieved by removing the clothing. (Useful in asthma.)

The pains in the thorax are chiefly such general sensations as accompany the asthma and the fatiguing cough just described.

No heart symptoms.

In the sacral region, pain at night which hinders turning in bed.

Contracting and constricting pain in the sacrum, and thence into the sides and back and the interscapular region.

Lassitude and pain as if beaten; dragging and bearing down in the pelvis.

In the extremities, lassitude, heaviness and aching and drawing pains.

We come now to the

GENERAL ANALYSIS.

On the functional activity the action of Nux vomica is well marked. It affects the sensorium but little in comparison with its effects on other parts of the nervous system, offering a marked contrast to Stramonium, which produces tetanic convulsions resembling those resulting from Nux vomica, and at the same time produces violent mania; whereas during the convulsions of Nux vomica the mind is not affected.

In this respect of profoundly affecting the organs and functions of nutrition and locomotion, while the mind and senses are but little affected, Nux vomica resembles Veratrum, Camphor and the poison of Asiatic cholera.

The reflex function of the spinal marrow is unquestionably the great seat of action of Nux vomica, as the symptoms of convulsion or of semi-paralysis in the limbs and trunk, together with the spasmodic affections of the face, jaws, throat, œsophagus, intestinal and urinary tracts, and the respiratory organs, particularly the larynx, plainly show.

It is an error, however, to regard the action of Nux vomica as restricted to this region. It acts with hardly less vigor upon the organic substance of the body; and this more particularly in the entire intestinal tract and in the urino-genital organs, modifying the secretions in both quantity and quality, and causing not only perversions of function but also changes of structure, as we see in the aphthæ and in the hæmorrhoids which it produces and cures.

The sphere of action of Nux vomica will be seen thus to be quite extensive, involving most of the functions and organs of animal and vegetable life. The sensorium is not deeply affected, save secondarily. The skin, bones and glands are not primarily affected by Nux vomica.

Periodicity. There is a well-marked periodicity in the action of Nux vomica. As a general rule,

STRYCHNOS NUX VOMICA.

it may be stated that its symptoms are aggravated in the morning.

Peculiarities. Among the peculiarities attending almost all the symptoms, and which serve as characteristic indications, are the following:

The symptoms are worse in the morning; they are made worse by motion and by exertion, and by exposure to cool air, being ameliorated by repose and by warmth. In all these respects Nux vomica is the opposite of Pulsatilla.

The sleep of Nux vomica is peculiar. Instead of being wide-awake in the evening, as under Pulsatilla, the prover falls asleep in his chair, is very heavy, and on going to bed sleeps immediately. On the other hand, an hour or two before day-break the prover wakens and then cannot sleep again, or, rather, he dozes after a while in a semi-conscious state, and then wakens more tired and inert than before he dozed.

Under Pulsatilla there is difficulty in falling asleep in the evening, but the sleep is sound till morning, and, on waking, the patient is languid.

Many of the symptoms occur or are aggravated immediately after eating; whereas under Pulsatilla they did not occur or were not aggravated until several hours after eating.

The symptoms are aggravated by mental exertion or by sedentary habits, to which nevertheless, the Nux vomica patient is disposed.

The disposition is irritable, choleric, impatient. If there be despondency it is of the impatient kind.

PRACTICAL APPLICATIONS.

Hahnemann says in the introduction to the proving: "There are a few medicines, the greater part of whose symptoms are analogous to the principal and most common diseases to which mankind is subject, at least in Europe, and which, consequently, are most frequently employed in homœopathy. The term polychrest may be applied to them.

"To this class Nux vomica especially belongs. The use of it was formerly dreaded because it had been tried only in very large doses; and in cases with which it did not correspond it could not fail to injure. But in a moderate dose it is the mildest and most precious of medicines in instances where its symptoms accord with those it excites in healthy persons.

"Nux vomica is chiefly successful with persons of an ardent character, or a temperament disposed to anger, spite or deception. If the catamenia occur several days too early, or are too abundant, Nux is perfectly adapted to meet the consequences."

In this respect Calcarea carbonica is similar to Nux vomica. Pulsatilla and Sulphur are opposites.

"This medicine (Nux vomica), taken some hours before going to bed, acts more mildly than at any other time of day. Any case of immediate necessity must of course be excepted.

"It is best for very sensitive persons not to take it fasting in the morning or on first waking, because its most powerful symptoms are then called out. Also, it should not be taken immediately before or after a meal, or when the head is much exercised, nor should the patient, after taking this (or any other) medicine, directly employ his faculties in writing, reflecting, or reading, or reciting. He must wait at least two hours to avert ill consequences.

"Among the diseases in which Nux vomica is especially efficacious are many chronic affections; for instance, those caused by excess of coffee or wine, especially in persons of sedentary habits; or those proceeding from too protracted literary application. It is also a remedy for many epidemic disorders and acute fevers, chiefly those in which cold is preceded or accompanied by heat. It frequently prevents the bad effects of chills.

"It is more particularly suitable when the patient is worse in the morning than at any other time of day; when he awakes about three A. M., and remains wakeful with a multitude of ideas crowding his mind, and when, just at day-break, he falls involuntarily asleep, filled with busy dreams, from which he wakes tired and indisposed to arise. It is also adapted to persons who, several hours before bed-time, fall asleep in their chair."

Vertigo..Headache...Gastralgia...Flatulent colic ...Constipation...Diarrhœa...Dysentery...Hæmorrhoids...Hernia...Coryza...Bronchitis...Laryngesimus....Asthma....Bad effects of coffee and wine.... Intermittent fever.

ALOES.

THE *Aloe spicata,* the inspissated juice of the leaves of which is the part used in medicine. It has various names denoting the origin of the specimen.

1. Socotrina, the finest kind, called also Turkish or Indian Aloes, of a garnet red color with a golden or yellow red when powdered.

2. Hepatic, similar but less brilliant.

3. Cape Aloes, the most abundant, derived from the Cape of Good Hope, greenish and dull.

4. Barbadoes Aloes, strong, dark brown, used for horses.

Aloë has been used in medicine since very early days. Its great bitterness has given it reputation as a tonic, but its chief use has been as a cathartic.

The ancients ascribed to it a special power to purge off the bile, and to cure affections of the abdomen and of the head, supposed to depend on a disordered state of the biliary secretion.

Aloë is a drug in very frequent use in our day. Very few purgative pills are ordered by practitioners which do not contain a portion of Aloes. It is the standing ingredient of the so-called anti-bilious vegetable purgative and other pills known as "patent medicines." Likewise of certain of officinal mixtures, about the names of which there has gathered from the days of our childhood a certain odor of antique sanctity, to wit, the tincture of aloes and canella, known as hiera picra (or sacred bitters), and the tincture of aloes and myrrh, known as the elixir proprietatis (or, more commonly, elixir pro).

Trousseau and Pidoux give an excellent summary of the action of Aloë:

"Administered in small doses (one-half grain to one grain) once or twice a day, it provokes moderate colics, followed by the expulsion of one or more diarrhœic stools. It is remarkable that the action of this purgative is very slow, the stool rarely follows within six or seven hours after the dose, and often not till twenty-four hours after it. The first effect, then, is to augment the number of the stools, or simply to facilitate their evacuation, and it likewise stimulates the functions of the stomach, but only where the slowness of digestion is not accompanied by symptoms of chronic gastritis. If the use of Aloes be continued for a long time, there soon ensue symptoms of sanguineous congestion of the pelvic organs, such as heat, itching, sensation of weight toward the extremity of the intestine, excitation of the genital organs, and frequent need to evacuate the bladder. In women, pain and heaviness in the uterus, in the groins and in the loins, increase of the leucorrhœa, uterine colics, more painful during the menses, increase of the menstrual flow."

Aloë has been known, in numberless cases, to produce congestion of the lower part of the rectum, with hæmorrhage from the hæmorrhoidal veins. And the tendency to this action is a great objection to the customary long-continued use of this drug as an habitual palliative in constipation. Nevertheless, Aloë has been successfully used by Eberle in the treatment of hœmorrhoids.

By reason of its power to cause congestion of the pelvic organs, Aloë has been used by the old school as a derivative in cases of severe cerebral congestion, also in amenorrhœa (particularly the tincture aloes et myrrhæ or elixir pro).

Our direct knowledge of Aloes is derived from a proving conducted by Dr. Hering (and published in his "Amerikanische Arzneiprufungen," vol. i.).

A most excellent, accurate and spirited translation of this admirable proving will be found in the appendix to vol. v. of the "American Homœopathic Review." It was executed by Prof. T. F. Allen, A. M., M. D., of New-York, and is a model of philological discrimination, avoiding at once the indefinite and flippant gracefulness of modern English, and the corduroy roughness of colloquial German; combining the acerb crispness of rugged Yorkshire with the Amherst softness of highly civilized southern Saxony.

As already stated, the action of Aloes is chiefly exerted upon the pelvic organs, in which it produces functional changes (in so far as the secretions are concerned in frequency and manner), and organic in this that the organs are gorged with blood.

The action upon the head I believe to be secondary upon the action on the pelvis. I have never seen it disassociated therefrom.

The peculiarities of Aloes will appear in the special analysis.

SPECIAL ANALYSIS.

On the sensorium Aloë produces a singular combination of anxious restlessness, despondency, indisposition to mental or bodily exertion, and confusion of the intelligence. These conditions alternate, but the depression is predominant.

Considerable vertigo is produced, which, however, coincides with constipation or other disordered condition of the intestine and its functions.

It resembles the vertigo of Chelidonium, which coincides with pain in the right hypochondrium and at the angle of the scapula, and with icteric complexion and bilious urine.

The headache of Aloes is chiefly a confused feeling of heaviness or pressure in the anterior part of the head, a weight pressing down the middle of the forehead to the root of the nose. The pressure sometimes extends to the vertex, sometimes to the temples. Sometimes throbbing. Most provers note that this headache accompanies or alternates with colic or constipation, or with the kind of diarrhœa peculiar to Aloes.

The scalp becomes sensitive to touch. Respecting the eyes, we not here only a symptom which often accompanies the pressing frontal headache, viz., pressure on the eyes from above and a feeling as if it were necessary to contract the eyes and make them very small in order to see (symptom 172). I have prescribed on the authority of this symptom Aloes for a patient whose other symptoms were not very clearly indicative of Aloes, and thereby succeeded in permanently curing a chronic headache.

I call attention to the ear symptoms in the published proving, because Dr. Hering has found Aloes to be a good ear remedy. I have no experience with it as such.

Hypochondria. In the hepatic region we find pressure and tension, discomfort, a sensation of heat, pressure, and single not severe stitches. These symptoms, along with the sickly expression of face and the bitter taste, point to some derangement of the liver, though, from the absence of fever in the Aloes proving, it cannot be acute inflammation. Eberle signalizes the efficacy of Aloes in certain forms of jaundice.

(Lycopodium has tension and pressure, but these are felt in the left as well as in the right hypochondrium, and are aggravated by pressure on the epigastrium. China has symptoms in the right hypochondrium, similar to those of Aloes, but is distinguished by the fever symptoms and others. The Chelidonium liver symptoms are accompanied by pain under the right scapula, and generally by cough.)

The abdomen is somewhat distended with flatus. There is head fullness, a sense of weight and dragging, particularly in the hypogastrium, and the abdomen is tender on pressure.

The heaviness extends into the rectum and into the region of the bladder. Flatulent colic accompanies the pelvic congestion.

As regards stool, it is first, by very small doses, retarded and diminished. Then it is more free; finally there ensues a half-fluid, light yellow, moderately offensive stool, and at last a yellow watery diarrhœa.

The peculiarities of the evacuation characterize this drug. The diarrhœa comes on early in the morning, say at five A. M. The desire for stool wakens the patient, and he can hardly rise with sufficient rapidity. In this respect Aloë resembles Sulphur, Thuja (and Bryonia).

Croton tiglium has a morning diarrhœa, light yellow, watery, almost painless, very abundant, gushing out in an instant, imperative, leaving prostration.

Sulphur diarrhœa is white mucus, watery, painless, containing undigested food; the patient has to get up to go to stool.

Thuja, pale yellow, forcibly expelled, with much

wind. It returns at the same hour but is not imperative.

Bryonia, dark and putrid, smelling like old cheese. Only A. M.

But with Aloes there is throughout a peculiar sensation of weakness in the rectum, and particularly in the sphincter ani, as if the latter would be suddenly relaxed in spite of the patient's will, and would permit the escape of fæces.

The diarrhœa rarely continues later than ten A. M. The disposition is always brought on by eating, *e. g.*, at the breakfast table.

So treacherous does the sphincter ani seem to be that the emission of flatus is dreaded as sure to be accompanied by the escape of fæces. (Similar to Phosphoric acid.) So likewise the patient dreads to pass water lest the slight exertion and bearing down involved in that act should also move the bowels.

A very similar state of things obtain with regard to the sphincter of the bladder.

At the same time there is a frequent disposition (as with Nux vomica) to evacute the bladder and rectum.

At the extremity of the rectum, burning, itching. Bleeding from the rectum.

In the perinæum, a sensation of weight and a feeling as if a plug wer wedged in between the symphisis pubis and the os coccygis.

Hepar sulphuris, Thuja and Causticum have similar sensations pointing to affections of the prostate gland.

In the pelvis, heat, weight, pressure and dragging downward.

The menstrual flow is augmented and hastened.

The practical applications of Aloes follow clearly from the statement of symptoms. Experience has thus far established its value in the treatment of diarrhœa, headache and vertigo depending on pelvic congestion, hæmorrhoids, prolapsus uteri and menorrhagia.

The symptoms which have seemed to me the most characteristic are those of the head and of the abdomen, stool and urine. They are those on which my use of Aloes in practice has been based. Chief among these are those of the stool.

From symptoms 512 to 860, we gather that Aloes produce a diarrhœa consisting of light-colored semi-liquid fæces, preceded and accompanied by much gurgling and flatus in the abdomen; that the diarrhœa occurs especially in the morning, say from two A. M. to ten A. M.; that the desire for stool is sudden and extremely urgent, being felt in the hypogastrium and in the rectum, and being so urgent that the patient can scarcely retain the fæces long enough to effect the necessary strategic "change of base;" that, during this brief interval, he fears to evacuate wind by the anus or to make any physical exertion, or even to strain to pass water, lest he should have an involuntary evacuation of the bowels. This sensation of the uncertain tenure by which the fæces are held in the rectum is a very well marked characteristic of Aloes, as shown by the following symptoms:

"The evacuation takes place without any exertion on the part of the patient; it seems, as it were, to fall out of the rectum (765). At stool a constant feeling as if there were more fæces to be passed (769). Involuntary passage of fæces when emitting flatus (824). Disposition to stool when passing water (826). Fæces and urine seem inclined to pass and do pass simultaneously (827). When passing water feeling as if a thin stool were about to pass (828). When standing, sensation as if fæces would pass (833)."

There is also a similar frequency or urgency of the desire to pass urine, with a similar uncertainty in the tenure of that excretion, as we perceive from the following symptoms:

"Frequent desire to urinate (990). Increased desire—quantity not increased (992). So urgent a desire he can hardly retain the urine (993). On rising he was obliged to run quickly to urinate (996)."

And the similarity of the affection of the urinary organs and the intestines is shown in symptom 1001:

"At stool, urination; when urinating, desire for stool."

In connection with these two series of symptoms, those of the pelvis deserve notice. Among them we find, "heaviness, pressure downward (865, 861). Feeling as if a plug were wedged in between the symphysis pubis and the os coccygis (860)." This is equivalent to a weight upon the perinæum. Viewing it in combination with the symptoms of stool and urine above referred to, we are justified in saying of Aloë, in regard to this portion of its sphere of action, that it srikes the patient equally "between wind and water."

It is understood, of course, that this is not the only action of Aloes upon the abdominal organs. It is believed, however, to be that variety of action which is most characteristic of the remedy and least likely to be confounded with the effect of any other drug. In the frequent desire for stool; in the frequent, pappy, not very abundant stool; in the pressure downward in the back and pelvis; in the abundant formation of flatus in the abdomen, which rumbles and gurgles, producing pinching pain in the lower part of the abdomen just before the stool, the action of Aloes very closely resembles that of Nux vomica, a remedy so useful in diarrhæa and dysentry. It is distinguished, however, by the peculiarities of the evacuation of stool. Nux vomica produces very frequent desire for stool, with inability to evacuate the fæces. Under Aloes, on the contrary, the difficulty is to retain the fæces as long as the patient desires to do so. Aloes seem to paralyze the sphincter ani to a certain extent, Nux vomica to excite in it a spasmodic action of exalted power. In this action on the sphincter, Aloes resemble Hyoscyamus.

Among the symptoms of the head I am inclined to regard as characteristic of Aloes, those which described a heavy, confused dullness in the front part of the head extending to the root of the nose, with inability to think; a pain in the forehead which compels the patient to close the eyes or, if he wishes to look at anything, to constringe the eyes, making the aperture of the lids very small. It must be admitted, however, that symptoms so similar to these are found under other remedies, that these symptoms alone could not be regarded as a sure indication for Aloes.

The following cases will show how I have prescribed Aloes, and will suggest some reflections upon the mode of selecting remedies in practice.

Within the last three years I have treated about thirty-five cases which so closely resemble each other in their characteristic elements, that the description of all may be given in that of the last of the series, which came under my care a month ago.

A young man applied for relief from a diarrhœa which had persisted about two weeks in spite of various remedies which had been prescribed for it, and among which were Calcarea, Nux vomica, Bryonia, and the inevitable Arsenicum. He described his stools as being light yellow, pappy, somewhat frothy, and tolerably abundant. They were preceded by flatulent rumbling in the abdomen and by pinching pain in the hypogastrium. The necessary for a stool awakened him from a sound sleep about three A. M. From this hour to nine A. M. he had from four to six stools of the character above described. None at any other period of day or night. When the desire for stool was felt, the urgency became instantly so great that he was compelled to spring from the bed and hasten to the water-closet. Yet this urgency was not of the nature of tenesmus, but rather a sensation of weakness in the sphincter, as though he could not prevent the fæces from falling out. During stool, which passed freely in a mass the instant the restraint of the patient's volition was withdrawn from the sphincter ani, there was a slight burning in the rectum. After stool, cessation of pain, but a very slight general sensation of weakness and lassitude.

During this period, from three to nine A. M., the patient was compelled to avoid all rapid or severe exertion of body, and especially straining to pass water. The penalty of such exertion or straining was sure to be an involuntary evacuation of fæces.

I prescribed one powder of Saccharum lactis containing two globules of Aloes^{200} to be taken dry on the tongue at ten A. M. (the hour at which he called on me). From this time he had no diarrhœa. The next morning he slept until seven A. M., and at nine had a natural stool as was his habit in health.

During the winter season, a gentleman about seventy years of age applied for relief from a dull, heavy, frontal headache, which incapacitated him from mental labour. He could give me no more definite nor characteristic description of his ailment.

It was felt as soon as he waked and lasted all day. From such a description as the above, it would be impossible to prescribe with any certainty of selecting the right remedy. I set myself, therefore, to investigate the patient's previous history, in the hope of getting some help from the Anamnesis to which Hahnemann and Bœnninghausen attach so much importance. I learned that this headache was no new affliction. It had for years annoyed this gentleman, rather more during the winter season, whereas during the summer he was comparatively free from it. No peculiarity of diet or regimen could explain this fact.

On the other hand, I learned that during the summer season my patient was very frequently attacked with diarrhœa, the disease coming on suddenly, waking him at two A. M., with a pinching, flatulent colic, and so urgent a call to evacuate the bowels that he would be compelled to seek the water-closet instantly, experiencing, meanwhile, the greatest difficulty in retaining the fæces. From this time till ten A. M., he would have four or five stools, pappy, copious, light yellow, great difficulty in retaining the fæces for even a moment after the desire for stool was first experienced. Desire for stool provoked by eating, so that he was compelled to leave the breakfast table. Involuntary stool when straining to pass water. When comparatively free from headache he was inclined to diarrhœa, and *vice versa.*

I have long been persuaded that a most

important condition of success in the treatment of chronic diseases, consists in the practitioner taking such a view of the case as shall combine the various ailments of which a chronic patient may complain at different periods of time and in different organs, even though these periods and organs be remote from each other and apparently disconnected. In no other way, it has sometimes seemed to me, could the characteristic indications of the remedy for such a case be found.

Acting upon this persuasion in the case in question, I regarded the headache which predominated in winter, and the diarrhœas which predominated in summer, as in some sort complementary series of symptoms, and as making up, both together, the "totality of symptoms" for which I was to seek, in the materia medica, the *similimum*.

The symptoms of the headache—indeed of the entire winter affection—presented nothing that was characteristic of any one remedy to the exclusion of all others. Carbo vegetabilis, Sabadilla, Sulphur, Aloes, Nux vomica, and several others, might be regarded as about equally well indicated.

When, however, to the head symptoms of the winter I came to add the diarrhœa symptoms of the summer, regarding the sum total as one disease, it was then impossible to avoid perceiving that the diarrhœa symptoms were strikingly characteristic of Aloes, and could not indicate any other remedy. This furnished the clue to the prescription. On studying the head symptoms of Aloes, it was seen that they corresponded to the head symptoms of my patient quite as well as the symptoms of any other drug. Aloë^{200} was given, and it afforded a relief which my patient had sought in vain from other remedies taken on the strength of the head symptoms alone. The headache returned a few times afterward with very much diminished severity, but yielded at once to Aloes. Latterly, my patient has been entirely free from it, nor did the diarrhœa return as it used formerly to do whenever the headache ceased to prevail.

In a third case I have given Aloes for incontinence of urine in an old gentleman who has enlarged prostate. The prescription was based on the fact that he is very subject to a diarrhœa, presenting all the characteristics of the Aloes diarrhœa. The peculiarities of the incontinence, moreover, correspond to those of the Aloes urine symptoms. Thus far, the success of the treatment leaves nothing to desire. But as the patient has been but a few weeks under the treatment, it is too soon to express a decided judgment or to entertain sanguine expectations of a cure.

SULPHUR.

WE use the sublimed Sulphur (flores sulphuris), triturated with sugar of milk, and then prepared in dilutions, *in modo Hahnemanni;* or alse a tincture prepared with alcohol. It is an ancient remedy, first mentioned as employed to purge the cities of Sodom and Gomorrah.

Ulysses used it to purify his palace by fumigation, after his terrible slaughter of the suitors who infested it.

(And perhaps the modern Ulysses may be able in like manner to purify the White House of the office-seekers and parasites who haunt it.)

Hippocrates and Pliny mention it. Pliny praises it in lumbago, and in lichen and prurigo of the face. And he says it cures cough with purulent expectoration and dyspnœa. Dioscorides speaks of its power to cure cutaneous eruptions, and especially itch.

Modern allopathic writers hold it in very moderate esteem. They ascribe to it first an exciting, but ultimately a depressing action; the peculiarity of exciting diaphoresis, and of producing semi-fluid stools; also, according to Giaccomini, brownish spots on the skin, and various ephemeral cutaneous eruptions. Its virtues as a specific for scabies they consider to depend upon its power to kill the acarus scabiei.

Hahnemann's extensive proving, published in the fifth volume of his chronic diseases, has been singularly confirmed by an elaborate proving made by the Austrian Homœopathic Society, under the leadership of Dr. Wurmb, and published in 1857.

We proceed at once to the

SPECIAL ANALYSIS.

Sensorium. Vertigo. This is most apt to occur in the morning, and is often accompanied by nose-bleed, although sometimes, like many other Sulphur symptoms, it occurs in the evening or at night when the patient is in bed. It is produced or aggravated by stooping and by walking in the open air, and by looking upon objects in rapid motion.

Much confusion and bewilderment of the sensorium. The memory is weakened.

Head. Headaches are not of an acute character. Sulphur unquestionably produces congestion of the head, and the headaches correspond to this condition. The pains are:

Heaviness, making every motion irksome, not only walking and stooping, but even motion of the head when sitting and lying. Pressing generally in the forehead and over the eyes; sometimes general, as if the head were encircled by an iron hoop; generally worse at night. Mercurius has a similar symptom. The headache is often attended by nausea. The hair falls out. The forehead is covered with acne.

Eyes. The lids swell, the margins are inflamed, are thickened and sore. They burn, are worse after washing. This aggravation after washing is characteristic of Sulphur. In the eye, heat or a biting burning, as from Ammonia. Moderate photophobia. The conjunctiva is reddened. Vision is perverted; there are sparks before the eyes and a red wheel appears to encircle the candle flame. White or dark spots float before the eyes, and objects are not seen distinctly.

Ears. Tearing pains in the ears. Stitches which likewise involve the parotid gland. Ringing, hissing and swashing noises in the ears. Transient deafness. Sometimes connected with the heavy headache there is over-sensibility of the auditory nerve.

Mouth. The gums swell; sometimes bleed. The teenth seem too long and loose, and pain in biting. Similar to Carbo vegetabilis and Lycopodium. Burning pain in the tongue, and burning vesicles upon it. Sometimes it is covered with an aphthous deposit. The tongue and mouth are coated with saltish mucus. There is dryness with thirst. (Unlike Pulsatilla.)

Throat. Burning, sensation of swelling, and constriction of the fauces.

Taste. Sweetish or flat, sometimes bitter, which is relieved by eating.

Appetite. Impaired. Aversion to meat and bread. Great and continued thirst.

Gastric Symptoms. Oppression after eating. Flatulence, lassitude, eructations putrid or sour, or tasting of the food. Waterbrash is a common symptom. Nausea and sometimes vomiting.

Stomach. Sulphur produces (and cures) a kind of stomach cramp; severe, griping pain in the epigastrium, with tenderness of the stomach and liver.

Abdomen. Pressure, stitches, in the upper part and sides of the abdomen; the stitches are aggravated by deep inspiration, by walking, and are conjoined with a sensation of burning.

In the region of the liver stitches from within outward. Feeling of tension and pressure in hepatic region and throughout the abdomen, with great depression of spirits. Burning in the abdomen worse by motion. Sensation in the abdomen of soreness or of internal rawness; worse on motion and deep inspiration, as well as at night.

Sensation of pressure downward and outward in region of the abdominal ring, with soreness and bruised sensation, not suffering the pressure of the hand.

Pressure in the hypogastrium and public region.

Stool. Before the stool, aching in the abdomen and intestines.

During the stool, nausea, heavy headache, painful pressure in the rectum.

After the stool, sensation of soreness and weakness in the intestines; general lassitude; pressing pain in the rectum and at the anus.

Sulphur constipates, with frequent ineffectual tenesums, both before and after stool, and constant pressing, even at night, followed by aching and sticking pain in the rectum and anus, often very severe and distressing. It appears, then, that, instead of inaction of the lower bowel, we have congestion, irritation of the muscular fiber and irregular, inharmonious action, resulting in tenesmus, and likewise hyperæsthesia.

Sulphur has a yellow or whitish mucus or watery diarrhœa, painless, almost involuntary, compelling one to rise early in the morning, and containing undigested food. Similar to Aloes, Bryonia and Podophyllum. Moreover, it produces a diarrhœa consisting of mucus streaked with blood, and preceded by colic, and attended by tenesmus and pain (like dysentery). It is characteristic that the blood is in thread-like streaks. Thus, it appears that whether the mucous membrane of the rectum and colon discharge bloody mucus or be unnaturally dry (whether there be constipation or the so-called diarrhœa), the inharmonious muscular action, irritation and hyperæsthesia are the same. The character of the evacuation does not afford a basis for division of symptoms into primary and secondary, and for a law of dose resting upon it.

There is also constipation, which, however, is always attended by fullness heat or itching at the anus and in the lower part of the rectum, whereas the constipation of Veratrum and Opium is simple inaction of the rectum, without concomitant symptoms.

In the rectum, burning and throbbing, with moist hæmorrhoids; itching and soreness.

Urinary Organs. The secretion is increased in quantity; evacuation frequent at night. The desire comes suddenly, and is imperative; if not gratified, the urine passes involuntarily; the stream is forcible.

This resembles Aloes.

Hepar sulphuris has the opposite, which is highly characteristic of that drug, and often an indication for it in affections of other organs of the body, *e. g.,* the stream of urine is slow to start, and very feeble and sluggish, falling in a right line rather than describing an arc.

The act of micturition is often preceded by cutting pains in the hypogastrium.

At the end, and after the act, cutting in the urethra. Also burning, tearing and biting in the urethra during the act.

Sexual Organs. Male. Inflammation of the orifice of the urethra and of the prepuce, which is thickened and red, and burns. In the testes, stitches and tension; sexual desire is increased.

Female. Menstruation appears to come too soon, and to be increased in quantity. It is preceded by various pains and symptoms, *e. g.,* dry, evening cough, colic, toothache, and accompanied, by abdominal cramps.

SULPHUR.

This, however, is not the only action. Menstruation is likewise delayed or suspended, and this symptoms, if accompanied by the night restlessness, constipation and other symptoms characteristic of Sulphur, affords a very valuable indication in practice. I have often found Sulphur successful where menstruation was suppressed, whether by cold during a previous period, or by unknown causes, and where Pulsatilla had been given without effect. Indeed, I think it more frequently indicated in amenorrhœa than pulsatilla.

Concomitants of menstruation are nose-bleed, rush of blood to the head, and pressure in the epigastrium.

Leucorrhœa which follows menstruation is yellow and acrid and thick.

Respiratory Organs. Nasal Membrane. Sneezing and violent coryza, alternately fluent and dry. The dryness predominating, with a troublesome obstruction of the nostrils, relieved temporarily by the occasional discharge of masses of thick muscus.

Throat. Rawness in the fauces, with hoarseness amounting at times to aphonia; at the same time there is much mucus in the bronchi, and this moving, with the respiration, produces a disposition to cough.

Cough. In general it is dry; occurs at night as well as by day. It is provoked by irritation in the region of the ensiform cartilage.

It produces soreness and shocks in the epigastrium and in the hypochondria. Besides this dry cough, there is a loose cough, provoked by the movement of mucus in the air-tubes, the sputa being thick, yellow and sometimes sweetish. The cough is often forcible, causing headache and gagging.

Dyspnœa. Considerable, especially at night; comes on suddenly on turning on the left side, relieved by sitting up. Lassitude and great heaviness in the chest.

Like the congestions and orgasms of the blood in the head, are the corresponding affections of the chest. They occur at night, and are aggravated by motion, and accompanied by heat and burning in the chest. The chest is sore externally.

Back. Lassitude, heaviness, soreness; the pains in the lumbar region are worse on walking, and especially on rising from a seat, than when sitting or lying. In the lumber region, a peculiar stiffness and a sudden loss of power on attempting to move, have led to the successful use of Sulphur in certain forms of lumbago.

Rhus toxicodendron and Petroleum have similar symptoms. Ruta and Staphysagria are indicated in a lumbago which is worse in the morning, before rising, and better after rising. That of Staphysagria compels the patients to get up at an unreasonably early hour.

Extremities. Lassitude, heaviness, burning. Induration of the axillary and inguinal glands; swelling of the hands and feet, with heat and tingling; soreness, tension in the muscles, and especially in the aponeuroses, and inability to move them. The pains are worse at night. The skin of the extremities, especially of the hands, presents a vesicular eruption, which discharges a yellowish water, and itches, being very sore when scratched. The skin chaps, and cracks at the joints. Ulceration at the sides and roots of the nails. Itching pustular eruption upon the elbow joints and backs of the hands.

PRACTICAL APPLICATIONS.

In the case of Sulphus has been made the first and only successful generalization in the way of indication for treatment based on pathological anatomy. It was made by Dr. Wurmb, of Vienna, in his studies of pneumonia (1852).

Speaking of Sulphur in pneumonia, he says:

"If the pneumonia be not complicated with other diseases, then generally there comes a period when the febrile storm subsides; the pains, the dyspnœa, etc., cease. In short, the patient feels himself greatly relieved so soon as the infiltration has become complete. At this period Art can have no other problem than to support Nature while she, for the sake of removing the exudation, increases the activity of the processes of absorption; or, on the other hand, to oppose Nature, in case she shows a disposition to get rid of the pneumonic infiltration by a purulent degeneration.

"Now, in our view, no remedy yet proved corresponds so well to these indications as Sulphur; none compares with it in point of certainty and celerity of action.

"Sulphur penetrates the entire organism even in its finest and most recondite portions. It increases the activity of vegetative life generally, and of the processes of secretion and absorption in particular. It accelerates the interchange of elements and makes it more pervading; in a word, it fulfills all the demands upon which the removal of an abnormal product is conditional. Upon these grounds we apply Sulphur to the removal of pneumonic infiltration, of serous exudations and of old as well as recent deposits in the skin, the parenchyma, the joints and the bones."

This masterly generalization is justified by the results of practice. It is a mode of seeking indications that is warranted by the facts, that provings on the healthy—the only absolutely certain source of indications for reating the sick—can never furnish us analogues of the exudations and infiltrations referred to by Wurmb. We must in such cases fall back on generalizations based jointly on pathology and pathogenesy.

This generalization will give us an explanation of the beneficial action of Sulphur in the second stage of exudative inflammation throughout the body; as in meningitis, ophthalmia, otitis, peritonitis, hæmorrhoidal tumors, pleuritis, pneumonia, periostitis, ostitis, adenitis, pericarditis.

But the generalization does not exhaust the subject of the applications of Sulphur. In puerperal peritonitis, at the very commencement of the disease, Sulphur is, I think, our most efficient remedy.

Even here there is an analogy to the second stage of an idiopathic inflammation. For it may be considered that the storm of invasion was exhausted by the labor of which the peritonitis is a sort of a sequel. And perhaps this view accounts in some measure for the asthenic character of this disease from the outset.

The skin diseases for which Sulphur is appropriate are papular, vesicular, or pustular eruptions, with the peculiar sensations already described.

As regards itch—scabies—if we restrict the term to the vesicular affections caused by the acarus, we must doubt the power of Sulphur to cure it specifically. If we use the term as Hahnemann and his contemporaries used it, to embrace impetigo, tinea, etc., Sulphur is one of our most efficient remedies.

Sulphur cures an unhealthy state of the skin in which it cracks, and in which slight scratches ulcerate and are slow to heal.

The kind of lumbago caused by Sulphur has been described.

In the second stage of acute articular rheumatism, where deposits are to be removed and where the feet in particular are affected, it is of great service.

In certain forms of paraplegia of children it often effects a cure.

Never prescribe this or any other drug without carefully comparing the symptoms of the case with those of the drug.

GENERAL VIEWS.

The limbs go to sleep easily; sensation of lassitude, weariness and soreness in the limbs and bone pains, as if the flesh were off the bones.

Prickling and itching of the skin, at night in bed. Old scars and spots begin again to itch; soreness but not burning.

A scabious, eczematous eruption like cow-pox.

Jerking spasms of individual limbs and attacks like epilepsy, preceded by a feeling in the arms and back as if a mouse ran up them.

Ebullitions of blood, the veins of the hands swollen and burning, and from this restlessness throughout the body. Cannot sit in one posture; must stretch out the hands, limbs and toes.

Sleepiness by day; in the afternoons; recurring after meals.

Late sleeping in the morning, not refreshed on waking. Sleepy in the evening, but cannot go to sleep for a long time; and during the night, wakeful, with excitement and restless tossing, and pressure of blood to head and chest. Wakes in affright. Lively and anxious dreams. Many symptoms come at night; burning in mouth, with thirst; nightmare; pains in hip joint; cramps in calves.

Fever. Mixed. Cold predominates.

Heat. Partial, and in the head and chest.

Excited, hasty, going from one subject to another; depressed and despondent.

GRAPHITES.

THIS remedy belongs exclusively to the Homœopathic Pharmacopœia. It was classed by Hahnemann among the "Antipsoric Remedies," as being more especially adapted to the treatment of chronic diseases. We shall see that it is sometimes called for in acute affections.

In his introduction to the proving, Hahnemann says:

"The purest Graphite is a kind of mineral carbon. Its slight contingent of iron may be regarded rather as an admixture than as an essential constituent, as was fully proved by Davy's conversion of the diamond into Graphites by treating it with Potassium."

He continues:

"The first idea of its use in medicine was given to Dr. Weinhold, during his travels in Italy, by some workmen in a looking-glass factory in Venice, whom he saw using Graphites as an external application for the removal of eruptions. He imitated them and described the result in a little work, entitled "Graphites as a Remedy for Eruptions. 1812."

Hahnemann's proving is published in the "Chronic Diseases."

The action upon the sensorium is not marked. Upon the head, confusion and pressure, chiefly in the forehead, and a drawing pain from the forehead extending down the face to the throat. So, liwewise, the pain of constriction extends down the occiput to the nape of the neck. The headache is often very violent every morning, causing cold sweat and faintness.

Externally, the action of Graphites is noteworthy. Scabby eruptions, exuding moisture, appear on the scalp; they are sore when touched, and cause the hair to fall out. This furnishes an indication for Graphites in tinea capitis. We meet here the first example of the skin affection of Graphites,—a moist, scabby eruption. Lycopodium has a dry, scaly eruption. Mezereum, a thick, hard scab, from under which, when it is pressed, thick pus exudes. Hepar sulphuris, a scab easily torn off, and which leaves a raw and bleeding surface.

Viola tricolor in tinea capitis is indicated by the peculiar odor of the urine of the patient. It smells like cat's urine.

Face. The complexion is pale and sallow; the eye sunken. The muscles of one side of the face are contracted, and speech is difficult. Externally, a kind of erysipelas, with a burning, sticking pain.

In acute facial erysipelas, in which Belladonna and Rhus are so often indicated and serviceable, Graphites or Euphorbium or Apis may be required.

If so, they are particularly indicated by symptoms of other organs. So may Carbo animalis.

Eyes. Paralytic heaviness of the lids. Vision is so affected that myopia results. Photophobia, heat, biting lachrymation, and pressing, aching pain in the globe which extends to the head. Also stitching pains in the eye from looking on white objects. Ulceration of the margins of the lids. Where hordeola recur frequently, although each one is relieved by Pulsatilla, Graphites or Staphysagria may be indicated by the general symptoms, and each has been beneficial in many cases.

Ears. Various noises in the ears, rushing, ringing and hissing. These noises and a clucking or cracking noise are produced by stooping and rising again, by eructation, by eating, and generally by moving the jaw. These symptoms point (analogous to Silicea, Lachesis and Gelseminum) to an affection of the Eustachian tube (and perhaps the meatus externus). Graphites has been of service in many cases of deafness. Itching of the external ear and of the cheek in front of the ear. Where the parts have been scratched lymph exudes, and "a raw" is established.

In a crevice behind the ear a crack, raw, moist and quite painful, similar to the cracks in chapped hands.

Similar cracks are observed in this locality in children during the age of dentition or after it. Graphites is a valuable remedy. So is Calcarea carbonica, which may be indicated in preference by other symptoms.

Nose. Increased acuteness of the sense of smell. Scabs in the anterior nares; occasional epistaxis, with fullness of head and heat of face.

Mouth. Around the mouth and on the lips and chin, eruption and scabby ulcers; swelling of the sub-maxillary glands. The breath is offensive, or smells of urine.

Gums swollen and sore. The toothache is worse in bed and from warmth.

A kind of spasm in the throat, as if deglutition were impossible.

Digestive Tract and Function. The tongue is much coated; the taste is bitter, there is much hiccough and eructation of bitter or sour green water.

Aversion to meat and to sweets; much thirst; nausea, even when there is strong hunger. Graphites produces many symptoms after eating, such as headache, sleepiness, waterbrash, burning in the eyes, colic, fullness in the abdomen. Cutting, burning and drawing pains in the abdomen. Especially, however, is the abdomen tense, as though distended with flatus, which appears to be incarcerated in various parts of the abdomen. Pressing toward the abdominal ring before discharge of flatus. These symptoms—the abnormal sensations and accessory symptoms after eating, the accumulations of flatus—indicate slow and imperfect digestion, a condition which is demonstrated by the stool so characteristic of the Graphites diarrhœa, viz., pappy, half-digested brown stool, of a most atrocious odor.

Rectum. In the rectum, violent stitches, a smarting or cutting and sore pain; also much itching. The anus is swollen, the veins enlarged, protruding and sore. These symptoms have led to the successful use of Graphites in that painful affection, "fissure of the anus," which can be cured by homœopathic remedies speedily and permanently, and needs no surgical intervention. Ignatia, Nitric acid, Platina, Plumbum, Pæonia alba, and Ratanhia, are other remedies that may be required, and have proved successful in "fissure of the anus."

Stool. Two conditions obtain. Constipation,—the stools are hard, lumpy, and evacuated with effort, and often accompanied with mucus or blood. There is sometimes ineffectual tenesmus. On the other hand, there is diarrhœa; stools not frequent, generally in the forenoon; pappy, brown, containing half-digested food, and of an atrocious, almost putrid odor, not attended with pain, but often accompanied by discharge of flatus. I cannot say which of these series of symptoms is primary and which secondary. In reference to a recent much-pushed theory, I am constrained to say that, as regards the dose, it makes no difference which is primary and which secondary. With the 200th I have cured constipation, and with the 200th I have cured diarrhœa.

Urine is diminished in quantity. A cutting pain accompanies the evacuation. Urine is dark and has a white or a reddish deposit.

Male Sexual Organs. The sexual appetite is decidedly increased, but the power is diminished, ejaculation of semen taking place before the erection is complete. By virtue of this action, Graphites has been of service in sexual weaknesses, consisting of lively desire with incomplete erection, and too rapid or too early discharge of semen, such as sometimes follows the habit of masturbation, acquired in boyhood and abandoned early.

Testes Swollen. It is noteworthy that Graphites has been successfully used in treating hydrocele. Other remedies are Clematis, Rhododendron, Aurum and Spongia.

The Female Sexual Organs present many symptoms that point to Graphites as a remedy for corresponding maladies.

Menses are delayed and are scanty; they are imminent for several days before the flow fairly sets in. The onset is accompanied by a variety of accessory symptoms (as with Sepia), such as hoarseness with dry cough, headache evenings, swelling of the feet and painless swelling of the cheeks, chilliness, colic-like labor-pains, backache.

Hahnemann says that Graphites is often indispensable where obstinate constipation and delayed menstruation are wont to occur together.

Leucorrhœa copious and thin, causing a biting, smarting sensation in the vagina.

GRAPHITES. 399

Upon the respiratory organs the action of Graphites is not marked. It produces coryza, hoarseness toward evening, attended by headache; rawness in the chest and a tickling in the throat, provoking a dry cough, the peculiarities of which, however, are not apparent. There is some dyspnœa.

Externally, the nipples are painful and tender, and disposed to become fissured.

Clinical experience has shown Graphites to be a valuable remedy in "sore nipples" of nursing women. The end of the nipple presents cracks and fissures from which exudes a limpid serum. This disposition to fissures or cracks in the integument seems characteristic of Graphites.

In the extremities, besides aching and drawing sensations and the indefinite feeling of lassitude, common to so many drugs which act profoundly on the system, we have no marked action save that on the skin, viz., erysipelas of the hands, eczema of the fingers, eczema and impetigo on the lower extremities and toes. There are sticking pains in these eruptions and much soreness. Eczema between the lower extremities and upon the male genitals is an effect of Graphites.

The feet sweat profusely; the sweat is not offensive as under Silicea, but moderate walking causes soreness between the toes, so that the parts become raw. Finally the sides and roots of the finger and toe nails become sore, uncerate and swell and are exceedingly painful.

GRAPHITES.

Graphites is one of our best remedies in that painful affection loosely called "the ingrowing toe-nail." Silicea and Hepar sulphuris are also of value, and must be chosen in preference if general symptoms require it.

As regards sleep, Graphites produces great sleepiness by day; and the patient goes to sleep early in the evening, but during the night there is wakefulness, tossing, heat and 'anxiety (symptoms much like those of Sulphur). Dreams are anxious and terrifying. At last patient sinks into a profound and dull morning sleep. (This is not like Sulphur.)

Fever has been observed. Coldness predominates —a daily paroxysm—in the evening. It begins with shivering followed by heat of the face and cold feet, followed by sweat in the morning.

Generally a moderate exertion brings on sweat.

The disposition is excited and irritable

The action on the skin is very marked: moist eruption, eczema, impetigo, and fissure or cracks on the fingers, at the corners of the mouth, on the nipples, at the anus and between the toes.

Already-existing ulcers become tender to touch and motion, with tearing and sticking pains.

The action of Graphites on the skin, the digestive apparatus and the male and female sexual organs, is of great importance. It is eminently a "polychrest."

LACHESIS.

VENOM OF LACHESIS TRIGONOCEPHALUS.

IT was procured by Dr. C. Hering, and proved under his auspices. The results were published in "Archiv," and in his monograph "Schlangengift."

The symptoms given by him are both those of the bite and those produced by internal use. There is an evident correspondence between the two varieties of symptoms, the latter presenting finer shades of subjective symptoms than could be observed under the severe effects of the bite.

Sensorium. Absence of mind, inability to think; has to think how words are spelled; errors in writing and reading; vertigo; giddiness, especially on closing the eyes, on sitting or lying down (Theridion); vertigo, with staggering; deadly paleness (nausea and vomiting sometimes).

Head. Pains deep seated in various parts of the head, worse on the left side. In the left frontal protuberance a sore pain, worse early in the morning—worse on pressing the parts; sore aching above the eyes, extending to the root of the nose and down the nose; heaviness on waking, with nausea and vertigo, such as is produced by exposure to the heat of the sun; curative in sunstroke; pressing pain in the forehead from within outward; bursting throbbing and undulating pain in the forehead, generally worse after sleep and on stooping, attended by vertigo and sometimes by nausea and by weakness of the limbs and of the mind.

Scalp. Sensitive, especially the left side, as if it had been burned by the sun.

Eyes. Most of the symptoms are subjective, and consist of pains above the eyes; aching and pressure in the eyes, worse on touch and motion; and itching and stinging in the eyes.

Given on the strength of these symptoms, and others affecting other organs, Lachesis has been curative in inflammation of the margins of the lids, and in ulceration of the cornea. Vision is affected; it becomes weak—objects are not easily discerned; there is a mist before the eyes, also black flickering objects before the eyes, and a bright ring around the candle flame.

Ears. Soreness of the mastoid region; swelling between the ear and mastoid process, with stiffness, pain and throbbing; stinging and piercing pain deep in the left ear, with a disagreeable sensation between the ear and throat. The ears feel obstructed, and there is deafness; at the same time abnormal sounds are heard in the ears—chirping, roaring and the hammering sensation or sound which is peculiar to Lachesis. These sounds cease for a while after inserting the finger in the external meatus and shaking it. They probably depend upon obstruction of the Eustachian tube.

Nose. Epistaxis is a frequent symptoms both from bites and from internal use. It precedes the menses, accompanies the headache, occuring especially early in the morning, and is often induced by blowing the nose.

Soreness with discharge of water, and the soreness remains long after the coryza has ceased. Obstinate coryza, alternately fluent and dry, breaking out suddenly.

Lachesis has proved a valuable remedy in obstinate coryza, in complaints seeming to depend on suppressed coryza, and in the sequelæ of influenza; also is ozœna with suspicion of a syphilitic taint.

Face. Complexion pale, yellow, earthy. Eyes sunken.

Prosopalgia. Tearing above the orbit. Drawing and tearing in the malar bone, extending to the ear. Digging and screwing around in the malar bone. Swelling of the face, closing the eyes, worse on the left side.

Erysipelas of the face, worse under the left eye; swelling of the lip, distortion of the face.

Teeth and Jaws. Tearing and throbbing, especially about the roots of the teeth, worse after sleep and by cold or warm drinks, with swelling of the gums (ending in discharge of pus). An excellent remedy in periodontitis from dead never pulp in the fang of decayed or plugged molar, which must end in abscess. The gums bleed easily.

Mouth. Burning in the mouth and soreness of the roof of the mouth.

Ptyalism. Burning as from pepper. Tongue white, yellow, blackish. Tongue stiff, difficult to protrude. It trembles when protruded. Paralysis of the tongue.

Tongue swollen; ulcerated.

Gangrene of the tongue. Difficult speech, as if the tongue were too heavy. Unintelligible talking after an apoplectic fit.

Inflammatory swelling of the velum pendulum palati.

Pharynx and Œsophagus. Feeling of hollowness in the throat, as if the pharynx had disappeared. (Phytolacca decandra.) Rawness in the pharynx. Sensation as of a lumb in the pharynx, generally on the left side, impeding deglutition, worse on deglutition, and a sharp pain then goes into the ear. Constant desire to swallow, as if a sponge or a button adhered to the left side of the pharynx worse from swallowing food. Lumps dark red, with ulcers or gangrenous spots. Fetor of breath.

Difficult deglutition. Abnormal contractions of pharyngeal muscles; food returns by the nose. As if a piece of dry skin were in the pharynx.

(Tonsillitis beginning on the left side. Lycopodium where it begins on the right side. Lippe.)

Taste. Bad, bitter, putrid, flat. Loss of appetite, but faintness from fasting. Empty, faint feeling in the stomach. Weakness of digestion, distress from food, especially in drunkards.

Stomach. Regurgitation of food. Nausea and vomiting with vertigo and faintness. Tenderness in the epigastrium. Gnawing before a meal. Pressure toward the heart. All the symptoms are worse after sleep. Sensation in the stomach and abdomen, as if a lump were accumulating.

Hypochondria. Cannot bear tight clothing about hypochondria (characteristic). Pain as if ulcerated on coughing. Pain in the liver as if forming a lump, as if something had lodged there.

Abdomen. Tension. Pain as if diarrhœa would set in. Stitches in various directions, as from the right os ilium through the abdomen and chest as far as the shoulder. Stabbings during the menses, soreness and sharp pain in the left ovarian region, cannot lie on the left side because it hangs and rolls over. Sensitive; cannot, when standing, bear down weight and pressure of clothing; must hold it up, it produces pressure on the uterus.

Painful swelling and induration in the right side of the abdomen, between the crista ilii and umbilicus; burning, pulsating, etc., and pains extending to the hip joints, etc.

Stool. Constipation. Hard fragments like sheep-dung; difficult evacuations, as from spasm of the sphincter; feels as if fæces press against it without passing.

Stools light colored, and alternately loose and dry and hard.

Cadaverous odor of diarrhœic stool. Blood and pus.

Drawing and hammering in the anus. Urging as of stool, worse when sitting; makes lame, cannot rise. Prolapsus ani, with bleeding.

Urinary organs. Micturition frequent. Urine scanty and dark, and turbid with dark sediment.

Male sexual organs. Depressed condition.

Female. Menses scanty and inclined to delay, preceded and attended by many accessory symptoms (nervous attacks). Leucorrhœa *before* menses, copious and acrid and thick. Uterus very sensitive to contact. Cannot bear external pressure on the uterine region nor the weight of clothes.

At the climacteric period flashes of heat. Pain in the uterine region, increasing day by day till a bloody discharge appears, then ceasing, to re-appear in a few days.

Larynx and Cough. Pain when touching the larynx and on lying down. Throbbing and sensation of narrowness. Swelling sensation, rawness, scraping and desire to swallow. Sensation as of a plug which moves up and down, with short cough. Hoarseness, worse in the evening, and with a sensation as of something which ought to be hawked up.

Cough generally dry, spasmodic, provoked by tickling in the throat, by smoke, by pressure on the larynx as by touch, throwing the head back, etc.; worse every time he wakes; worse from eating; has always to leave the table. Sometimes mucus and bloody (latter generally when sympathetic with heart trouble), again thick yellow sputa in suspected phthisis pulmonalis.

Chest. Dyspnœa on exertion, or attending other symptoms. In paroxysms, suffocative fullness. Cannot lie down; must have windows open. Stitch in the left side, with dyspnœa, worse when coughing or on inspiration; neglected pneumonia.

Spasmodic pain about the heart. Constrictive sensation in the region of the heart. Irregular beating of the heart; every intermission attended by strange sensation in the heart, and as if the circulation were restored by coughing a little. Palpitation, with anxiety and weakness; spasmodic, suffocative feeling, with palpitation on exertion.

Trunk. Pain in the loins. Stiffness from the sacrum to the loins, and extending down the thighs (with tenderness in the right ileo-cœcal region). Drawing pains and stiffness in the back and nape. Beating in the back and anus as with little hammers.

Great painfulness of the neck to touch and pressure. Outer swelling with inward inflammation and soreness. Swelling and pain in the submaxillary and parotid region.

Lameness, tension and *numbness* in the hands and feet. Limbs weak, weary and trembling.

Ulcers bluish, livid, worse in the evening, surrounded by smaller ulcers, and burn when touched.

Sleep. Drowsiness and stupor all the time. At night easily disturbed, not refreshed, always worse after sleep.

Fever. Not regular, periodic. Fever of low type; prostrate with stupor; muttering; sunken face, dropping of the jaw, red or black tongue, cracked and bleeding, and which trembles when protruded.

Skin. Ulcers, etc. Gangrene traumatic, of an ashy gray color and very offensive.

General symptoms. Languor, weariness, pains. Aching in bones. Awkward stumbling gait, numbness of the hands and feet, paralysis, mental and bodily languor. Constant desire for rest. Faintness. trembling. Vertigo.

Disposition. Depression, melancholy. Anxiety about her illness, nervous irritability. Inertness.

APPLICATIONS.

Lachesis, in common with other serpent poisons, produces, first, direct weakness of the heart's action; second weakened respiration and difficult deglutition; third, an incoagulable condition of the blood, and third, as Mitchell proved by experiment with Crotalus venom, actual disorganization of the muscular tissue. Locally it produces gangrene.

From this we may have, first, death from syncope or suffocation; second, ecchymoses and death from blood disorder; third, local gangrene.

Again, we have special peculiarities of heart and throat symptoms, etc., with characterize Lachesis.

The throat action begins, according to Lippe, on the left side, and extends to the ear, accompanied by tightness in the larynx. Internally, deep red or purple; externally, swelling as though the cellular tissue were infiltrated; external tenderness, no coating of tongue like mercury; no defined sharp prick like Hepar sulphuris, nor fever, etc., like Belladonna, which has bright redness.

Scarlatina, two applications; first, in the foudroyant style of invasion; second, when there is infiltration and threatened sloughing of the throat and gangrene.

Typhilitis. Hæmorrhoids. Diseases of women. Cough, etc.

In neglected pneumonia, or when resolution lingers, or after whooping cough.

Heart affection, weakness of action, palpitation, irregular beats, aching, etc., but especially cannot lie down, and cough sympathetic. Ulcers. Paralysis.

[This paper is supplemented by an additional one on the same drug in the second volume.]

LECTURES

ON

MATERIA MEDICA.

FIFTH EDITION
(*SECOND INDIAN*)

BY

CARROLL DUNHAM, M. D.
AUTHOR OF "HOMŒOPATHY THE SCIENCE OF THERAPEUTICS."

CONTENTS.

		PAGE.
I.	PRINCIPLES OF HOMŒOPATHY—PRINCIPLES *vs.* PRACTICAL KNOWLEDGE	1
II.	SYMPTOMS, THEIR STUDY; OR "HOW TO TAKE THE CASE"	25
III.	THE ANAMNESIS	49
IV.	PULSATILLA	57
V.	CYCLAMEN EUROPÆUM	80
VI.	EUPHRASIA OFFICINALIS	98
VII.	ALLIUM CEPA	105
VIII.	MATRICARIA CHAMOMILLA	108
IX.	IGNATIA AMARA	122
X.	PLATINA	129
XI.	SEPIA	138
XII.	MUREX PURPUREA	158
XIII.	KREASOTUM	164
XIV.	SECALE CORNUTUM	169
XV.	JUNIPERUS SABINA	175
XVI.	ACHILLÆA MILLEFOLIUM	177
XVII.	ARSENICUM ALBUM	178
XVIII.	HYDRARGYRUM	208
XIX.	CUCUMIS COLOCYNTHIS	231
XX.	PODOPHYLLUM PELTATUM	239
XXI.	LACHESIS	243
XXII.	LYCOPODIUM CLAVATUM	256

CONTENTS.

		PAGE.
XXIII.	NATRUM MURIATICUM	266
XXIV.	VERATRUM ALRUM	272
XXV.	HEPAR SULPHURIS CALCAREUM .	280
XXVI.	DULCAMARA	287
XXVII.	CALCAREA CARBONICA	307
XXVIII.	CAUSTICUM	317
XXIX.	NITRIC ACID	320
XXX.	CARBO VEGETABILIS	325
XXXI.	CARBO ANIMALIS	332
XXXII.	APIUM VIRUS	333
XXXIII.	PHOSPHORUS	338
XXXIV.	COCCULUS INDICUS	346
XXXV.	CONIUM MACULATUM	362
XXXVI.	CINA	367
XXXVII.	THE ART AND MODE OF PRESCRIBING	386
XXXVIII.	PATHOGNOMONIC SYMPTOMS AND CHARACTERISTIC SYMPTOMS . .	392
XXXIX.	VALEDICTORY ADDRESS	402

PRINCIPLES OF HOMŒOPATHY.—PRINCIPLES vs. PRACTICAL KNOWLEDGE.

IN entering upon the general consideration of any subject involving a number of topics, it is expedient always to seek to obtain at the very outset a clear view of the scope, and extent of the subject to comprehend what it involves and to perceive what are its limits and what its relations with other kindred subjects. Let us begin our course by doing this with reference to homœopathy, the principles of which it is my duty to lay before you.

You all know that by homœopathy is generally understood that system of practical medicine, in accordance with which the physician seeks to cure his patient by giving him a remedy which has been known to produce in the healthy subject symptoms similar to those which the patient presents. It is a system claiming to be the only scientific system of medicine, inasmuch as it possesses a "law of cure" as it is termed; or, as it might be more correctly expressed, a law for the selection of the remedy in any concrete case of illness; the law expressed by the now familiar formula—*"Similia similibus curantur."*

You will hear also that homœopathy is called the science of therapeutics, and I will add that it is the only therapeusis which exists possessing the elements of a natural science; that it is the only science of therapeutics. Now, by therapeusis or therapeutics, we mean the science of treating diseased persons by means of drugs.

We thus arrive at a view of the limits and scope of our subject, homœopathy. It is a therapeutics. It deals with the science and method of treating the sick by means of drugs. And this is its whole scope. As homœopathists strictly, and confining yourselves to the application of the science of homœopathy, you will perform your entire function when you accurately select and rightly administer a suitable drug to your patient.

But you will go forth from these halls as doctors of medicine. Shall you have no other professional duties toward your patients than to administer drugs to them? Assuredly you will. Then you must be homœopathists and something beside.

The injuries and accidents to which men are exposed, involving destructive injury to limb or tissues, may require the interference of the operative surgeon. As such you will act under the law of mechanics, guided by your knowledge of anatomy and physiology, and governed by the traditions and maxims of surgery. It is true that few surgical cases occur which do not sooner or later involve the entire organism in such a way that the patient's condition demands the co-operation of the therapeutist; and as you will combine in your own person the function of operative surgeon and therapeutist, you, who have when operating, acted outside of your office as homœopathist or therapeutist, will now select and administer a drug suited to the condition of your patient, in accordance with the therapeutic law. You will, thus, in treating this case, act in a double capacity. You will be both an operative surgeon and a prescriber of drugs. It is in the latter capacity only that you will be a therapeutist, that you will practice homœopathy. It is true that your possession of a science of therapeutics will make the intervention of operative surgery much less frequently necessary than it is deemed to be by our allopathic brethren, who have no science of therapeutics. For homœopathy gives us the means of curing many diseases formerly supposed to require mechanical treatment; and in so far your function as homœopathist will encroach on that of surgeon. Yet the two are in a scientific aspect entirely distinct, and may not be confounded, unless you would introduce confusion into your views of the principles of medicine.

So, likewise, as obstetrician, you are called upon to superintend the physiological process of parturition, to prevent accidents or to remedy them; to anticipate or to cure diseases that may complicate the process. Some of your interference will be mechanical, as when you turn the child or use instruments. Such interference does not come under the scope of homœopathy. It belongs to another department of science and art. Another kind of treatment for the abnormal conditions which may supervene during parturition, consists in the administration of drugs in accordance with the homœopathic law. In doing this you are acting of course within the limits of the science of homœopathy, being therapeutists. Thus in the practice of obstetrics you fill a double office; you are therapeutists, and as such, homœopathists, and may also be operative surgeons, exercising another art.

Here again homœopathy puts us in possession of remedial means which, in a great many cases, obviate the necessity of resorting to mechanical interfernce, because they enable us to prevent the occurrence of morbid states which lead to conditions requiring such interference; and thus the function of the homœopathic therapeutist circumscribes that of the operative obstetrician, as it is laid down in the text-books of the allopathists. And it should be our aim so to develop our therapeutic science as still further to circumscribe its limit and do away with the necessity for operative interference. For instance, if I may venture to spend a moment on this subject, homœopathy, as a system of therapeutics, educating our powers of observation and sharpening our clinical foresight, enables us to anticipate the recurrence of uterine hæmorrhage as an incident of parturition, and so to prescribe that we prevent or control it; thus making the mechanical appliances so frequently resorted to by the allopathists at least so seldom requisite that some homœopathists have affirmed that the tampon, etc., can never be required. In the same way and to the same extent of rarest use or absolute disuse has homœopathy brought the entire apparatus of pessaries and supporters and bandages for the treatment of uterine disease. In these cases, as in other similar cases, it will be for you, in the exercise of a sound judgment, to determine whether the best interests of your patient demand that you shall act solely as operative surgeon, or solely as therapeutist, or whether you shall combine these functions. You cannot exercise this sound discretion aright unless you are fully instructed in both departments of science, unless you know all that can be effected by therapeutics from the stand-point of the homœopathist, and know also the resources and limits of operative surgery. The point which I wish to make is that as doctors of medicine you combine in yourselves the functions of therapeutist, surgeon and obstetrician; and that in the latter capacity you do not, cannot, and are not called upon to act as homœopathists, inasmuch as the homœopathic law applies only to the selection of drugs for diseased conditions.

Once more, hygiene is that department of medical science which includes the prevention of disease, and the removal or cancellation of material causes which induce or perpetuate disease. The advances of physiology and pathology, chemistry and natural history, within the last thirty years, have given to sanitary science a scope and importance which were not heretofore imagined. Many epidemic diseases have been shown to be dependent upon the conditions in which the individual, the family and the community live—conditions which by knowledge and care might be obviated. I refer in general to improper drainage of the soil, deficient ventilation, unwholesome food and drink, lack of light and heat, injurious occupations, improper social habits and relations. Surely the doctor of medicine can have no more important business than the prevention of disease by diligent endeavor,—whether as a public officer or as the medical adviser of a family or of an individual,— to modify unfavourable conditions, and thereby remove material causes of disease, and place those with whose care he is charged under circumstances most favourable to health. In doing this you will apply the principles of chemistry or of mechanics or of vegetable physiology; and although fulfilling one of your most important vocations, you, who will style yourselves homœopathic physicians, will not be acting within the scope of homœopathy; will not be applying its law of cure. You will, as hygienists, have nothing to do with homœopathy.

Furthermore, it has been ascertained by modern research, that certain diseases depend for their perpetuation, if not wholly for their origin, upon parasitic vegetable or animal growths, the removal of which by chemical or mechanical means is an essential condition of speedy cure. While you effect this removal by such means, you are fulfilling your duty as those intrusted with the care of the sick, just as faithfully and fully as when you administer, in accordance with the homœopathic law, the remedy which shall so change the vital processes of the patient as that his body shall no longer be a favorable nidus for these parasitic germs. But remember that when you seek the aid of chemistry or of mechanics to remove these parasites, you are not exercising your vocation as homœopathists, because you are acting as hygienists, not as therapeutists; you are not combating disease by drugs.

I lay stress upon these instances. I desire to show clearly, and impress upon your minds the fact, that homœopathy applies only to the treatment of the sick by means of drugs; because, unless your minds are clear upon this point, unless you perceive plainly that as curators of the sick you have other functions beside that very important and essential one of administering drugs, you may err as many do who strive to apply the homœopathic law of cure to their every action as medical men; and to make it cover not only their treatment by drugs, but also the surgical, obstetrical, hygienic, chemical and mechanical expedients and procedures. They come into the dilemma, that either dreading to prove recreant to their guiding principle, which they cannot perceive to lead them in any of these procedures, they neglect something which is essential to their patient's safety or recovery, and thus fail of their duty as doctors; or else, resorting to measures which their common sense and experience show to be necessary, they attempt to explain them in such a way as to bring them under the homœopathic law, and thus make themselves ridiculous and bring ridicule upon the science which as therapeutists they profess and honor.

Remember, then, the scope and limits of homœopathy. It is the science of therapeutics, and concerns only the treatment of the sick by means of drugs. Do not misunderstand me, and think me to say, inasmuch as I am a homœopathist, that therefore I believe diseases are to be treated only by drugs. Being a science, the elements of which are natural phenomena, viz.: those of the sick and the phenomena of drugs in their relation to the living human being, homœopathy takes rank with the other natural physical sciences.

For the better understanding of our subject let us take a general view of the nature and elements of a physical science. The physical sciences are variously arranged. There are sciences of classification, and sciences which are pursued with a view to the practical application of the knowledge they afford us to the affairs of daily life. But all of them deal with the phenomena of the physical universe as we observe them by means of our senses, aided by the resources of art. Let us study for a moment the science of astronomy, the most perfect and least complicated of the physical sciences. It deals with the phenomena of the bodies which compose the universe. We observe these phenomena, which consist of the movements of the heavenly bodies in space and upon their axes; and our observation is assisted by whatever instruments the ingenuity of man has contrived for the purpose, every successive invention enabling us to discover some new feature of these phenomena. In observations of the movements of the heavenly bodies we observe their movements in relation to each other. This is obvious, since the motion of one body is perceptible only in relation to some other body. Our object is to understand the relations of the heavenly bodies to each other in respect of their phenomena, and then to be able to foresee and predict what will be their relations and relative positions at some future time. We accomplish this object when, by virtue of our studies of the phenomena of the heavenly bodies and their relations, we are able to foretell the occurrence of eclipses at definite times, and to indicate, years beforehand, the position of the heavenly bodies at a given time.

I ask you now to notice several facts respecting this science.

First: In all its processes we never think of bringing in the question—what is the *cause* of the motion of the heavenly bodies? Such a question must present itself of course to every reflecting mind; but its consideration belongs to the speculative or metaphysical sciences, and has nothing to do with astronomy proper, or celestial mechanics, —is certainly in no sense and to no degree a basis of it. Out opinions on this point may be most various; yet this variety will not prevent our perfect agreement in the processes and conclusions of astronomy when considering the relations of, say two heavenly bodies.

Second: Astronomy deals with two series of phenomena, viz.: those of the two heavenly bodies, or systems of bodies, under consideration. And this science reckons the effects of one body or system of bodies upon the other in accordance with some law or formula which is general, applying to all bodies, and which expresses the mechanical action of bodies upon each other as regards mass and distance; in other words, their mechanical relations to each other.

Third: This law or formula, expressing the relation of bodies to each other, was perceived in a single instance. The mind which perceived it formed at once the hypothesis that it was a general formula expressive of the relation which exists between all bodies. A vast number of experiments and observations having confirmed this hypothesis, it is now universally accepted as the law of the mechanical relations of bodies.

Fourth: Observe that this law, which is a bare statement that bodies attract each other directly as their mass, and inversely as the square of their distances, is not based upon any theory of the nature of attraction—how it is that one body attracts another. Myriads of hypotheses on this subject might be framed, defended and overthrown, yet this formula would remain unshaken. It expresses the relations of phenomena which we observe, and nothing more—the relations therefore of what we know. For, what besides phenomena can we know—phenomena or things which are apparent to our senses, which may be seen and touched, smelt and tasted and heard. How disastrous would it be if in our science of astronomy the phenomena were limited by a law or formula based upon a theory of the cause of attraction. Phenomena we see and apprehend, and may be said to know, but the causes of them no man has seen or touched. Causes are hidden from our senses. We can reach them only by the action of the mind in hypothetic speculation. It must needs be that with every advance in observation a new hypothesis would spring up, overturning former doctrines of causation, and with them whatever laws or formulæ might be based upon them; and if the central formula of the science rested on them, it would be overturned to give place for a brief interval to some as short-lived successor. Progressive knowledge would be impossible on such a basis.

Fifth: Observe, finally, that one great object of the cultivation of this science is, that it affords us the means of prevision; it enables us to foretell events within its domain. And this is true of all the natural sciences when constructed on a sound basis. It would, therefore, furnish a test of the soundness of a science so called. For, on ultimate analysis, every natural science (save those of classification) consists of two series of phenomena connected by a law expressive of their relation to each other. Now, in the application of the science to the purpose of prevision the problem is this: Given one series of phenomena and the law of relation to find the other series of phenomena, to foretell what they will be. This problem is continually applied in astronomy, and the results uniformly attest the accuracy of the method.

In conclusion, then, this episode enables us to state understandingly the elements of a natural science. They consist of two series of phenomena (the results of observation) and a law which expresses a uniform and invariable relation between these series of phenomena. The phenomena must be susceptible of indefinite exploration, study and elaboration without disturbing the law of relation.

The law must be such as will enable us to foresee and predict future events. One series of phenomena and the law being given, we must be able to indicate the other series of phenomena; and this in advance of any observation of them or of any experiment.

Such must be the structure and the elements of the science of therapeutics, the only possible science the elements of which are capable of being developed independently by study and experiment and observation without detriment to the science as a whole, and which in its integrity will enable us to foretell the future, will put it in our power, having one series of phenomena and the law, to predict the other series.

Therapeutics being the science of treating the sick with drugs, it must deal with two series of phenomena, viz.: those of the sick and those of the drug as it affects the living human body; and it must present us with a law expressive of some constant and general relation between the phenomena of the sick and the phenomena of the drug as it acts on the human body. And by means of this law we must be able to foretell events. If we have the phenomena of the sick and the law, we must be able to tell correctly what shall be the phenomena of the drug which will cure the patient, even though no such experience has ever been had. Or, conversely, having the phenomena of the drug as it acts on the human body and the law, we must be able to tell what phenomena of disease that drug will remove, even though none such have ever been witnessed or experimented with. Now, gentlemen, homœopathy is just such a science of therapeutics. It has again and again submitted to this test, and has come forth triumphant. It possesses this law, which is not interfered with by the indefinite expansion of the phenomena with which it deals. I proceed to state it in detail in the light of what has been said.

The object of your study as medical practitioners is of course the patient—the sick person who sends for you. Your first care is to ascertain if he be really sick. He states perhaps that some organ is the seat of pain, that some function is not properly performed, or that the unusual appearance of some part of his body has attracted his attention and excited his alarm; and now he asks your opinion, advice and assistance. He wishes to know what ails him, what will be the issue of his sickness, and how long it will last, and finally he wishes you to assuage his sufferings and restore him to health as quickly, safely and gently as you can. The first question is this, Is the patient sick? Is any organ or tissue in an unnatural condition? Is any function arrested, or performed in an unnatural manner? You compare the patient with your recollection of a sound and healthy man. Your knowledge of anatomy will enable you in this comparison to detect abnormal conditions of organs or tissues. Your knowledge of physiology puts it in your power to discern the abnormal performance of functions. In a word, you observe whatever of a material character is wrong with your patient. Where it is possible you assist your senses by instruments. The functions of respiration and circulation are inspected by means of the stethoscope; the tissues of the eye by means of the ophthalmoscope; of the ear by the otoscope; the tissues and, to some extent, the functions of the larynx, by the laryngoscope; the renewal and waste of tissue, to some extent, by the thermometer; to some extent, by chemical examination, the excretions and secretions. These examinations, which are made by the aid of a comparison of the patient with our recollection of a standard, healthy, living human being, furnish us with the objective phenomena which the patient presents. Besides these there is another class of phenomena. Rarely are any tissues or functions in an abnormal state without the existence of some sensations in various parts of the body complained of by the patient, unless he be in such a benumbed condition that he cannot feel nor describe. Such phenomena, since they are perceived only by the patient, are called subjective phenomena; we cannot verify them. The patient may deceive us in stating them. He may not be capable of describing them so that we can understand him or get a distinct idea of what he feels, or, he may be dull or comatose and take no note of them. These objective and subjective phenomena together constitute that in which the patient differs from a healthy man. He wants to know what ails him, for the purpose of forming an idea whether and how soon he can get well. You from your dignosis by means of your knowledge of the relation of phenomena to lesions of tissue; and you give your prognosis from your knowledge of the history of the course of diseases under treatment. You have not come to your duties as therapeutists until your diagnosis and prognosis have been made and pronounced.

This having been done, your great duty as curers of the sick lies before you. Is the case one in which it will suffice to order a change in the mode of life, abstinence from some hurtful article of food or drink, change from a noxious habitation to a more wholesome one, substitution of suitable for injudicious raiment, of a nutritious for a scanty diet, of a healthy for a baneful occupation? If so, you will have done your whole duty when, from the stand-point of hygiene or sanitary science, you have cared for these things, and have placed the patient under the conditions which are requisite for the normal performance of the functions of the body and mind. But we will assume that, these things having been attended to, the patient remains ill; and that we need to apply to his organism some special stimulus which shall bring him back to a healthy condition. A drug is such a stimulus.

We are now in a position to apply the science of therapeutics. The phenomena of the patient with which we deal, are the subjective and objective phenomena of which we have already spoken. We include these under the general term "symptoms," and we consider that, practically, the aggregate of the symptoms constitutes the disease under which the patient labors. A great outcry has been raised against homœopathists because of their alleged exclusive attention to symptoms. It is affirmed that they prescribe on symptoms only, not taking cognizance of the disease, and this is made a reproach to them.

In part this reproach springs from the failure to start on a mutual understanding of the term symptom. The old school does not give it so extensive an application as we do. For we include among the symptoms of the patient every deviation from a healthy condition of mind or body which the physician can in any way discover or perceive, or which the patient makes known by his statement or complaints, or which the attendants of the patient have observed and can communicate to the physician. Now, this definition includes every possible deviation from a healthy condition of tissue or function whether objective or subjective, which it is possible to have. And what is called a disease in contradistinction to such an aggregate of symptoms, is simply abstraction, a mental conception devised for the purpose of expressing this aggregate in a single phrase. For example, the patient has heat of skin, a hard frequent pulse, rapid and short respiration, a quick, dry cough or cough with rusty sputa. These are objective symptoms which the physician may observe. The patient in addition complains of oppression of the chest, of sharp pains through the lung on coughing, or of rawness behind the sternum. The physician, by physical exploration of the chest, discovers, on percussing a certain part of the chest, dullness, or a fine crepitation. Let this collection of symptoms constitute all there is about this patient which is a deviation from his condition when in health. These phenomena, being the results of positive observation, are known; there can be no error or uncertainty about them. Now, if we wish to express to another physician the condition of our patient, it may be and is convenient to have a brief term which will include and imply the presence of these phenomena. But does it add anything to our knowledge if we designate this aggregate of symptoms by the name pneumonia or inflammation of the lungs? The fallacy is that we are in danger of including under the given name cases agreeing in anatomical lesion, but differing in symptoms, and requiring different treatment.

It has been objected to the use of a collection of symptoms as the basis of a prescription, that, if we depend on symptoms alone, we may fail to discover the existence of latent disease. But if disease be really latent, not manifested by any symptom whatever, by any deviation from a healthy condition, why then it must be so completely latent, must lie so hidden, that in no way is it discoverable.

Let us remember that Hahnemann taught, and that we believe and teach, that the aggregate of symptoms, which we regard as identical with the disease itself, includes and comprises everything which the physician and attendants discover or have observed about the patient as different from his condition in health, and every deviation from health of which the patient is conscious. Let the physician avail himself of all the appliances of the modern accessory medical sciences, the most approved methods of research and observation;

whatever he observes in any way in the patient which is a deviation from health, is a symptom in the sense of the homœopathist, and the aggregate of these symptoms constitutes for him the disease. I may say that the most recent and most enlightened writers of the old school, Virchow, Carpenter, Bouchut, express themselves much in the same sense.

These symptoms, then, these phenomena of the patient, constitute one series of the phenomena with which the science of therapeutics deals.

The other series of phenomena are those of the action of drugs upon the living body. Let us come to an understanding of what we mean by a drug. The condition of a sick person is this: The organs which, while the patient was in health, have been performing their functions regularly and normally, under the action of the general stimuli of light, heat, aliment, etc., on which we all depend, have in some way, through some cause, come to act abnormally. Now we seek for some special stimulus which is capable of modifying the action of the organism; and if we can hit upon that stimulus which will modify them in just the right way and to the right extent, we shall have the means of modifying the organism back from its perverted action to a healthy action. To hit upon this special stimulus, this is the therapeutic problem.

We gather from this statement that any substance whatever which has the power to produce in the living organism a definite deviation from its healthy, normal action, may come under the designation of a drug. Thus almost every substance in the world, provided it have the power, as most substances have, of producing a definite and constant modification of function and tissue in the organism, may be a drug, and may be used to cure disease if we only know how to use it. Those who deny the possibility of curing disease affirm that a pathological process once begun cannot be arrested;—why not as well as a physiological process? As a matter of course, almost as early as men began to record observations of nature, in however rude a way, they began to note the effects produced upon the organism by natural objects taken into the system accidentally or by design. And these observations were the foundation of the science of pharmacodynamics, or the effects of drugs upon the living organism. Subsequently systematic observations and experiments began to be made, with a view of extending our knowledge of pharmacodynamics and making it exact. It was not however until a very recent period that these experiments were instituted on the proper basis and in the proper way to secure permanent and valuable results.

At first, and indeed until a very recent date, experiments and observations with drugs upon the human organism, were made in the case of sick persons in the way of endeavors to cure them. Now in this way we could not arrive at any certain knowledge of the action of the drug upon the organism, because of the organism being already in abnormal action under the influence of the cause of disease, whatever it might be.

When we add the modifying influence of the drug, the result would be a kind of action due to the combined influence of drug and morbific cause. Nor could we know how much or what deviation to ascribe to each of these influences. Such an experiment could give us knowledge of nothing save the action of the drug upon an organism already affected by disease, precisely as the subject of the experiment is affected. But when we consider how very rarely two identically diseased conditions occur, it will be very apparent that such knowledge would be of but little practical value to us. It would not afford us the constant quantities we seek. It was apparent to some of the most clear-headed of the earlier physicians, after the restoration of learning, that in no way could a knowledge of the properties of drugs in relation to the human organism be obtained except by observations of their action upon the healthy subject. Although this conviction was expressed with more or less clearness by several, and notably by Haller, it was reserved for Hahnemann both to demonstrate its truth, and to illustrate it by undertaking and accomplishing a gigantic series of experiments with drugs upon the healthy organism; experiments of which the results constitute the bulk of our materia medica; and which form the most splendid and enduring monument of scientific acumen and philanthropic devotion of which humanitarian science can boast.

The remarks which were made in relation to symptoms as compared with abstract conceptions supposed to be represented by them, apply to observations of the action of drugs; since the effects of drugs are really artificial diseases. The phenomena observed by the prover or his friends upon him, whether subjective or objective, constitute facts; constitute what we know about the action of the drug. Speculations about its mode of producing these symptoms are certainly interesting, and may lead to further discoveries, and certainly do stimulate to closer observation; but they are no part of the positive facts which constitute this second series of phenomena of our science of therapeutics.

We have now two series of facts or phenomena; the symptoms of the patient and the symptoms produced by drugs upon the healthy It is reasonable to believe that if we knew how to bring the latter action to bear upon the former we might arrest the morbid action of the organism; might modify it back to a healthy action, if, among all the drugs which act with such a variety of difference upon the organism, we only knew how to select the right one.

Wanted, then, a law of selection; a rule for selecting the right drug for each patient; a formula expressing the relation between the symptoms of the patient and the symptoms of the drug which would cure that patient, the law of the interference of symptoms.

This law, of which others had had vague glimpses, was discovered by Hahnemann to be the general law of therapeutics. It was expressed by the phrase "*Similia similibus curantur;*" or "Likes are to be treated by likes." It is the law for the selection of the drug. It expresses nothing concerning the *modus operandi* of the cure. It ventures nothing of hypothesis. It is a bare and as general a formula as that of celestial mechanics.

Discovered by accident, supported by multitudes of instances, established by direct experimentation and clinical demonstration, it interferes in no way with the growth of either series of phenomena,—either the phenomna or symptoms of disase, their causation and connection, or the phenomena of drug action; and yet it affords us the means of prevision that have already been most fruitful of blessings to mankind, as in the case of cholera in 1831.

Let us for a moment, in conclusion, suppose the science of therapeutics otherwise constructed, first on the rationalistic, and then on the empirical basis.

On the former, the symptoms are observed and a cause is assumed for their existence. The action of a drug is observed and a theory formed of the cause of its action. Here two theories come in to introduce two possible points of error. The science cannot progress, because advancing knowledge must continually change the hypotheses concerning the cause of symptoms and of drug effects upon which the treatment was based. Take for example the use of mercury in liver diseases. It was assumed from observation in disease that mercury increases the formation and discharge of bile. In certain diseases then, which were supposed to depend upon a diminished secretion of bile, mercury was administered. But subsequent experiments showed that mercury does not increase the flow of bile. Then all observations and conclusions based on this treatment must be thrown away as worthless, and we must begin again; and so on *ad infinitum.*

The empirical method simply records that A. has cured a patient sick with B., and concludes that A, is a remedy for B. But diseases occur alike so very rarely that the results of treatment based on such experience never agree. Nor does this method afford means of prevision, a defect which is fatal to its claims as a science. Nothing remains but the science as we have explained it, and of which we shall proceed to study in detail and in a practical way the different elements.

The subject of the next lecture will be: "Symptoms; or, How to take the Case."

SYMPTOMS, THEIR STUDY; OR, "HOW TAKE THE CASE."

IN my last lecture I endeavored to define the scope, nature and limits of the science of therapeutics, and to show that homœopathty constitutes this science. I tried to explain to you how it is that, by analysis, every natural science may be reduced to two series of phenomena, connected by a law or formula which expresses the relation of these two series of phenomena to each other; and how the practical problem which the science enables us to solve is this: Given one series of phenomena and the law of relation, to find the other series of phenomena; and that, in this problem lies a test of the soundness of whatever claims to be a natural science, viz.: that it furnishes us a means of prevision or foreseeing and predicting that which is to be observed or discovered; points which I illustrated by a reference to the history and structure of the simplest and most complete of the natural sciences, astronomy or celestial mechanice. Finally, I explained that the two series of phenomena which are the subject of a natural science, must be each capable of independent and indefinite expansion and development as a separate department of natural history; and that no expansion of either must destroy the applicability of the law of relation. I then showed you that in the science of therapeutics or homœopathy (as it is more familiarly called) the two series of phenomena are respectively the phenomena of the patient on the one hand, and the phenomena produced by the drug upon the healthy, living, human being, on the other hand; while the formula which expresses the relation between these series of phenomena is the well-known therapeutic law, *"Similia similibus curantur'*,, "Likes are to be treated by likes."

I showed you that, in our practical application of the science of therapeutics, the constant problem before us is that which is the problem in every natural science, viz.: Given one series of phenomena and the law, to state the other series. Given the phenomena of the patient and the law, to find the phenomena of the drug which bear to the phenomena of the patient the relation expressed by the law. Or if we are studying a drug, and have the phenomena which it produces in the healthy, living, human being, then, having the law, to find the series of phenomena in the sick which, bearing a certain relation to the phenomena of the drug, will be canceled by the latter in the terms of the law. In other words, our constant problem is: Given the symptoms of a case, what drug known to us will cure according to the law, or what must be the effects of such a drug, not yet known to us, as will cure such a case. Or, conversely: Give the effects of a drug, what case, as yet seen or never yet met with, will that drug cure? Such prevision as this homœopathy has again and again in notable cases enabled us to exercise; and by this test she has justified her claim to be entitled the science of therapeutics.

After this general view and analysis of the subject, it remains for us to study in detail the elements of which the science is composed, viz.: the two series of phenomena respectively and the law.

I shall therefore ask your attention now to the first series of phenomena, those of the patient; or briefly to the subject of "symptoms," or how to take the case.

And, here, at the very beginning of the subject, let me say that much unnecessary confusion exists in the minds of our own school, and of our opponents, because we have not agreed upon the meaning we shall attach to the word symptom.

By the old school and by some homœopathists who have gone astray after the "strange gods" of the physiological school of medicine, a very restricted meaning is given to the word symptom; and this being done it is made a reproach to homœopathists that they take note only of symptoms, as though we disregarded some important phenomena presented by the patient. Assuming that homœopathists understand by symptoms only the subjective phenomena or sensations which the patient experiences and describes, "How, then," exclaims Prof. Bock, "can they prescribe for a typhoid patient who neither hears, sees, tastes, smells nor feels, and who could not express his sensations if he were conscious of them, but lies in a passive apathy, as indifferent as a log!" Well, the fact that he lies there and cannot express his sensations, if he have any, and that the avenues of communication between his brain and the world about him, his special senses and the general sense namely, are closed, constitutes a most important series of symptoms. For, gentlemen, in accordance with Hahnemann's instructions, no less than with the common sense of the matter, we include under the term "symptom" every phenomenon presented by the patient which is a deviation from, or an addition to, his condition when in average health.

Whatever we can ourselves observe by careful scrutiny of the patient, bringing to our aid every instrument of observation which the ingenuity of man has contrived; whatever the patient can tell us as the result of his observation of himself or of his sensations; whatever his friends and attendants have noticed concerning his appearance, actions, speech and condition, physical or mental, which differs from his condition and actions when in health,—all these phenomena together constitute what we call the symptoms of the patient.

I conceive that it would be a waste of time to examine the alleged distinction between symptoms and "the disease." Since we have made the term symptom cover every phenomenon, whether it be felt by the patient, or observed, seen, handled or heard by the physician, it is manifest that we can know nothing of any disease except by the presence of symptoms; that its presence is announced by the manifestation of symptoms; that when the symptoms have all disappeared we cannot know that any disease exists, and that therefore by us, for all practical purposes, the totality of the symptoms must be regarded as equivalent to, and identical with, "the disease." Let, then, the bugbear of a disease as distinct from the totality of the symptoms never more haunt your path-way in practical medicine.

Hahnemann directs us to acquaint ourselves with every deviation from the patient's normal, healthy condition which we can observe; to gather from the patient's friends and attendants all of a similar character that they have observed; to listen to the patient's statement of everything of the kind which he has noticed and of all unusual sensations and pains which he has experienced, and all unusual phenomena of which he has been conscious, whether of body or mind.

You will perceive that here are two classes of phenomena referred to, viz.: such as may be observed by the physician or attendants and friends, and such as are perceived and can be stated only by the patient himself. The former, which may be the objects of study and observation by the physician, are called *objective* symptoms. The latter are the subjects of the patient's own consciousness, and are styled *subjective* symptoms. We may notice and study the spasmodic twitching of the facial muscles, the alternate flushings and pallor in a case of facial neuralgia, but the patient alone can make us aware of the sensation which he experiences simultaneously with those twitchings and flushes. In a case of pleurisy we may detect a friction sound denoting dryness or roughness of the pleura, or the dullness denoting effusion; we may observe the deviation from the natural symmetry of the thorax; the labored and hurried breathing, the short, dry cough and the expression of suffering which accompanies it, but the patient alone can tell us that he suffers from a stitch in the side, where it is, what direction it takes, what provokes and aggravates and what relieves it.

The physician and attendants may notice and observe the accelerated yet unsustained pulse, the dulled perceptions and sluggish or perverted intellection, the red, or dry, or cracked and trembling tongue, the elevated and uniformly fluctuating temperature of body, the tympanitic abdomen, the tenderness about the cœcum caput coli and the enlarged spleen which characterize a typhoid fever; but only the patient could have made known to us the failing strength of body, mind and will, the peculiar headache and the desolate sense of illness which, perhaps many days preceding the commencement of the doctor's attendance, began to take possession of him.

We meet with few cases which do not present throughout their course, or at least in some portion of it, both subjective and objective symptoms. If there be an exception, it is that of some chronic affections, consisting exclusively, so far as our observations enable us to speak, of pains and abnormal sensations. I say so far as our observations enable us to speak, for I can hardly conceive of an abnormal sensation except as coincident with some structural change of tissue, although this be so fine as to elude our present means of research.

On the other hand, we meet cases presenting at first view only objective symptoms, as for example, chronic, cutaneous affections and heterologous formations. And yet I believe that in every such case, if we take a broad enough view of it, including the history of the case, we shall find a tradition of subjective symptoms. However this may be, and whatever may be their relative number, and what comparative importance we may be disposed to attach to them, these are the two varieties of symptoms which patients present to us.

Now we may study symptoms under two views, with two different objects: First, we may study the science of symptoms as a branch of medical science, as a department of the science of biology,—much as we study physiology, which is the other department of biology,—without any view to a practical application of the results of our study, without any reference to a proposed application of the therapeutic art, without considering how we shall remove the symptoms by interposing the action of a drug; and Second, we may study symptoms with reference to the practical application of our knowledge in bringing drug action to bear upon the patient's symptoms.

Let us first consider the study of symptoms as an independent department of science. It is one, let me say, which has not received the attention to which its great importance entitles it.

The patient is before us, the object of our observation and inquiry, just as the healthy human being is before us when we study his constituent tissues and organs and their respective functions in pursuing the sciences of anatomy and physiology. We observe his objective symptoms and learn from him his subjective symptoms.

A fact of prime importance for us to remember at the outset of our inquiry is this: that as in nature there are no accidents, so there can be no symptom which is not directly the result of some immediate cause operating in the organism of the patient; no abnormal appearance or condition of any tissue or organ which does not proceed from a modification of its cell structure, its nutrition, or of the normal proportion of the tissues which compose it; no abnormal sensation experienced by the patient which is not the result of some change, either appreciable in some tissue of the body, or assumed to exist therein, or referred to the indefinite realm of dynamics, the convenient habitat of functional derangement for which we have not as yet discovered any structural substratum.

No symptom, then, is to be passed over as unimportant. We know not how important that which now seems most trivial may to-morrow be proved to be. This we know, that everything in the human organism, as in the universe, moves and occurs in obedience to Law; and when we observe the phenomena of nature, we fail of the reverent spirit of the true and faithful student, if we pass over any phenomenon assuming it to be of no account, just because our faculties are so little developed that we cannot see that it has any significance. If it be true, as the Lord of Glory tells us, that of two sparrows which are sold for a farthing not one falls to the ground without our Heavenly Father, that the very hairs of our head are numbered, how can it be that changes of tissue or of excretion or secretion should occur, that abnormal sensations should be experienced save in accordance with some law of the organism? The noble sentiment of the Latin poet, "I am a man: Nothing that is human can be alien to me," is true in a physical no less than in a moral sense.

It is our object to observe everything that is a deviation from the healthy condition. We must then keep up, during our observation, a constant recollection of the condition of organs and tissues, and the performance of function in the healthy subject; and our observation will be a sort of running comparison.

Our object is to note every deviation. We must necessarily follow some method in our investigation, otherwise among such a multitude of objects some would surely escape us. If it be necessary for a dog in hunting to scour a field according to a certain method of lines and angles, surely method must be needful when we are beating up this complicated field of the human organism, and that too in search of game which does not start up at our approach.

We may adpot the *regional* method and survey the whole body, passing from region to region in anatomical order. This is a valuable method and indispensable to a certain extent. It fails, however, to give us sufficient information respecting organs and tissues which, from their situation, are entirely removed from our physical examination or exploration, as, for example, the kidneys and the ovaries. The anatomical method of investigation must be supplemented by what I may call for a moment, somewhat incorrectly, the physiological method. By this we seek to arrive at the condition of an organ or its tissue, or of the parts of an apparatus by examining how it performs its functions. Thus, by examining the excretions of the kidney we form some conclusion respecting the condition of that organ. If we find albumen and certain microscopic objects in it, we may be certain that a portion of the kidney has become changed in a very definite way, which, however, we could not otherwise recognize during the life of the patient. The same is true of many other organs.

This knowledge has been obtained by accumulated

observations of the symptoms of diseases, and of the results of diseases as noticed after death. But so difficult is the are of observation, and so hard is it to obtain from patients all of their subjective symptoms, for the reason that patients have not been trained to the observation of natural phenomena, and are not good observers even of themselves, that we should hardly succeed in getting all the symptoms of a case if we did not add to the regional and the physiological another mode of observation. The history of disease has taught us that when certain symptoms are present in some one organ or apparatus of the body, there are almost sure to be present certain other symptoms, objective or subjctive, in other organs often anatomically quite remote, and of which the patient probably is hardly aware until his attention is called to them by the physician.

I may cite as examples the fact that certain pains in the head, persistently experienced by the patient, are found, by observation of a great many patients, to co-exist with certain uterine affections, of the existence of which the patient was hardly aware; and the immediate symptoms of which would probably have been overlooked in the recital. Another noteworthy instance, a recent discovery, is the coincidence of a certain morbid condition of the retina with a form of Bright's disease of the kidney, to which attention may thus be called at an earlier stage than that at which the kidney symptoms would have discovered it.

To recapitulate, then: we observe the changes in form and structure which are open to our senses, we use whatever methods we possess to discover others; we illuminate the interior of the eye, the rima of the glottis, the canal of the urethra, the meatus of the external ear. We sound the thorax and the abdomen by the methods of percussion and auscultation; we analyze the secretions and excretions, and reason from the results—through our knowledge of the history of disease—to a conclusion respecting the condition of organs and tissues hidden from our observation. Thus we obtain our complete series of objective phenomena.

We then address ourselves to the task of taking the subjective symptoms of the case. Availing ourselves of the regional method which investigates in topographical order one region of the body after another; the physiological method which traces sensations from one organ to another, and leads us to look for sensations or even objective symptoms in some part of the body because we know them to exist when certain others are present; and, finally, employing our knowledge of the history of disease to trace symptoms, both subjective and objective, from one organ and apparatus to another, we make up our series of subjective phenomena.

Now, it may occur to some of you that when I speak of the modifications of tissues and organs found in the patient, and of the necessity of exactly observing and studying them, I am advocating the study of pathological anatomy; and that in showing how a study of the connection of symptoms in the patients may greatly facilitate the discovery of symptoms by showing their mutual connection, dependence and succession, just as the study of physiology anables us to grasp the phenomena of the healthy organism, I am defending the study of pathology. And so I am. For just here we have the province of pathology and pathological anotomy, which are indispensable instruments in the study of symptoms. Let us not be frightened from their legitimate use for the reason that they have been put to a false use.

If we disregard these auxiliary sciences, our collections of symptoms must be for us incomplete lists of unmethodized and unarranged observations. How can we imagine that any department of medical science can exist and be pursued which would not be a useful auxiliary to the physician?

Let us turn now from this glance at the independent study of symptoms as a science, to their study as the means to a practical end. As practitioners of medicine, what is our object in collecting and studying symptoms?

If we regard our duties to our patient in the order in which they were stated in my last lecture, that we are to ascertain for him where and what he ails, whether and how soon he can recover, and finally what will cure or help him, we study symptoms, first of all, to form our diagnosis. Viewed with this object. the symptoms we have obtained from the patient at once classify themselves in our minds. Certain symptoms take front rank as indicating the organ which is chiefly affected, and the kind of deviation from a healthy state which exists in it. Such a symptom is called pathognomonic; and is entitled to that epithet if it be found only when a certain diseased condition exists, and always when that condition exists. We cannot pronounce a symptom to be pathognomonic, nor recognize it as such, unless we are acquainted with the history of disease. Then we require to form our prognosis. Here again we must have a knowledge of the history and course of disease, that we may recognize any symptoms which indicate a lesion so extensive that recovery is unusual or impossible. We must know, likewise, the history of disease, as its course is capable of being modified by medical treatment, and by different varieties of medical treatment.

Third: Our object in the study of symptoms is to get into position to ascertain what drug shall be applied to cancel the symptoms and effect a cure. The is the practical end.

The homœopathist obtains his series of symptoms, and then, in accordance with the law, *similia similibus,* he administers to the patient the drug which has produced in the healthy the most similar series of symptoms.

Now, in speaking of the independent study of symptoms as a science by itself, I have urged the necessity of eliciting all of the symptoms, both objective and subjective, bringing every auxiliary science to aid in the search for symptoms. But when we come to the practical application of the law, *Similia similibus curantur,* when we come to place side by side the two series of symptoms, those of the patient and those of the drug respectively, it is manifest that those of the patient to which we find nothing corresponding in the symptomatology of the drug, are of no use to us in the way of comparison. Practically, then, unless the observation of symptoms as produced by drugs in our provings is developed *pari passu* with that of symptoms as observed in sickness, there will be much of which practically we can make no use. And you will find this view to explain much that is said in disparagement of the study of pathology and pathological anatomy, and of any aid which they may afford to the practitioner.

The difficulty resides in the present imperfection, respectively, of the sciences of pathology, symptomatology and pathogenesy.

Of the symptoms which we have obtained from our patients, the question of their relative value must occur to you. I have mentioned pathognomonic symptoms and their supreme value as determining the diagnosis. Are they as valuable when we are in search of the right remedy? To answer, let us see what we are doing. We are seeking that drug of which the symptoms are most similar to those of the patient. We may have seen in our lives a hundred cases of pneumonia. Every one of these presented the symptom which is pathognomonic of pneumonia. And yet the totality of the symptoms of each patient was different, in some respects, from that of every other pneumonia patient. And this must necessarily be so, because the diseased condition of each patient is the resultant of two factors, the morbific cause, assumed to be the same for all, and the susceptibility or irritability to that cause, which susceptibility may be assumed to be different for each; the resultant must be different for each. We must look, then, for the symptom which shall determine our prescription in some other symptom than the pathognomonic, in some symptom which from the diagnostic point of view is far less important, in some subjective symptoms, or in a condition which individualizes.

Is it essential that the pathognomonic symptom of the case should be present among the symptoms of the drug? Theoretically, it certainly is. Practically, in the present rudimentary condition of our provings, it is not. We attain a brilliant success if not a certain one, where it has never been observed; although I think we are bound to assume, and are justified in assuming, that were our provings pushed far enough it would be produced. This subject will come up again hereafter.

Recalling now the practical division made of symptoms into objective and subjective, the question presents itself: Do we, in the practical use of our symptom series, make use of objective symptoms as in the independent study of symptoms? Unquestionably, wherever the character of our provings has made this possible, and indeed wherever clinical observation has supplemented the provings.

In skin diseases, wherever we meet the well-defined, smooth erysipelas of Belladonna, or the vesicular erysipelas of Rhus, or the bullæ of Euphorbium, or the cracks of Graphites, or the lichen of Clematis, or the intertrigo of Lycopodium, or the hard scabbed ulcers of Mezereum, from the edges of which thick pus exudes on pressure,— do not these symptoms almost determine our selection of these remedies? Or the white tongue of Pulsatilla, the red-tipped, dry tongue of Rhus, the moist trembling tongue of Phosphoric acid, the broad, pale, puffed and tooth-indented tongue of Mercurius solubilis, the yellow coat at the base of the tongue of Mercurius proto iodatus, or the patchy tongue of Taraxacum,—do we not recognize these symptoms as most important indications for these remedies respectively? Shall I further mention the objective symptoms,—sandy grains deposited in the urine, or a red deposit which adheres to the vessel, or the various peculiarities of feculent excretion and of sputa, which are well-known and universally admitted indications of certain remedies, or the radial pulse, or the heart rhythm?

It appears, then, that objective symptoms are valuable indications for the remedy, just in proportion as they have been observed in proving drugs, so as to afford a ground of comparison; and just in proportion as the observation has been precise and definite, enabling us to distinguish one case from another, or, as we term it, to individualize the case.

Such is the value of objective symptoms. But, our object being to individualize the case, it frequently, indeed generally, happens that the distinctive symptoms are subjective.

How now shall we examine the patient to get his symptoms? Do you say that this is an easy matter? Gentlemen, it is the most difficult part of your duty. To select the remedy after a masterly examination and record of the case is comparatively easy. But to *take* the case requires great knowledge of human nature, of the history of disease, and, as we shall see, of the materia medica.

We see the patient for the first time. If the case be an acute one, it may be that at a glance and a touch we shall observe certain objective symptoms which, at least, help us to form our diagnosis, and constitute the basis of the picture which leads us to the choice of our remedy.

Further examination reveals other objective symptoms. For others, as well as for subjective symptoms, we must depend on the testimoney of the patient and his attendants. We have then to listen to testimoney, to elicit more testimoney by questioning and cross-questioning the patient and his friends, and to form conclusions from their evidence. We have to weigh evidence, and here we encounter a task which is similar to that of the lawyer in examining a witness, and success in which requires of us obedience to the rules for the collection and estimate of evidence. We must study our witness, the patient; is he of sound understanding? may we depend on his answers being true and rational? He may be naturally stupid or idiotic, he may be insane, he may be delirious under the effect of the present illness. Or, putting out of view these extreme suppositions, is the patient disposed to aid us by communicating freely his observations of himself, or is he inclined to be reticent? You will be surprised at the differences in patients in this regard. Some meet you frankly, conscious that by replying fully, and by stating their case carefully, they are aiding you to help them. Others act as if they felt that in meeting the doctor they have come to an encounter of wits, in which they are determined that their cunning shall baffle his shrewdness. Others again are morbidly desirous of making themselves out very sick, and and will unconsciously wrap their statement of their symptoms so as to justify their preconceived notion of their case; and if you question them, however you may frame your question, they will reply as they think will make out the case you seem to apprehend. Others, on the contrary, so dread to give testimiy which, they fear, may make it certain that they have some apprehended disease, that they cannot bring themselves to state facts as they are, but twist and misstate them as they fain would have them.

I might pass without mention the case of those who deliberately conceal or deny the existence of symptoms which would betray the presence of diseases of which, with abundant reason, they are ashamed because, I take it, you will be minded to have no dealings with those who refuse to their physician their unlimited confidence.

There is another class whose statements are plus or minus what exactness would require. Almost all of our descriptive language is figurative. We describe sensations certainly according to our idea of what effect would be produced by certain operations upon our sensory nerves, *e. g.*, burning, boring, piercing. This involves an act of the imagination. We are differently endowed with the imaginative faculty. Some persons cannot clothe a sensation in figurative language, and are therefore almost unable to describe their subjective symptoms, and are very difficult patients. Others, again, naturally express themselves in this wise, and, where imagination is controlled by good judgment, are excellent patients, because they describe their symptoms well. This is a matter dependent upon natural endowment, and not upon education or culture. Some persons who cannot construct a sentence grammatically will give us most graphic statements of symptoms; while others who have borne off the honors of a university are utterly at a loss for the means to express what they feel.

Finally, some persons have a natural fervor and tropical luxuriance of expression, which leads them to intensify their statements and exaggerate their sensations. And some, like the Pharisee who believed he should be heard for his much speaking, think to attract our attention, and excite us to greater effort in their behalf, if they magnify their sufferings and tell us a pitiful tale. Others, on the contrary, of a more frigid temperament, give us a statement unduly meagre in its Arctic barrenness; or else, fearing to seem unmanly if they complain with emphasis of suffering which is perhaps the lot of all men, understate their case and belittle their symptoms.

In estimating your patients in these regards, judging while the tale is being told what manner of man you have to deal with, what allowances you must make, what additions, what corrections, you will have full scope for your utmost sagacity and *savoir faire;* and of the value of this estimate of your patient I cannot speak too highly. I have often seen the thoroughly scientific man led astray and bamboozled, where one far inferior to him in scientific knowledge detected the peculiarities of the patient, made the necessary corrections, got an accurate view of the case, and then the prescription was easy. Why, sometimes the patient will, in good faith, state a symptom so incompatible with others that we know and must declare it impossible, and so it is finally admitted to be by the patient.

If it be necessary to make this estimate of the patient, so must we likewise of his friends, who, besides having the peculiarities already spoken of, may be unfriendly to us or to our mode of treatment, and may thus be reticent or reluctant witnesses, or may even mislead us willfully.

We make this estimate of our patient and his friends while he and they are stating the case to us; and this statement we should as far as possible allow them to make in their own way, and in their own order and language, carefully avoiding interruption, unless they wander too far from the point.

We must avoid interrupting them by questions, by doubts, or even by signs of too ready comprehension of what they are telling us. It will of course happen that they skip over important details, that they incompletely describe points that we need to understand fully. But we should note these as subjects for future questions, and forbear breaking in upon the train of our patient's thoughts, lest once broken he may not be able to reconstruct it. When he has finished, we may, by careful questioning, lead him to supply the deficiencies. We must avoid leading questions, and at the same time must not be so abstract and bald that for lack of an inkling of our meaning, the patient becomes discouraged, and despairs of satisfying us. It is never our object, as it may be that of the lawyer, to show our own cleverness at the patient's expense, and to bamboozle him. We must, on the other hand, make him feel, as soon and as completely as possible, that we are his best friend, standing there to aid him in so reviewing his case that we may apply the cure. And so we must encourage his diffidence, turn the flank of his reticence, lend imagination to his matter-of-fact mind, or curb the flights of his fancy, as may be required.

We want a statement of the case in graphic, figurative language, not in the abstract terms of science. It does not help us to hear that the patient has a congestive or an inflammatory pain (however correct these conceptions may be); but a burning or a bursting pain is available. Nor does it specially enlighten us to know that the patient feels now just as he did in last year's attack, unless indeed we attended him then.

Having received the patient's statement and made our own observations, we have a picture of the case, more or less complete. What are we to do with it? What is the next step? We have now one series of phenomena. The law tells us that the drug which will cure that patient must be capable of producing in the healthy a similar series of phenomena.

Seeking the means to cure the patient then, we look among drug provings for a similar series of phenomena. Let us suppose that we find one which corresponds pretty well. Not exactly, however, for here are certain symptoms characteristic of that drug, of which the patient has not complained. We examine the patient as regards those symptoms. No! his symptoms in that line are quite different. We try another similar drug, comparing its symptoms with the patient's, and questioning the patient still further; and thus the comparing and trying proceed until we find a fit. This is a mental process, so expeditious sometimes that we are hardly aware how extensively we engage in it. But it shows how difficult it is to take a case unless we have some knowledge of the materia medica, and how much an extensive knowledge of materia medica aids us in taking the case; and this explains why the masters in our art have given us such model cases. (In consultations, a doctor will send his taking of the case. We cannot prescribe from it. We must take the case ourselves.) In thus fitting the case and the remedy be honest with yourselves, just as in getting shoes for your children. Do not warp or squeeze to make a fit.

And now, before we go further, let us ask what are the symptoms generally which give the case its individual character, and determine our choice of the remedy. Are they the pathognomonic ones? They cannot be unless we are to treat every case of disease named by a common name with one and the same remedy. Are they those which are nosologically characteristic? No, for the same reason. They are the *trifling* symptoms, arising probably from the peculiarity of the individual patient, which make the case different from that of the patient's neighbor. They may be a sensation or a condition. If it be metrorrhagia, the mere fact that the flow is worse at night may determine the choice between two such remedies as Calcarea and Magnesia.

THE ANAMNESIS.

IN my last lecture I tried to explain the nature or the series of symptoms which make up a case of sickness; the different kinds of symptoms, and how to observe and get a knowledge of them; the different value of symptoms, depending on the object which you have in view when you are studying them. I endeavored to show the importance of an independent study of symptoms as a distinct branch of the science of biology, without reference to the practical application of the art of curing. And, finally, I showed how the totality of the symptoms when obtained, was practically made available for the selection of the remedy, by being compared with the symptoms produced by drugs in the healthy subject; that drug being selected which had produced symptoms most similar to those of the case; and I showed how it must be that sometimes it is apparently trivial symptoms which determine the choice between one and another drug.

It may have occurred to some of you, as it must have occurred to all who, having had practical experience in the homœopathic treatment of disease, did me the honor to be present at my lecture, that I took no notice of a very important feature in the examination of the case,—a most important element of the case,—viz.: the previous history or the anamnesis, at it is called

As a matter of course, in our investigations for the purpose of forming a diagnosis and a prognosis, the previous history of the case and of the patient before he became ill must have received our earnest attention. But it has not yet appeared, from what I have said, what part the history of the case is to play in enabling us to select the appropriate remedy. To this subject, as it is both very important and not always clearly understood, I shall devote much time this morning.

You will please bear in mind that the process by which we accomplish the selection of the remedy for a case of sickness, is a process of comparison. We compare the symptoms of the case with the symptoms which drugs have produced in the healthy; and we select the drug of which the symptoms are most similar to those of the patient. We seek a parallelism between drug symptoms and those of the patient.

You will remember also that the symptoms of a case of sickness, like the physiological phenomena of persons healthy, are not always and during all time the same; they vary from day to day, from hour to hour, or from minute to minute. Indeed it might properly be said that life is, in so far as every physiological process is concerned, a series of oscillations within physiological limits; now action is vehement, now mild; waste is now in excess, now in deficit. Just so is it with morbid phenomena or symptoms, whether they be of natural, or of artificial or drug, disease. We are then instituting comparisons between, so to speak, oscillating and continually shifting series of phenomena. Now, the point of importance here is that this oscillation and shifting require time, and that therefore our summary of the symptoms must cover not merely the moment of time at which we observe the patient, but also some previous time during which the symptoms may have been different from those of the present time. This remark applies both to the drug and the case. It is necessary not simply for the purpose of getting a full picture of the case, but also to make certain that there is a complete parallelism between the case and the drug we think of giving the patient.

Two lines, each an inch long, may appear to be parallel. If we would be certain whether or not they are so, let us project each line until it is a foot long. We shall then more easily see the divergence or convergence if there be any. Just so, at some paticular moment, the symptoms of a case and of a drug may appear to be very similar; but if we compare the succession and order of the symptoms, for the space of a day or two, with the succession and order of the drug symptoms, we may notice a marked difference. This is illustrated by comparing the symptoms produced by two drugs in the healthy prover. There is a period in the action of each, when, to my mind, the symptoms of Aconite and Carbo vegetabilis are very similar, and yet, taking a broader view of these drugs, we can hardly find any more unlike.

Shall I shock any of my hearers by stating this necessity for taking into consideration the course and succession of symptoms in selecting a remedy; and shall I be told that strict homœopathy requires that a prescription shall be made for the symptoms that are present, the remedy to be changed when the symptoms change? I believe that some conscientious physicians too closely follow this method— too closely for the best success. Let us take a practical instance; a case of intermittent fever. The patient has certain symptoms which precede and usher in the chill. Then, for two hours or more, he has the symptoms which constitute the chill; then, after an interval those which constitute the hot stage; then those of the sweating stage; after which comes a period of from ten to forty hours, constituting the apyrexia, during which the patient probably may have some symptoms which serve to characterize his case, and individualize it. We may see the patient during one or all these periods. His symptoms at the different times are certainly very different. Is it our custom, is it good practice, to give the patient a different remedy, corresponding to each of these stages; or, would the nicest faculty of selection lead us to select for

THE ANAMNESIS. 53

each stage the same remedy, to which a survey of the whole case would bring us? The former is not our custom. It would not be good practice. We could not so select. On the contrary, we extend our lines of symptoms—unless they correspond with the complete paroxysm and apyrexia—and then we can judge of their parallelism. We seek a remedy which produces just such cold, hot and sweating stages in just such order and with just such concomitant symptoms, and that likewise produces such symptoms in the apyrexia. Do you point me to cases in which no such parallelism is found, and yet a successful prescription is made? I reply that, as I said at first, we are like the Israelites, and must make bricks whether we have straw or not. We must prescribe from our materia medica as it is. Where we can do no better, we must prescribe on a few symptoms, on an inference or an analogy, rather than refuse to prescribe at all. Yet nobody will deny the greater certainty of the prescription when such a parallelism can be established. In such a case, then, we follow the patient along a series of violent oscillations between cold, heat, sweat, and the normal state again. And this we do, to a greater or less extent, in very many illnesses in which the oscillations are not so violent.

I believe that a broad enough consideration of this subject would lead physicians to abstain from alternation of remedies even in the few instances in which Hahnemann sanctioned it, and would deter them from the error, as I deem it, of leaving a patient several remedies to be taken, variously, as different phases of sensation or objective phenomena succeed each other. But to be able to prescribe in this large-viewed way for your patient, you must have studied the materia medica in the same comprehensive way; you must have studied the connection and succession of the symptoms. A mere repertory study for the case in hand will not suffice. You must have made a systematic study of each drug and of each group of drugs.

Now I see no reason, especially in chronic diseases, why this method of taking into consideration the oscillations of symptoms should be limited to a few days or a week. If a patient present himself, having a fever at night and chilliness by day, we comprise these oscillations in one group, and seek a remedy which presents a parallel group. If, now, we find a patient who has a certain set of symptoms in the summer, which uniformly gives place to another set in the winter, and these again are replaced in turn by the summer set, why should we of necessity restrict our view in the summer to the symptoms of that season only, and in winter the same, when we might by a broader view comprehend both under one prescription? It is a practical question. Can it be done? I answer from experience, it can; and let me tell you an advantage. The symptoms of one season may be so vague and indefinite that you cannot find a remedy for them, just as in the intermittent the

THE ANAMNESIS. 55

symptoms of one stage may have so little about them that is characteristic that you cannot select a remedy. But, perhaps, the symptoms of the other season, the summer, are so characteristic as to leave no doubt of the remedy. Then, if you believe in this unity of disease, you may in the winter prescribe on the strength of the summer symptoms, although these disappeared months ago and will not recur for months to come, and you may effect a radical cure. I shall presently illustrate this by a case.

Let me say further, that if this be a correct method of prescribing, we may extend it, and instead of requiring a succession of oscillations, even at so distant intervals as summer and winter, we may regard an acute attack of illness and the chronic condition which follows it as one series of phenomena, and prescribe as for one present malady, even though years have passed since the acute attack of illness was merged into the chronic affection. I shall illustrate this point by two cases.

I come now to a third kind of case, in which a family predisposition to the recurrence of a certain form of disease at a cretain period is so marked, that we may consider indefinite and vague symptoms as indications that the tendency is working to development, and may prescribe for it in anticipation. I should not venture upon this statement had I not a case to present in illustration of it. Let me repeat that the advantage of these methods lies in the fact alone that they give us data for a sure prescription, whereas otherwise we should be unable to find a basis for a prescription. I will now relate cases.

1. E. W. D. Headache in winter, nondescript diarrhœa in summer, indicating Aloes. I prescribed Aloes in the winter, on the strength of the summer diarrhœa, and cured both.

2. The case of G. W. W., jr. Deafness from milk-crust. I prescribed Mezereum for the milk-crust, and the deafness never returned. He is now attending to business.

3. A case of epilepsy. I prescribed Platina, on the strength of previous strong passion and peculiar disposition; imperious and high stepping.

4. The case of Mrs. B. was one of supposed uterine disease; she had been treated by caustics, etc. She complained of aching in the heels, and I suggested Agaricus. The whole family had spinal meningitis; two brothers had died, and a sister was paraplegic. Agaricus cured the uterine disease.

PULSATILLA.

ANEMONE PRATENSIS. PULSATILLA NIGRICANS.

I HAVE chosen this drug to commence a course of lectures on materia medica, as well because it has been very thoroughly proved and verified by clinical experience, as also because it is one of our chief polychrests.

Polychrest is a term applied to a number of the remedies that are the most frequently used in practice, and that have an extensive range of application.

It would be an error, however, to suppose that a polychrest, which is called for every day, is any more useful in any given case than a drug that we are required to give only once a year will be in the case which requires it. It must never be forgotten that every case requires just the identical remedy which is most homœopathic to it, even if it be a rare and seldom used remedy; and that no other remedy, however popularly or however constantly in use, can be as good as, or can take the place of, this homœopathically indicated remedy.

But just as some disease are very common, being met with every day. such as dyspepsias, bronchial catarrh, diarrhœa, ephemeral fever, etc., so there are certain remedies which produce, when proved upon the healthy, series of symptoms similar to those of these frequently recurring diseases. It is obvious that these remedies will be frequently indicated in practice, will be often used and in many cases. These remedies are our polychrests. We must know them well; although it is of great importance that, in bending ourselves to the study of them, we neglect none of the other remedies of our materia medica.

In studying Pulsatilla and all other remedies, we shall follow Hahnemann's anatomical order, stating the symptoms of each region in succession; and calling attention to the conditions of aggravation and amelioration, and to the simultaneous manifestation of groups of symptoms in different regions. We shall then take a general view of the remedy, endeavoring to appreciate its characteristics and its special spheres of action. Finally, we shall consider its more obvious applications to diseased conditions frequently met with, its resemblance to other remedies, and the differences between them.

We begin with the

Sensorium. Pulsatilla produces vertigo or dizziness, which occurs while sitting, but is relieved while walking or sitting in the open air; dizziness when directing the eyes upward, and especially when stooping, when it seems as though the head were to heavy; a drunken dizziness, the head feeling hot inwardly, and the face pale. The vertigo occurs or is worse in the evening or after eating. We here meet conditions which we shall find to pervade the Pulsatilla proving, and to be characteristic of the drug, viz.: occurrence or aggravation of the symptoms in the evening, after eating, during repose, and amelioration from motion and from being in the open air; also paleness of the face, even with sensation of internal heat.

Head. The headache is chiefly in the forehead and supraorbital region, and in the temples. The pains are a heaviness, a bursting sensation in the temples, and throbbing. These sensations are aggravated by stooping, by mental exertion, and in the evening, and by rolling the eyes upward. Occasional stitching pains in different parts of the head, frequently confined to one half of the head. Indeed, this is a peculiarity of Pulsatilla pains generally, that they are often confined to one half of the body, like those of Ignatia, Thuja, Spigelia, Valeriana and Silicea.

[Helonias dioica has a pressing pain in one or both temples (in a small spot), a "burning sensation" in the top and front of the head, which is entirely dispelled by motion and mental exertion. It comes on immediately when either the motion or mental exercise is desisted from.—S. A. JONES, M. D.]

It may be added that a Pulsatilla headache is generally coincident with disturbances in other regions of the body, as, for example, the digestive tract, or the genito-urinary organs, especially the latter in females.

Eyes, Eyelids. The margins are inflamed; hordeola form upon them. Further, the lids are dry and scurfy—in the morning they are agglutinated. In the eyes themselves the pains are: stitching, and especially itching and severe aching, with a sensation as if a foreign body were in the eye, or a veil before it which could be winked away. There is great lachrymation in the open air, and considerable photophobia.

Vision is obscured, but it is to be noted that this observation is conjoined with vertigo and nausea, whence we may infer that it is functional and not dependent upon organic lesions of the eye. The same may be said of the other symptoms of vision; fiery circles, and starry apparitions, and double vision. Nevertheless, these symptoms are not to be ignored, for they individualize and characterize the disturbance in other organs and systems with which they coincide in occurrence.

Ears. Internally, itching, stitching and tearing sensations; also, violent pain like a distending or outward-pressing ache. The external ear is hot, red and swollen. Discharge of pus from the ear.

Deafness as though the ear were stopped. Murmur and rushing noise isochronous with the pulse.

In front of the ear an eczematoid eruption, with a burning-biting pain, and swelling of the cervical glands. Stitching pain in the parotid.

In ordinary catarrhal otitis, Pulsatilla is our best remedy; *i. e.,* the symptoms of such cases most frequently indicate Pulsatilla. Silicea resembles it closely.

In deeper-seated inflammation of the cellular tissue, Mercurius or Silicea or Rhus is called for. Tellurium corresponds to a peculiar affection of the meatus auditorious externus and the external ear.

Chamomilla indications differ from those of Pulsatilla in the symptoms of the disposition, and especially in the great intolerance and impatience of pain.

The same may be said of the Arsenicum ear-indications.

Nose. Superiorly near the inner canthus of the eye, an abscess like a lachrymal abscess. The alæ nasi are ulcerated, so have the nares internally a sensation as if ulcerated. There is in the nose a smell as of an old catarrh. (It is perhaps this symptom which first induced a trial of Pulsatilla in ozæna simplex.)

Mouth. Tongue covered with tenacious mucus. A white-coated tongue is an indication for Pulsatilla.

Yellow coat at the base of the tongue, Mercurius protoiodatus.

Teeth. Two varieties of pain—a stitching or digging, worse in the evening or early night; and a drawing, tearing sensation, as if the nerve were drawn tense and then suddenly let go.

PULSATILLA.

The toothache is renewed always after eating, and whenever anything quite warm is taken into the mouth. Aggravation by eating and by warmth.

Chamomilla toothache is aggravated by cold or warm food or drink.

Coffea toothache is controlled by ice-water constantly in the mouth. (Published by Hale, confirmed by me)

Mercurius toothache is aggravated by cold water in the mouth, but relieved by warm.

Carbo vegetabilis. The whole row of teeth too long and very tender; he cannot bite.

Causticum. Gum swollen; feeling as if the tooth were being crowded out of the alveoli; tooth too long, aggravation in the evening and by eating.

Lachesis. Swelling corresponding to the external fangs of the upper molar, with swelling of the cheek; the skin feels tense, hot and crips, as if it would crack; throbbing in the cheek. Periodontitis.

Throat. Sensation, on deglutition, as though the uvula were swollen. Apart from the deglutition, a feeling as if raw and sore in the throat, as if the submaxillary glands pressed inward and were sore. Sensation of great dryness of the mouth, palate and lips; these parts coated with tenacious mucus; a bad taste in the mouth.

Digestion. Manifold symptoms. The taste is variously perverted and altered—seldom bitter, except just after eating or drinking. More frequently a sour taste. But more characteristic of Pulsatilla is the taste of the food returning to and remaining in the mouth long after eating. In fact, Pulsatilla makes digestion very slow.

Hahnemann gives us a symptom in parentheses: (Food tastes as if too salt). On the strength of this symptom I gave Pulsatilla^{200} with entire success to a patient convalescent from Charges fever who had become well enough to sit up and walk about his room, but had a slight chill every afternoon, followed by a flush of fever and a sweat at night; no appetite, depression of spirits, little thirst, irritability and peevishness in place of his usual amiability, and a perverted taste so that all food prepared for him tasted as if saturated with salt. A single dose of Pulsatilla removed the latter symptom, and within six days all the others had vanished, and he rapidly regained strength and vigor, and has as yet (ten years) had no return of fever.

Appetite. Moderate; often a gnawing sensation in the stomach as from hunger, and yet no desire for any special kind of food.

Thirst. An almost complete absence of thirst is characteristic of Pulsatilla; Sabadilla resembles it in this absence of thirst.

Nausea or qualmishness at the thought or smell of food, especially of fat or rich food, or on attempting to eat. The sensation is somewhat as if a worm were crawling up the œsophagus; the nausea comes up from the stomach.

Vomiting of food, especially at night or evening; waterbrash and gulping up of water or of food into the mouth (regurgitation).

Epigastrium. Feeling as if a stone lay there. (Bryonia has the same.)

Throbbing in the epigastrium, perceptible to the hand laid thereon. A contracting sensation in the œsophagus, as if one had swallowed too large a morsel of food; the same sensation extends over the hypochondria, then up over the chest, and impedes respiration.

Abdomen. Sensation of tension and fullness throughout the abdomen, and involving the thorax up to the mammary region. Pinching and cutting pains, especially around the umbilicus, worse toward evening.

Much flatulence, as might be expected where digestion is so slow as under the action of Pulsatilla. Flatus moves about in the intestines, causing pinching pains, and with rumbling noise; worse on waking or just after supper.

Externally. The abdominal walls are tender to the touch, when sitting, or when coughing, especially after an alvine evacuation.

Stool. A twofold action (which yet we are hardly justified in designating as primary and secondary effects). Difficult stool, with much backache and urgency, or frequent desire for stool with insufficient evacuation or no fæces, but instead thereof, yellowish mucus, sometimes mixed with blood. On the other hand, Pulsatilla produces diarrhœa at night; stool consisting of green and acrid burning mucus, preceded by commotion in the bowels.

PULSATILLA. 65

In the frequent desire and effort for stool, and the difficulty of evacuation, Pulsatilla resembles Nux vomica. The difference is found in the general symptoms.

The diarrhœa of green mucus occurring at night resembles that of Dulcamara, which likewise is nocturnal, and but slightly painful. It, however, is ascribable to dampness, and is accompanied by rheumatic symptoms; while that of Pulsatilla follows errors of diet, especially pork and fat food generally. It is not a free purgation, but rather a catarrh of the intestine, with spasmodic action of the muscular coat.

Pulsatilla has painful blind hæmorrhoids, with itching and sticking pains and soreness.

Urinary Organs. Pressure upon the bladder, as if from flatus. Frequent pressure to urinate, and cutting pain during the act of micturition. (This differs from Cantharides in that the latter has pain after micturition.) Involuntary discharge of urine, drop by drop, at night, or on making exertion, as walking, coughing, etc. The urine is sometimes clear and abundant, and again, scanty and with a red or brownish deposit.

Burning in the urethra during micturition.

Genitals, Male. Itching of prepuce and scrotum. Testes swollen, hanging low, and painful; tensive and tearing pains.

Mucus discharge from the urethra, with burning during micturition. Increase of sexual desire.

Pulsatilla has been of service in hydrocele, also

in gonorrhœal orchitis, but it is not so often called for in orchitis as Rhododendron, Clematis, Spongia, Aurum, or Belladonna.

Sometimes indicated in gonorrhœa by general symptoms rather than local ones.

Genitals, Female. The decided action of Pulsatilla upon the female genital system has been shown by a large clinical experience. In the hypogastric zone, drawing, pressing or constricting pains, like labor pains, converging toward the pudenda. Such pains are relieved by crouching forward. They come, generally, just before the menstrual period, are attended by a feeling of weight, like a stone, in the hypogastrium, and accompanied by chilliness, stretching and yawning. The menses are delayed, difficult and scanty, or even fail altogether.

Before the menses, labor-like pains as above.

During the menses, many symptoms, such as weight and downward pressure in the abdomen and sacral region; nausea; getting black before the eyes; stomachache and faintings; all worse in the warm room and by much exertion, better in the open air.

Leucorrhœa, of a thick mucus resembling cream. It is sometimes acrid, producing a burning pain, sometimes bland; most profuse after menstruation.

Pulsatilla appears to stimulate the action of the uterus during labor, when the pains diminish and become inefficient.

Comparisons. Cyclamen and Sepia resemble

PULSATILLA.

Pulsatilla in relation to the menstrual function. Nux vomica, which is so analogous in many respects to Pulsatilla, resembles it in the scantiness of the flow, but, true to the spasmodic character which distinguishes it, brings on the flow too early, and keeps it up for too many days, although the total amount of fluid lost is not excessive.

The aggravation of Sepia is before menstruation; of Pulsatilla, during menstruation.

Under Nitric acid, menstruation gradually passes into a leucorrhœa which is brown and thick, and finally in a few days becomes a thin, watery, flesh-colored, offensive discharge, sometimes acrid.

Kreosote has a leucorrhœa for five days succeeding menstruation, thick mucus, exceedingly acrid, causing the pudenda to swell and itch, and excoriating the thigh. Micturition exceedingly painful. The leucorrhœa smells like fresh green corn.

Borax is indicated by leucorrhœa, acrid, just midway between the menstrual periods, with swelling of the labia and inflammation, and discharge from the glands of Duvernay.

Respiratory Organs. Coryza. From the first, a discharge of thick yellow mucus from the nose. Sometimes it is green and offensive. Loss of taste and smell.

Throat. Roughness and dryness. Sudden hoarseness, without much oppression or cough, and equally sudden relief.

The hoarseness for which Pulsatilla is so efficacious is capricious, coming and going, and without apparently adequate organic cause. That of Causticum comes on, or is much worse, from five P. M. to midnight, and is accompanied by a teasing, dry cough. That of Phosphorus is more constant, and conjoined with soreness and rawness of the larynx and behind the sternum, and a weight upon the chest. That of Carbo vegetabilis has ulcerative soreness in the larynx, and a burning pain in the lungs after a hard cough.

[I do not say that these are all the conditions and concomitants, but they are frequently met, and are characteristic.]

Pulsatilla produces two varieties of cough; one with abundant sputa, consisting of thick yellow mucus, sometimes bloody, often of a bitter taste; the other dry, occurring chiefly at night. The feeling which provokes the cough is a tickling in the trachea. I have, for years, hesitated to give Pulsatilla for a loose cough, even though it seemed well indicated, it seeming to change the loose cough into the dry, hard night cough. It produces dyspnœa and asthmatic oppression, especially at night, with palpitation, especially when lying on the left side.

The sensations in the chest are chiefly tension and constriction, in conjunction with the dyspnœa and asthmatic symptoms. In the middle of the thorax a pain, which frequently occurs in the Pulsatilla proving: that of an internal ulcer.

The mammary glands are swollen and tense. Itching of the nipples.

Back. In the sacral region, pains on assuming the upright posture, or on bending backward, as well as after sitting, so that one can hardly stoop or straighten up. Aching as from fatigue, and a pressing as from within outward. Finally, in this region, a pain as if luxated when moving; and when sitting, a bruised pain, relieved by motion.

Considering the action of Pulsatilla upon the female sexual organs, causing weight and bearing down, with leucorrhœa, etc., it is reasonable to ascribe the aching and some other sacral pains to this action, and experience justifies this view. Other pains are analogous to the rheumatic pains of the extremities.

In the back, drawing, tensive and stitching pains, which seem to impede respiration and interfere with free motion.

Extremities generally. First, we note tearing pains, as for example, in the shoulder-joint, where it compels one to move the arm, and is relieved by lying on the painful side. Again, in the muscles and bones of the arm, and even in the fingers, where it seats itself in the tensor tendons. In the lower extremities it appears as a jerking, tearing pain, from the hip-joint to the knee when lying in bed, or only in the knees when sitting; or in the ankles and extending to the heel, the sole and the great toe, where it is a tearing pain.

Observe the characteristic: compelling the prover-to move the affected part, which is equivalent to relief by motion; and by pressure, which is analogous to motion.

Then, drawing pains, affecting the whole length of the extremities, occurring at night and during repose (often associated with chill).

Stitching pains occur in the upper extremity, especially on moving the arm, as in the shoulder-joint and in the deltoid muscle. Likewise a feeling of heaviness and paralysis in the arm when trying to raise it. Indeed the tired, heavy, aching sensation such as comes from fatigue, and yet is not relieved by repose, but is rather aggravated thereby, is marked in the Pulsatilla proving.

Burning itching in the soles of the feet after getting warm in bed. This symptom led to the successful use of Pulsatilla for effects of frost-bite. See Petroleum and Agaricus.

Fever. Pulsatilla produces many symptoms akin to one or other stage of fever. Chilliness predominates. It accompanies the evening pains of whatever kind, as well as the abdominal pains, the gastric disturbances, and especially those of the female sexual system. It occurs frequently after a meal, and early in the morning. But, in and by itself, as an independent symptom, chilliness occurs generally in the evening. It may be general or partial, affecting the extremities. When heat follows the chilliness, if it be only a sensation of heat with no objective warmth, there is no thirst; but if the heat be, as it sometimes is, both objective and subjective, it is then attended by thirst. Remember this, because absence of thirst is said to be a characteristic of Pulsatilla, and presence of thirst, therefore, to contra-indicate. This is true, with the limitation stated.

Frequently the fever symptoms are complex, and much mixed up; chilliness and heat rapidly succeeding each other, or occurring simultaneously in different parts of the body, or on the different sides of the body; but these complex symptoms occur almost always in the evening or at night.

Ruckert calls attention to the fact that though the Pulsatilla symptoms generally are not attended by thirst, yet sometimes thirst is present when the hot stage is strongly marked; and he has had excellent success in puerperal fever and other fevers when thirst was present, the mass of the symptoms having indicated Pulsatilla.

Moreover, the cheeks are often hot and red while the back is chilly and the feet cold—a state of things often observed when the menses are retarded in young women. Again, flashes of heat over the whole body, producing great discomfort and anxiety. In short, a condition of erethism such as may co-exist with a depressed nutrition,—an approach to the erethistic form of chlorosis.

Sweat is abundant, chiefly in the early morning, sometimes throughout the night; often, like, other symptoms, the sweat is semilateral.

Sleep. Certain peculiarities of sleepness and sleep are characteristic of Pulsatilla. Sleepiness in the afternoon, such not being the habit of the prover. Sleepiness after even a moderate meal. The prover does not feel sleepy in the evening; on the contrary, wide awake; ideas throng, the fancy is brilliant; he (or she) does not wish to go to bed, and, on going to bed, does not fall asleep for a long time. The sleep is somewhat troubled and restless, with talking, frequent waking, with frightening dreams, until toward morning, when sleep is more quiet and profound, and is most sound just when the time is come to get up. The prover wakens dull and inert, although not with aggravation of any other symptoms.

This is a great characteristic of Pulsatilla, and is almost always present when Pulsatilla is clearly indicated by other symptoms. When, therefore, a doubt rests upon the selection of Pulsatilla, it is safe to be inclined toward it if the sleep symptoms are such as have been described, viz.: wide awake in the evening; does not want to go to bed; first sleep restless; sound asleep when it is time to get up; wakes languid and not refreshed.

Pulsatilla contrasts strongly with Nux vomica in the sleep symptoms, as in some others. Under Nux vomica, the prover is very sleep and dull in the evening, cannot sit up long; goes to bed early, and goes to sleep immediately; sleeps well until about three A. M., then wakes and lies awake, thinking, etc., with mind quite clear and active till five A. M.; then dozes and sleeps an hour, and wakes more tired than when he woke at three A. M., and often with a headache. Sulphur, again, has the evening sleepiness of Nux vomica, but the night is full of unrest, tossing, nervous excitement, orgasm of blood; pains of various kinds, and but little sleep throughout.

The sleeplessness of Cocculus is from pure mental activity, chiefly of memory, and is well described by Walter Scott. ("Lady of the Lake," I., p. 33.)

Disposition. The disposition is affected by Pulsatilla in a very characteristic manner. The prover complains of anxiety or distress, as though some great evil were impending and this distress appears to him to come from the epigastrium; and with these symptoms come palpitation, chattering of the teeth, and flashes of heat; also, undue anxiety about the health or about household duties. In addition, there is a marked irresolution, the prover cannot determine which of two is the better course to pursue; this is akin to the well-known characteristic of Pulsatilla, the yielding disposition, which gives way under slight opposition, and manifests its concious feebleness by the readiness with which tears come to the eyes on slight provocation.

The disposition weep is certainly a strong indication for Pulsatilla, but two errors must be guarded against, in accepting and applying it. In the first place, it must not be considered that a lively disposition, and even a considerable amount of spirits and will, contra-indicate Pulsatilla; laughter and tears come often with equal readiness.

Again, let us remember that the desolate sensation of utter prostration which ushers in many a serious dyscratic disease disposes to tears, especially when it comes to a man or person in the midst of business or family cares, which he knows not how to neglect nor to delegate. If, then, a patient, in the incipience of a severe typhoid or a diphtheria, can hardly answer the doctor's questions for the tears and chocking that come, these must be looked upon as the physiological result of utter prostration of body and desolation of soul, coinciding with the consciousness of responsibilities and cares too heavy to bear and too precious to neglect. They are not especial symptoms of the morbid state, nor must they be taken as indications of Pulsatilla. I have dwelt upon these points because the error referred to is often made, and time is thus wasted which can never be regained.

GENERAL ANALYSIS.

1. The most marked disturbances of functional activity produced by Pulsatilla are: In the digestive apparatus; the genito-urinary of both sexes, but more especially the female; the respiratory, at least as regards the mucous membrane; and the articular synovial surfaces. The mucous membrane throughout the body is affected; as for example, in the middle ear, the eye, nose, throat, bronchi, stomach,

intestines, bladder, urethra, vagina, and uterus (probably).

2. Changes in the organic substance are effected chiefly in the secretions, and chiefly in those of the mucous membrane. The conjunctiva, chiefly the palpebral, secretes copiously, and the tears are augmented if not modified. The nasal membrane, after a brief period of unnatural dryness, secretes abundant mucus, which becomes thick, yellow or green, and offensive. It is probable that the secretions of the stomach and small intestines are modified, since digestion is so decidedly retarded by the action of Pulsatilla, and presents so many abnormal features; such as perverted taste, regurgitation of food or its flavor, flatus, pain, etc.; as well as that of the lower intestine, as witness the stool covered with mucus, and the mucus diarrhœa.

So, likewise, the mucous discharge from the bladder—as shown by the jelly-like sediment in the urine—and the discharge from the urethra, as well as the leucorrhœa, attest the modification of secretion.

The special function of menstruation is retarded in time, and the secretion (?) diminished in quantity. We shall be better able to explain this when we understand more about the pathology of chlorosis.

The testes are the seat of inflammation, pain and enlargement, and, although the ovaries were not similarly affected in any prover, yet, from analogy, Pulsatilla has been successfully used in ovarian affection, the symptoms otherwise corresponding.

The swelling and heat of the knee and ankle-joints, as well as of the small joints of the fingers and toes, together with the drawing, tense pain in them, and the accompanying symptoms of the digestive tract, suggest that Pulsatilla acts upon the synovial membranes and upon the nutrition much as one form of rheumatism does, and have led to its successful use, particularly in rheumatic gout, so called. The itching and biting tingling of the skin resemble those of measles.

Peculiarities and Characteristics. Our knowledge of Pulsatilla being derived wholly from provings on the healthy with moderate doses, we have no records of the effects of poisonous doses, and have therefore no data for constructing a theory of its pathological action on an anatomical basis; but, on the other hand, through the action of these moderate doses, under the clear observation of Hahnemann and his pupils, we have a quantity of characteristic symptoms, chiefly subjective, which furnish us indications for the selection of Pulsatilla more positive and precise than those of almost any other remedy.

Character of Pains. The pains are drawing, tearing pains, pains as of an internal ulcer, aggravated by touch; but the most peculiar pain is a tension, which increases until very acute, and then lets up with a snap. The pains occur or are much worse at night, before midnight.

They are accompanied by chilliness, but without thirst.

As the pains increase, the peculiar mental and moral Pulsatilla state is more pronounced; the patient loses courage and gets despondent, and inclines to tears, and as the pains diminish the spirits rise.

Certain parts of the body become very red or purple, without heat, the vessels becoming congested. This has led to the successful use of Pulsatilla in varicose conditions of veins.

As a general rule, the pains are relieved by motion and by cool air, but the abdominal pains are relieved by warmth.

The symptoms which occur when lying still on the back are relieved by sitting up and by motion. This relief is gradual, however, for the act of rising often for the moment increases the pain, and the more decidedly the longer one has been sitting still.

Long-continued motion also, like long sitting, provokes symptoms, which yet are, for a brief period, more evident on first coming to repose.

The general group of symptoms most characteristic of Pulsatilla, next to those of the disposition, is that of the sleep, which has been already detailed.

Clinical experience has shown Pulsatilla to be an excellent remedy for disorders produced by eating pork and fat food generally.

It is often indicated when the menses are scanty and delayed. Very frequently, when it fails to bring them on, Sulphur will succeed.

It is noteworthy that the pains of Pulsatilla often occur on one side of the body only.

Antidotes. For the sleepiness, lassitude, etc., Chamomilla.

For the restless anxiety, etc., Coffea.

Other symptoms, according to their similarity, may call for Ignatia or Nux vomica.

THERAPEUTIC APPLICATIONS.

In earache, toothache, headache, ophthalmia, palpebrarum, hordeolum, nasal catarrh, bronchitis, dyspepsia, nocturnal mucous diarrhœa, gonorrhœa, orchitis, vaginitis, prolapsus, rheumatic gout, varicose veins, measles and continued fever,—in all of these diseases when the symptoms correspond.

Remedies analogous to Pulsatilla may be named as follows:

As to its action on the eye, nose, bronchi and skin —Euphrasia, Dulcamara, Sulphur.

As to its action on the digestive organ— Nux vomica, Ignatia, Silicea, Sulphur.

As to its action on the female sexual organs—Sepia, Murex, Cyclamen, and, above all, Sulphur.

As to its action on the joints and ligaments—Rhus, Sulphur, Ledum palustre.

As to its action on the veins—Hamamelis, Zincum.

PULSATILLA MITTALIANA.

An American variety of the Pulsatilla has been proved by the Western homœopathists and others, and an excellent *résumé* published by Dr. Conrad Wesselhoeft in the "Transactions of the American Institute of Homœopathy," 1867. The following are the remarks of Dr. Wesselhoeft concerning the European and the American Pulsatilla:

"The resemblance is almost complete in every particular. * * * * The European has in a marked degree aggravation in the beginning of motion and amelioration during continued motion. The proving of the American Pulsatilla simply declares aggravation during walking, without saying whether the symptoms subsided during protracted walking."

CYCLAMEN EUROPÆUM.

SOW-BREAD.

THE student of materia medica should, at the very outset of his career, begin to guard against a danger which often besets the physician and leads him astray in practice—the danger of regarding certain remedies as favorite remedies and looking at them with a partial eye; of allowing the high estimate in which he has been led by his accidental experience to hold them, to incline him to see indications for these favorites where such indications do not exist.

You will sometimes hear an experienced practitioner speak of such or such a remedy as "a favorite" of his. To say the least, this is a dangerous way of regarding any drug. If it lead him to give it where a strictly impartial judgment would not pronounce it more exactly homœopathic to the case than any other known drug, it prevents his curing his patient in the quickest and surest way. Science has no partialities, and knows no preferences. Among the servants whom she puts at our disposal there is no possible position of honor for one above another. The drug which cures but a single case a year for us, because but one case in the year has demanded its administration, is as much entitled to our scientific regard as that which serves us every day.

Again, you should remember that your duty is, as scientific men, to judge impartially between the remedies which seem to be indicated in the case before you, and to choose, without fear or favor, that which is most homœopathic to it: without fear that because it is a remedy you have seldom used it may not act so well as the symptoms promise; without favor from an inclination to a drug that has often done good in many cases, and from which therefore you incline to hope for good, although it is not so homœopathic to the case in hand. This impartial judgment is very difficult but all-important. You will often find yourselves tempted to twist the patient's symptoms, ignoring some and perverting others, so as to bring the complex into a better resemblance to those of some drug from which you have often seen rapid beneficial action. It would relieve your mind so greatly if it would only turn out that the simile of the case is really to be found in Belladonna, or Bryonia, or Cimicifuga! And so you try to construe the symptoms in the direction of these drugs. Gentlemen, this is a delusion and a snare. If you thus deceive yourselves, and then give a drug which is not really indicated, you will get a little deceitful ease of mind for a few hours but no good to you patient. In these, as in all cases in life, look the truth right in the face, meet it squarely, and "do your level best!" You will find, perhaps, that not Belladonna nor Byronia nor Cimicifuga is indicated, but Silicea clearly, and nothing else. Now you get uneasy. What! Silicea a remedy for chronic diseases, for ulcers and abscesses—a drug of slow action! Can I dare to give it in this rapid-running and, if not arrested, speedily fatal phlegmasia, even though it be well indicated? Yes, give it, nothing doubting; and it will henceforth rank high in your esteem. It is my opinion that drugs which cure in chronic diseases appear to be slow of action because the morbid processes in such diseases are slow, and *vice versa.* In other words, I believe that the duration of action of a drug depends not so much on some inherent positive quality of the drug as upon the rapidity with which the physiological (and hence the pathological) processes are accomplished in the tissues involved and acted upon, which are slow in chronic, and rapid in acute, diseases. We shall have occasion to recur to this subject.

The value of Pulsatilla in measles having been mentioned, this is a suitable time to speak of another drug which, in its applicability to this same form of disease, is closely related to Pulsatilla; I mean the Euphrasia officinalis.

Moreover, the eminent value of Pulsatilla in certain forms of anæmia and amenorrhœa, makes this a proper place to treat of the Cyclamen Europæum, which is near akin to Pulsatilla in its physiological effects.

An immediate comparison of these drugs with their cognate, Pulsatilla, may bring sharply and clearly before your minds the resemblances and differences which constitute the elements of our decision in selecting or rejecting the remedy for a patient.

I shall proceed to treat of three drugs which, one in one point and others in other points, are related to Pulsatilla (but none of which is so well proved or so frequently called for in practice as that polychrest),—Cyclamen, Euphrasia and Allium cepa.

The Cyclamen Europæum, or Sow-bread, although no longer contained in the pharmacopœia of the allopaths, was extensively used in medicine by the ancients. Their descriptions of its properties are vague enough, but it is remarkable that they ascribe to it a power to affect the uterus and its appendages—which ascription was not physiologically verified until the most recent provings, which were made by members of the Austrian society of homœopathic physicians at Vienna. (Vol. ii.)

It used to be considered that the root of Cyclamen, applied externally, hastened difficult labors, and assuaged the pains. Also, that to touch Cyclamen, or take it internally, would produce abortion, or bring on premature labor. In less ancient times it was used as a remedy for amenorrhœa, and likewise to promote the expulsion of the placenta.

Our knowledge of the physiological action of Cyclamen is probably quite incomplete. It can offer no complete analysis of its effects. It was proved by Hahnemann and his pupils (Materia Medica Pura, vol. v.), and again by the Vienna society (Zeitschrift des Vereins, etc., vol. ii.).

SPECIAL ANALYSIS.

Sensorium. The sensorium is benumbed, the mind becomes inactive; lassitude and drowsiness oppress the prover, and yet he does not sleep inordinately. The memory is somewhat impaired; there is no disposition to mental labor. Cyclamen produces dizziness, which is perceived when one is standing still, and even when leaning the head against a support. It seems as if the brain were moving within the cranium, or as it does when one is riding in a wagon with the eyes closed. Objects move in a circle, or oscillate before the eyes. It is wors toward evening, and even is troublesome in bed, feeling as if the head were revolving. It is worse when one walks in the open air, is better in the room and when sitting.

Note the resemblances to Pulsatilla and the differences. The vertigo is worse in the afternoon and evening, as are Pulsatilla symptoms generally. But it is worse in the air and when in motion, and better in the room and when sitting quietly;

just the reverse of Pulsatilla in both of these conditions —air and motion. Confusion of the head and depressed feeling. Despondency, with irritation.

Head. The pains in the head are chiefly of a drawing, sticking or pressing character. Sometimes they pass from one side to the other, sometimes from the front to the back part of the head, but this is rare. They are located chiefly in the front part of the head, a stitching headache in the left temple being a strongly marked symptom. The semi-lateral character of the headache is marked, it occupies one side of the head or the other, the left temple being the seat of the pain almost always. In this Cyclamen resembles Spigelia, but the Spigelia pains involve the globe of the eye. Ignatia, Thuja and Silicea, among others, have semi-lateral headaches.

The pain is worse in the afternoon and evening. It is accompanied, when severe, by dimness of vision, or almost complete obscuration of sight; it is also accompanied by a sense of heat in the head, and this and the pain are relieved by the application of cold water.

The obscuration of vision accompanying the headache, when considered in connection with the pale complexion, rings about the eyes, depraved appetite and enfeebld digestion, and menstrual irregularities of Cyclamen, appears to be only a functional disturbance; but it is one which points to its use in certain forms of anæmia in women.

Eyes. The eyes look dull, lie deep, and have blue rings around them. The pupils contract and dilate alternately every few seconds. Dilatation is the more permanent condition. Glittering, as of a multitude of needles before the eyes. Obscured vision in all degrees, from the semblance of a cloud before the eyes to absolute (though transient) blindness. "It grows black before the eyes." Where there appears no obscuration, the strength of vision seems to be impaired.

It remains for clinical experience to show us the full significance of these symptoms and what relation they bear to diseases of the eyes attended by histological changes.*

Ears. Roaring and noises especially at night. Earache with the headache.

Nose. The sense of smell is blunted. Sneezing and profuse coryza. Frequent and forcible sneezing, with itching in the ear. Frequent but not copious epistaxis.

Face. The face is pale, but the cheeks are the seat of circumscribed redness and heat. Eruption on the face; many papules which often become filled with yellowish-white serum and then dry up; they are more abundant on the forehead.

Mouth. Much tenacious mucus in the mouth. Fauces red. Increased salivation. The diminution

---

* The sense of vision seems to be markedly modified, the pupils being greatly dilated, and the sight obscured even to absolute blindness; but it is to be noticed that these symptoms always accompany the symptoms of gastric disturbance and the headache, and they are unquestionably sympathetic with these affections, and are not idiopathic eye symptoms. [Taken from another paper on Cyclamen,— H. E. K. D.]

of the sense of taste in Cyclamen probably is closely related to the alteration of the mucous secretions of the buccal surface. Natrum muriaticum has complete loss of taste without such alteration, but coinciding with coryza. This coincidence is characteristics of it.

Tongue covered with a white coat, red at the tip, with several small vesicles which burn when she speaks or chews; salivation being abundant.

Taste. Pappy taste. The sense of taste is blunted; almost all food tastes alike (or is alike tasteless); nausea and bitter taste. The white-coated tongue, flat, pappy taste, aversion to fat and to bread and butter, remind is strongly of Pulsatilla. But the aversion to food after eating but little (although the first mouthful were enjoyed) and the great thirst, are different from the Pulsatilla symptoms.

Appetite. Diminished. Or good appetite, but one becomes satisfied after eating but little. Sudden satiety. Aversion to various articles of food, to bread and butter, to fat, and to meat. Great thirst; increased, even excessive thirst. Little or no thirst.

Stomach. The digestion is weakened; yet there is little or no change in the organic substance, although we might infer that a tendency to a change in the blood composition, similar to that in chlorosis, might result from a more thorough proving. Eructations of a fatty taste and smell; nausea, and accumulation of water in the mouth;

eructations tasting of the food last eaten. Nausea, with headache, vertigo, seeing of colors and double vision. The nausea is relieved by lemonade, as is also that of Pulsatilla, from fat food, especially pork. Oppression, as from too copious a meal. All of these symptoms are worse in the evening. Pressure and distention in the region of the stomach. Vomiting of mucus, after which sleep. There is much qualmishness and semi-nausea, as after eating fat food, with chilliness and depression of spirits.

Hypochondria. Stitches in the liver, and stitching pain in the intestines below the liver.

Abdomen. Fullness in the abdomen, distention by much flatus. Rumbling, with pain and nausea. The hypogastrium is very tender to pressure.

Stool. Much disposition to stool, renewed even after evacuation. While the rectum symptoms, tenesmus, etc., resemble those of Pulsatilla, the stool differs.

Stool first normal, then liquid, light yellow. Evacuation forcible, as if shot out. Diarrhœa yellow, pappy or watery, preceded by pinching pain in the abdomen. Pressure upon the rectum and anus, with itching, burning, and discharge of blood. Diarrhœa renewed by coffee.

Urinary Organs. Frequent copious discharge of whitish urine, stitching in the urethra, and dark-red urine. Scanty urine.

Sexual Organs. Men. Glans and prepuce sore.

Women. Menses too profuse and too frequent, with several labor-like pains. Discharge clotted, and black, and membranous. Cyclamen differs entirely from Pulsatilla. Instead of being scanty and retarded, the menses are too profuse and anticipate, while at the same time many constitutional symptoms are the same as those of Pulsatilla.

In the mammæ, a watery secretion, resembling milk, which leaves on the linen spots like a weak solution of starch. It flows spontaneously and can be pressed from the breast. This discharge followed and relieved a sense of fullness and tension and stitching in the mammæ, which were larger than natural, and felt as if a stream of air from the stomach and abdomen had been passing out through the nipples.

Thorax. Dyspnœa, oppression. Great lassitude; feeling as if she had not strength enough to darw a full breath. Pressure on the sternum. Stitches here and there in the chest. Palpitation of the heart. Irritated heart action. Pulse at first accelerated and double, then quiet and very weak.

Back. Drawing down the spine.

In the right side, in the region of the kidney, a deep pinching dull stitch, recurring every few seconds, worse on inspiration, which indeed is almost prevented by the violence of the pain.

In the glutæus maximus (left) rheumatic drawing extending to the sacrum. Drawing in the sacrum. Stiff neck. Tearing over the scapula, with paralyzed feeling in the arm.

Upper Extremities. Paralytic hard pressure, feeling as if it were in the periosteum and deep in the muscles, extending into the fingers and preventing writing. Painful drawing in the inner surfaces of the elbow and the wrist. Spasmodic, slow contraction of the thumb and index; it needs force to extend them again. Pricking itching as from needles betwen the fingers, relieved by scratching. Numbness in the right hand.

Lower Extremities. Cramp-like pain in the thighs. Numbness. Soreness of the heels and toes.

GENERAL ANALYSIS.

As regards functional activities, Cyclamen depresses the sensorium, as we have seen, producing confusion, vertigo, lassitude. Vision is enfeebled, and, for the time, under certain circumstances, suspended. Digestion is retarded and enfeebled, the taste blunted, appetite soon and suddenly satiated, desires, for food unnatural and restricted, thirst increased. The activity of the large intestine and of the female sexual system seems to be increased, diarrhœa and menorrhagia resulting. The organic substance is modified in so far as that diarrhœa is produced, the menstrual flow is increased, hastened, and changed to a dark, lumpy mass. The skin, too, is the seat of a vesicular or pustular eruption, itching, but relieved by scratching—this chiefly in the face. The scalp itches, the itching ceases on scratching, but immediately recurs in another place; the itching is a fine stitching or biting sensation.

The fever, in so far as fever is produced by Cyclamen, is partial in all its stages. Chill pre-dominates. The heat occurs at evening, and is without thirst.

Sleep is restless. It is hard to fall asleep in the evening. One goes to sleep late, has vivid dreams, wakens early, before day-break, but is very tired; lies awake, cannot sleep again, yet even at the usual hour for rising cannot get up because of lassitude and weakness. The pains, which ceased during sleep, re-appear soon after waking. This is different from the sleep of Pulsatilla, which begins late but is sound, and the patient sleeps till late in the morning. It is different from Nux vomica, which has early evening sleep. Sulphur has no sound sleep.

The peculiarities of Cyclamen are found in the fact that so many of the symptoms of various parts of the body, as for example the digestive and the female sexual organs, are accompanied by the semi-lateral headache (in the left temple) with nausea, vertigo and obscuration of sight, the face being pale and the eyes sunken.

The aggravations are at night and when at rest; from eating fat food, and while reposing. Ameliorations when moving.

If, now, we compare this record, scanty as it is, with the symptomatology of Pulsatilla, we are struck with the resemblance. The gastric symptoms are almost identical

We have the same white-coated tongue, the same qualmishness and disgust for food, especially fat food, the same absence of thirst and of febrile excitement, the same sympathy of the sensorium, eyes and head with these gastric symptoms. The peculiarities of the affections of the head and eyes are different, to be sure, from those of Pulsatilla; for Cyclamen produces semi-lateral headaches and absolute blindness, while the blindness of Pulsatilla is incomplete and only momentary, and the headache equi-lateral. But this very difference is a matter of congratulation, for there is a prospect that one or the other will cover most of the cases of sick headache and megrim that come before us for treatment.

But a large majority of such cases are the concomitants, if not the consequences, of menstrual irregularities, chiefly amenorrhœa, for they generally occur in women.

Now, you will have taken notice that in giving a summary of the action of Cyclamen just now, I said nothing whatever of its effects on the sexual organs of women.

What a pity, one cannot help exclaiming, that it does not act on these organs and affect their functions, for if it did, there could hardly be imagined a more admirably homœopathic remedy for the megrim that attends irregular menstruation. Failing such action, we might hardly be warranted in giving it. But does it not act on these organs and modify these functions? Hahnemann did not know that it did nor did his pupils. How could any one know? Only by the drug being proved by women on themselves!

No other form of proving, no other mode of investigation could give us this desired knowledge.

Not, therefore, until under the auspices of the Vienna Society, very imperfect provings were made by women, had we a knowledge of the fact that Cyclamen does indeed cause scanty menstruation, indeed cause absolute amenorrhœa, with megrim and loss of vision.

The only clinical indications for Cyclamen that I shall draw your attention to just now, follow directly from what has been said.

It promises to be, and has approved itself, a remedy of great value in those forms of menstrual irregularity which are attended by megrim and blindness.

In gastric disorders, the symptoms of which resemble those already described, and for which Pulsatilla seems to be the suitable remedy, but where the headache is semi-lateral rather than general, Cysclamen is likely to be service.

The remarks which have been made on the subject of our knowledge of the action of Cyclamen on the organism of women, lead directly to a subject of exceeding importance to all women who, in studying the profession of medicine, aim to be not merely apprentices to an art by the exercise of which they can make a living, but also, and more than this, students of a science fraught with blessings to the race, a portion of eternal truth, a science which it is the mission of the human race to elaborate and make perfect,—each student doing his or her appropriate work, and having a place to fill and a function to perform, indispensable to the perfection of the task.

Is it the ambition of any one of you to study science in this spirit? Will you work for a living, then die, and leave no sign? Or do you aim so to order your professional career that, while you gain an honorable livelihood by honorable toil, you may yet, when you pass away, leave science the richer for some facts or some generalization; adorned by some memorial of a life honorable to your art, which is eternal, as well as to your own ephemeral personality?

At the same time that you, in common with all students, may cherish this honorable ambition, do you more particularly, as women, desire to vindicate your enterprise in exploring the paths of medical science hitherto untrodden by your sex? Are you willing to enter upon a path of scientific investigation and research which the feet of man can never tread, the results of which, while they splendidly justify you in entering on the study of medicine, shall confer blessings unspeakable on that half of the race which is of your own sex, and thus on the whole race?

To those who are thus minded, to those women who can do for women what men have done for men, and would have done for women had it been within their power, I will indicate the way of self-sacrific which ends in honor.

All the facts stated in these lectures concerning the action of drugs on the human organism have

CYCLAMEN EUROPÆUM.

been derived from provings of drugs on the healthy subject. Although those provings have been extensively and accurately made only by homœopathicians, yet their necessity is urged and admitted by the leading authorities of every school of medicine.

The principle is this: We learn how a drug affects the healthy organism, and from this action we judge, according to a law of cure, what effect it would have upon a sick person.

Now, we have seen that drugs act differently upon different living organisms. We may not infer from the action of drugs upon animals their action upon man, because the organs of animals differ from those of man. Neither, then, may we infer from the action of drugs upon men their action upon women; more particularly as regards the action upon those organs which distinguish women from men.

Here, then I find a worthy and an indispensable work for women who are educated physicians, as worthy and no less indispensable than that of men.

Claim, if you please, for women an equal right with men to practice medicine and make money, I admit their right and would give them fair play, but I do not see any necessity, except it reside in their own desires and impulses. But as regards the work of perfectin the sciences of physiology and pathology and materia medica, I see so great a necessity for women to devote themselves to the labors of investigation and experiment, that I should never cease to a urge on them such a devotion of their gifts and of themselves, for the sake of science and of their own fellow-women whom this devotion would make science so much more potent to relieve!

I care not so much to shield women from what is called the rude attendance of rough men in the sick-room; but I do desire that women should prove drugs and ascertain their effects on the healthy, and what sicknesses they will cure, so that the medical attendant on sick women, whether he be man-doctor or woman-doctor, may know what drug to give and how to cure!

This is a mission which none but medically educated women can fulfill.

The students of our colleges and hospitals are all engaged, and are wont to engage, in drug provings. Will you do as much for your sex as men do for theirs? Will you engage in proving drugs? The mouths of those who rail against women's medical colleges would be effectually closed could we place in their hands an exhaustive proving by women of such a drug as Murex, or Cyclamen, or Caulophyllum!

The problem in drug proving is simply to ascertain the specific individual effects of the drug upon the healthy organism of the prover.

In order to get only the specific effects, uncomplicated with the generic effects, the prover must begin with very small doses, until the measure of his or her susceptibility has been gauged.

CYCLAMEN EUROPÆUM. 97

In order to be sure that the symptoms noted are in reality the effects of the drug experimented on, the prover must be always on the watch to discriminated between such effects and sensations to which he or she may be constitutionally subject; or the effects of unusual exertions, of changes in diet, of exposure to physical, mental or moral excitement or depression.

The symptoms of mind and disposition should be carefully noted.

The conditions of symptoms, viz.: the times and circumstances when and under which symptoms are aggravated or ameliorated should be most carefully noted.

Also the relations of symptoms to each other.

Inasmuch as changes in different organs in the body occur with very different degrees of rapidity, the prover should not hastily repeat doses, nor change the drug he is proving, nor relax the vigilance of his self scrutiny. For, though symptoms of the mind, or stomach, or lungs, may occur very soon after taking a dose of the drug, on the other hand, symptoms of the skin, bones and glands, may not occur for weeks or months.

I should recommend the proving of Murex purpurea as a drug that promises to be very useful, and would advise the provers to begin with the sixth dilution, taking a three-drop dose every night for four nights, and then awaiting results for a week. The class of provers may report progress every week.

EUPHRASIA OFFICINALIS.

EYEBRIGHT.

EUPHRASIA officinalis, or "Eyebright," is an annual, belonging to the family *Scrophulariaceæ*. It is common in northern Europe and in England, and is found in the northern United States. The Latin, as well as the English name, shows this plant to have had popularly ascribed to it healing virtues in diseases of the eye. Milton and Shenstone both speak of it as a well-known eye remedy. Since the year 1100 A. D. it has been mentioned as such in medical works. But, within fifty years, since it has become the fashion to ignore the specific properties of durgs, and to base prescriptions directly upon physiological and pathological hypotheses and the generic action of drugs, Euphrasia has been utterly neglected. Now, we may be sure that on substance ever gains, and for centuries maintains, over a whole continent, a high reputation for power to cure diseases of any organ, without there being something of solid foundation in fact for this reputation, whatever errors in degree, whatever absurdities in hypothetical explanation, may have grown up around this fact, and obscured and disfigured it. Hahnemann says that "it was not without reason that this plant received the name it bears," and that "it has fallen into unmerited disuse in the present day."

The same may be said of our own day. You will hardly hear of Euphrasia at the Eye Infirmary or at the hospitals, and yet you will there hear of no single remedy that will promptly and completely cure so many cases of catarrhal ophthalmia and of keratitis as Euphrasia will.

Our knowledge of the physiological properties of Euphrasia is derived from a proving of Hahnemann and is pupils, and one by the Austrian Provers' Society (Zeitschrift des Verein, 1857). These provings are not very complete, or if complete they show that Euphrasia does not embrace in its sphere of action the whole circuit of the organs of the body. I shall speak chiefly of the symptoms produced by it on the eyes and the respiratory organs.

The eyes appear to be affected in almost every part; eminently, however, the conjunctiva, the cornea, the lachrymal gland and sac, and the special sense. (Whether or not the retina be organically affected we cannot say positively, from absence of physical inspection).

The conjunctiva is reddened, the vessels enlarged, the mucous secretion at first disminished but speedily increased, and so modified as to become semi-purulent in character.

As necessary concomitants of these physical conditions occur the following subjective symptoms: A sensation as if dust or sand were in the eyes; pressure and tension of the globe; sudden and momentary obscuration of vision, relieved by winking, and evidently caused by the presence of opaque mucus upon the surface of the cornea; and nocturnal or rather morning agglutination of the lids. The secretion of tears is wonderfully increased in quantity, the eyes are constantly suffused; the lachrymal duct does not suffice to carry away this excessive secretion (perhaps its calibre is diminished through turgidity of its lining membrane), and the tears overflow upon the fact and run down the cheek.

The secretion of tears is not only increased in quantity; it is altered in character. The tears are very acrid, excoriating the lids, which swell and ulcerate on their margins, and causing inflammation and even suppuration of that part of the cheek which is kept wet by them.

It might be inferred from our knowledge of the natural history and course of ophthalmic disease, that where the globe of the eye is kept bathed in muco-purulent secretion and with acrid tears, as is the case under the action of Euphrasia, softening and ulceration of the cornea would speedily take place. We see this in cases of purulent ophthalmia, especially of a specific character; and we see it in cases where this condition of the eye is provoked, promoted or fostered by the constant injudicious application of hot fomentations and poultices to the eye.

From these facts it is a legitimate function of pathology which leads us to infer that the proving of Euphrasia would, if pushed further, develop ulcers of the cornea. Acting upon such an inference, or else guided only by the other symptoms of the case, homœopathic physicians early gave Euphrasia in cases of ulceration of the cornea; and the clinical record of its application is long and brilliant. It has been very successfully used in ulcers, both superficial and deep; and for the removal of obscurations and opacities of all grades.

Ulceration of the cornea is found also in cases not marked by the conjunctivitis and profuse discharges here described—cases of keratitis, or, as it was formerly called, scrofulous ophthalmia. The conjunctiva is even unnaturally bloodless, and the globe of the eye has a pearly aspect. The palpebral conjunctiva alone may be congested, striated, or studded with granulations. In such cases, when the photophobia is excessive, Conium maculatum is a remedy of exceeding value. It will, where indicated, be found to cover the symptoms of the depraved nutrition and innervation of the patient.

In other cases the lids are swollen and the secretions more abundant than where Conium is indicated, and the photophobia excessive in the morning and forenoon, so that the child buries its head in the pillow, while in the afternoon it will use the eyes freely. In cuch cases, the genral symptoms of the digestive tract and of the sleep almost always indicate Nux vomica, which cures the eyes as well, and very speedily.

As regards the special sense it is both exalted —photophobia resulting in a very marked degree, the patient being unable to endure the light— and it is perverted. The patient becomes very near-sighted. Again, the prover dreams of fire, lightning, flames, etc. Such dreams, if frequently repeated, are regarded as indications of deep-seated disease of the eye.

The nasal mucous membrane is affected much as the conjunctiva is. It is swollen, and secretes an abundance of water, and, later, of a mucopurulent substance, with sneezing and some degree of dyspnœa.

It is noteworthy that whereas the discharge from the eyes is acrid, excoriating the lids and cheek, that from the nose is bland, not excoriating the alæ nasi and lip.

Exactly the reverse is true of the discharges produced by Allium cepa from the eye and nose respectively. The tears are bland while the nasal discharge is acrid. This difference often serves to distinguish the indications of the two remedies.

The mucous membrane of the throat and bronchi is similarly affected. There is abundant mucous secretion, a loose cough, and a loud bronchial rale.

One prover speaks of a "red rash" upon the face, produced by Euphrasia.

The fever is not of a high grade. Chilliness predominates.

Among the clinical indications for Euphrasia I mention first, catarrhal ophthalmia; in fact, any inflammatory state of the eye which is characterized by congestion of the conjunctiva, or great photophobia conjoined with excessive lachrymation, the tears being acrid. Besides helping in these cases, it often removes chronic opacities; and it is said to have cured several cases of cataract. It is my belief that these chronic cases, which Euphrasia cured, once presented (viz., in their acute stage) the symptoms above described as indicating Euphrasia. And this statement of my belief induces me to call your attention to a mode of prescribing for certain chronic conditions which present no symptoms whatever to indicate a remedy. The method is to prescribe for the acute malady in which these chronic conditions originated. It can only be done when we can get a clear and trustworthy picture of the acute affection as it once really existed. As a striking illustration of this method of selecting a remedy, I venture to refer to a cure of deafness,* reported by myself in the "American Homœopathic Review," vol. i., and which I may add was a permanent cure. (1868).

Certain cases of measles present chiefly eye-symptoms, and these of such a character as to call to mind the symptoms of Euphrasia. Con-

---

* Deafness cured by Mezereum. See "Homœopathy the Science of Therapeutics," page 462.

joined with eye-symptoms are more or less of nasal and bronchial catarrh; and these symptoms find their analogues in Euphrasia.

As a matter of fact no less than of inference, Euphrasia is a remedy of prime importance in measles whenever the eye-symptoms are strongly pronounced as well as in ophthalmia, and is a valuable remedy in simple nasal and bronchial catarrh.

ALLIUM CEPA.

THE COMMON RED ONION.

WHY should not this peculiar and pungent vegetable, which contains notably phosphorus and sulphur, and of which the juice, even in the form of vapor, acts so promptly and so persuasively upon the conjunctiva and the Schneiderian membrane —why should it not produce physiological symptoms, and prove useful as a remedy?

Dr. C. Hering. of Philadelphia, to whom our materia medica owes so much of matter and of light, published a proving of a Cepa in his "Amerikanische Arzneiprufungen, 1857." The symptomtology is preceded by a most interesting *resume* of the history of Cepa. I propose to give a summary only of the action of Cepa upon the conjunctiva and the respiratory mucous membrane.

Biting and burning in the eyes with abundant secretion of tears; the eyes are constantly suffused with them. The burning is particularly felt in the margins of the lids. The tears are bland, not acrid, and do not scald the lid or cheek.

Under Euphrasia, on the contrary, the tears are acrid, while the nasal discharge is bland.

Coryza. Discharge from the nose watery; it drops from the tip of the nose. There is much sneezing, especially in coming into a warm room. It is worse in the evening.

Arsenic has sneezing in the cool air, after leaving a warm room; and its coryza is not attended by the laryngeal symptoms of Cepa. The coryza of Natrum muriaticum is characterized by entire loss of taste.

The nasal discharge of Cepa is very acrid, excoriating the upper lip, which becomes red and very sensitive.

Mercurius produces an acrid nasal discharge, but it is not so limpid, does not drop, and it excoriates the alæ nasi and columna, rather than the lip.

Along with this coryza there are roughness and rawness of the fauces and of the trachea. There is cough, dry and hoarse, or rough, provoked by a tickling in the larynx behind the pomum Adami. It is characteristic of Cepa that when in obedience to this tickling provocation the patient coughs, there results an extremely painful, splitting sensation in the larynx, as though that apparatus would be rent asunder by the effort of coughing. This pain makes the patient wince and crough, and brings tears to the eyes. No other drug produces this splitting in the larynx from cough in conjunction with acrid coryza.

ALLIUM CEPA. 107

The trachea feels rough and raw, and there is some dyspnœa, together with feverish heat and some acceleration of the pulse.

Prescribing in accordance with the above indications, I once succeeded in removing in the space of a few hours what I judged from physical exploration to be an extensive very recent congestion of the lungs, resulting from exposure to a cold north-west wind immediately after prolonged and violent muscular exertion.

MATRICARIA CHAMOMILLA.

THE name of this medicinal plant is derived from *matrix*, because of the specific action supposed by the ancients to be exerted by it on the uterus.

It was used by the ancients, by whom likewise and for similar reason the name Parthenion was given to it.

Culpeper says of it: "Venus commands this herb, and has commended it to succour her sisters; and to be a general strengthener of wombs; and to remedy such infirmities as a careless midwife has there caused."

It is found in most parts of Europe, in cornfields, waste grounds and by road-sides.

In medicine the whole plant is used; it is gathered when in flower, and the tincture is formed by expressing the juice of the whole plant, gathered fresh, and mixing it with twenty parts of alcohol.

By allopathic physicians the Anthemis nobilis has been substituted for the Matricaria chamomilla, their properties being assumed to be identical.

MATRICARIA CHAMOMILLA.

It is classed among the stimulant tonics. It contains an essential oil and a bitter principle. Its action is described as both stimulant and tonic. "In substance, or in a strong infusion, it produces a sense of warmth in the stomach, and, it is said, some acceleration of the pulse. It expels flatus, improves the digestion, does not confine the bowels, and is alleged even to possess emmenagogue virtues. In large doses it occasionally produces vomiting, looseness of the bowels, pain, with fullness of the head; and in certain idiosyncrasies it is even said to produce a sort of somnolent intoxication, with general depression and exhaustion."—Stillé, i., 557.

Our knowledge of the positive properties of Chamomilla is derived from Hahnemann's proving (Materia Medica Pura, iii., 1). This has been singularly corroborated with in a few years by proving conducted by Prof. Hoppe, of Basle.

Before proceeding to an analysis of the action of Chamomilla, it may not be amiss to quote at some length from Hahnemann's introduction of the proving. It is full of practical wisdom.

"This has been extensively used as a family medicine in complaints of all kinds, chiefly those that develop themselves rapidly. But physicians have held it too much in contempt, not considering it as a medicnie, but only as a popular remedy; and allowing their patients to use it, in conjunction with their prescriptions, in large handfuls, for infusions, teas, etc., and for external applications, while, at the same time, they were giving internal medicines; as if it were always a safe and salutary thing, never injurious, or at least quite unimportant. * * * * * *

"Thus we may see how far physicians have been blinded with regard to a plant belonging to a class of powerful medicines, when it was their duty to acquaint themselves thoroughly with its properties; not only that they might themselves make a wise and proper use of it, but a stop to the general abuse, pointing out when good effects might be expected from it, and, on the other hand, when it should be avoided.

"But physicians have hitherto not fulfilled this duty; they have rather rivaled the public in prescribing or permitting the use of this powerful remedy in all cases, without distinction, and in doses of all degrees.

"Yet is requires a very little ray of sense to perceived that no medicine in the world can be proper for all diseases; that each one has its circle of benefit strictly defined, beyond which every powerful medicine like Chamomilla must, of course, exercise injurious action in proportion to its energy; and therefore to avoid quackery the physician ought to know previously when Chamomilla may be useful and when prejudicial; as also how to proportion the doses, that they may be neither too powerful nor too weak. * * * * * *

"In fact no medicine, however polychrest it may be, can be useful and salutary in a tenth part of the existing diseases; neither can this prerogative belong to Chamomilla. But, admitting what is impossible, let us suppose it can cure a tenth part of the diseases of which mankind is susceptible, is it not clear that if it is employed universally it must be injurious to the other nine-tenths? Is it right to purchase success in one case to the injurty of the other nine? What do you mean by injurious effects? say the common practitioner; I see none that depend on Chamomilla. Certainly, I reply, so long as you are ignorant of the effects so powerful a medicine is capable of producing in a healthy person, you cannot perceive it to be the source of the mischiefs that are caused by the manner in which you employ it. These evils you consider to belong to the disease itself, and you attribute them to the malignity of that disease, and thus you deceive yourself, while you are doing harm to your poor patients.

"But cast your eye upon the mirror which I hold up to you; read the catalogue of the symptoms produced by Chamomilla, and then, if you fall back into your daily sin, if you put no limit to your habitual use of this plant, see how many among the apparent symptoms will be attributable to those belonging to Chammomilla, and judge of the distress and pain that will be caused to the sick by the abuse of this substance in those cases in which it is not suitable, and when given in large doses."

It may be remarked that the use of Chamomilla is

not so universal now as it was when Hahnemann wrote; but his observations apply with equal force to whatever drugs it may be the fashion to use in the same indiscriminate and reckless way.

GENERAL ANALYSIS.

1. On the *Vital Force,* the action of Chamomilla is shown:

In the fact that it exalts the general susceptibility, causing pains to be felt very keenly, so that a pain which might be supposed to be only moderately severe is, to the patient, intolerable. The disposition is impatient, intolerant, restless and very anxious.

In the prostration of general muscular power and in the lassitude, exhaustion and disposition to syncope which Chamomilla produces; in the peculiar modification of circulation which constitutes the fever of Chamomilla. This fever presents a compound of features above described. Though marked by excitement and increased sensibility, it is, nevertheless, not a well-developed inflammatory fever. The prostration is likewise represented. the heat is partial, confined for example, to one cheek, and is conjoined with profuse sweat of the head. The fever does not last long, but often recurs.

In the jerkings of isolated muscles, and in spasms.

In the special perversions of functions excited in the nerves of sensation of various parts of the body, and in the digestive and the urinogenital organs.

2. On the *Organic Substance*, Chamomilla does not act so vigorously nor so deeply as one might suppose from the nervous excitement which it produces. It acts:

On the digestive canal, increasing and changing the secretions, and provoking accumulations of flatus.

On the female genital organs, producing leucorrhœa, increased menstruation, and uterine hœmorrhage.

On the respiratory mucous membrane, increasing the secretion.

On the skin, producing a miliary eruption on the cheeks, isolated papules and pustules, and an unhealthy disposition of the skin, so that wounds do not readily heal, but become very painful.

Periodicity is in so far a property of Chamomilla action, that the pains recur in the evening, and are much worse at night before midnight, becoming then intolerable.

Peculiarity. It is a peculiarity of Chamomilla that pains are aggravated by heat: it is thus among a minority of medicines.

Hahnemann remarks that "a very small dose of Chamomilla seems to lessen very much excessive sensitiveness to pain, and the effects which pain produces on the mind. For this reason it relieves many of the morbid symptoms produced by excessive use of coffee and of narcotic substances; and it is also less beneficial to those who remain patient and composed under their sufferings."

SPECIAL ANALYSIS.

Sensorium. Vertigo, even to falling, especially after eating and when talking; or early in the morning on rising from the bed. Sometimes the vertigo is conjoined with a kind of syncope.

The intelligence is benumbed, or blunted, and distracted; not observant. In writing or talking the prover lets entire words and phrases drop.

Headache is felt even during sleep. The head is heavy. But the most frequent pains are tearing and drawing, generally anterior and almost always semi-lateral. The same is true of all the pains, they are semi-lateral.

Eyes. The pupils contract.

The margins of the lids feel dry, yet there is morning agglutination.

Pressure, heaviness and burning in the eyes. The conjunctiva is often deeply injected, without pain.

The special sense is somewhat affected. The sight is obscured,—there is a fluttering before the eyes.

Ears. The tearing, which is a characteristic symptom of Chamomilla, is felt in the ears;

sometimes also single stitches, especially on stooping, or a dull pressure. The ear seems stopped, and there is a buzzing of ringing in it.

Teeth. The affection of the teeth is a very prominent and characteristic action of Chamomilla, and has been turned to great practical account. The toothache rages chiefly at night, is accompanied by swelling of the cheek, and generally comes on or is aggravated after eating and drinking, and particularly after warm drinks. The pain is paroxysmal, is a drawing or tearing pain, with stitches towards or into the ear. The toothache, like the headache, is semi-lateral.

The taste is slimy, sour or bitter.

Appetite is extinguished. Food is repulsive.

Frequently there are sour eructations; and it is noteworthy that thereby whatever pains may be present are aggravated.

After eating, a sensation of fullness, nausea, and distention of the abdomen.

Nausea frequently occurs; frequently early in the morning.

Vomiting occurs sometimes, of food and bile.

Painful pressure is felt in the stomach, epigastrium and hypochondria, which sometimes embarrasses respiration; the pressure extends to the region of the heart. (Not only applicable in gastralgia but also in certain form of hepatitis.)

Flatus is generated in abundance. It moves about with rumbling and griping and a pressure downward, especially toward the inguinal canal.

There are likewise intolerable pains in the abdomen, cutting, pinching or taring; and particularly with a sensation as if the intestines were rolled up in a ball in the side of the abdomen.

The stool is diarrhœic, semi-fluid, sometimes yellow, sometimes green and watery, sometimes only white and slimy. It occurs most frequently at night, and is attended with cutting pains, which cause one to crouch together. It produces, likewise, blind and sometimes bleeding hæmorrhoids.

Chamomilla produces a yellow, acrid leucorrhœa. It causes also a uterine hæmorrhage, the blood being generally coagulated and passed with severe labor-like pains.

Before the menses there is produced a cutting colic and drawing in the iliac region, with frequent pressure to pass water.

The respiratory organs are affected chiefly in their mucous membrane.

The coryza is at first dry and obstructed; then the discharge is scanty and moderately acrid. There is hoarseness, produced by a tenacious mucus in the larnyx and trachea, with an almost uninterrupted tickling irritation, provoking a cough.

Along with this there is a kind of dyspnœa from pressure on the thorax and pressure on the sternum.

The mammary gland is affected. Indurations and nodosities occur in it, which are painful to the touch, and have, besides, a tearing and burning pain.

In the symptoms of the trunk we find

again the tearing and drawing pains of Chamomilla, worse at night.

From the lumbo-sacral region such pains extend into the thighs, like a kind of labor-pains (hence its use for after-pains).

Similar pains in the extremities, drawing and tearing, most violent at night, and seeming to have their seat in the ligaments and periosteum. They often extend from shoulder to finger, or from elbow to hand (and similarly in the lower extremity), and are conjoined with a paralyzed or numb sensation. The arms often go to sleep; there is a great disposition to cramps in the calves and in the toes.

The hands and feet becomes cold and stiff; and also at night the feet lose power, so that when attempting to stand the limbs give way.

Sleep. During the day there is great sleepiness with yawning, but at night sleeplessness with anxiety, inability to remain in bed, with prattling delirium.

Starting in sleep, weeping and complaints. Pain seems to be felt during the sleep.

Fever. The fever is partial in all its stages. The heat predominates. The chill is not always marked by external (objective) coldness; is attended by nausea, restlessness and tossing; often by burning heat of the head, or generally with internal dry heat. The heat is attended by thirst and dry tongue.

Sweat is partial, chiefly at night, generally on the upper part of the body.

118 MATRICARIA CHAMOMILLA.

The disposition is anxious, restless, impatient, intolerant of pain. There is easy starting, as if affrighted; easy vexing; irritability; disposing to anger; great sensibility to smells; and intolerance of music.

PRACTICAL APPLICATION.

The symptoms of Chamomilla, while their profound action on the nervous system and the excitement they show to be produced in the circulation, would lead us to expect benefit from Chamomilla in febrile affections, yet, nevertheless, show so little action upon the organic substance as to preclude the idea of relying on Chamomilla in parenchymatous inflammations, or in any purely and strictly inflammatory affection.

The fever is eminently one of irritation, and an attentive comparison of its phenomena with those which we observe at the besides, will show its similarity to fevers arising from a more or less permanent physical source of irritation, such as is supplied by dentition, or by the irritation of indigestible foreign bodies in the intestines.

The fever is partial; the nervous system is highly excited, and yet the sensorium is not perverted; pains are unreasonably intolerable; the patient cannot long retain one position; heat aggravates the entire condition, and yet, withal, the muscular strength is prostrated; twitching and jerkings of isolated muscles occur, and finally gen-

MATRICARIA CHAMOMILLA.

eral clonic spasms come on. This action of Chamomilla has led to its extensive and successful use in the diseases of dentition in infants. The diarrhœa which it produces is similar to that which so frequently accompanies dentition.

But dentition does not always so affect children that Chamomilla is indicated.

If the child be restless, irritable, wanting always to be carried about in the nurse's arms (muscular weakness), never content in one place, nor with anything that is done or said, one cheek red and hot, the other pale, with sweating head, hot mouth, tickling cough, green or yellow diarrhœa, with colic; with these, or most of these symptoms, but especially the disposition above mentioned, then indeed Chamomilla is indicated. But, if the disposition be mild and sluggish, the child disposed to be quiet, the bowels flatulent, to be sure, but costive, with frequent tenesmus, no matter if Chamomilla be recommended in forty books for dentition, give that child Nux vomica and cure it!

On the other hand, the fever may be really inflammatory, the pulse hard and full, and the sensorium excited with wild delirium, or dull and oppressed. In such cases we may except to find, on searching, that organic disease of some vital organ has set in, which must be sought and treated.

Chamomilla shows its adaptation to catarrhal affections of the eyes, ears, gastro-intestinal and urino-genital mucous membranes, and to similar affections of the respiratory mucous membrane. The secretions are moderately increased and are somewhat acrid.

For semi-lateral headaches, especially when they accompany otalgia, odontalgia or metrorrhagia, and when the disposition corresponds, Chamomilla is useful.

There must always be intolerance of pain, aggravation at night, and aggravation by warmth. This applies to the toothache, earache, facial and cervical neuralgia, and to the abdominal colic, and distinguishes it from the symptoms of Colocynth, which are diminished by warmth.

Chamomilla has been useful in bilious vomitings and in sub-acute hepatitis.

In mucous diarrhœas, frequent in summer, with abundant griping, yellow or yellow-green mucous stools, often produced by check of perspiration or crude food, it is a most valuable remedy. There is no great flatulence as in Colocynth, nor tenesmus.

Its action in controlling metrorrhagia is attested by both allopathists and homœopathicians.

The discharge is paroxysmal, the blood dark and coagulated.

In nasal and laryngeal catarrh its indications have already been pointed out.

As a remedy for after-pains Chamomilla enjoys considerable repute; likewise for certain forms of dysmenorrhœa, where pain precedes the period, which nevertheless is abundant when it does occur (which distinguishes it from Sepia).

Indurations in the mammary gland, with tearing, drawing pains, are often relieved by Chamomilla when other symptoms correspond.

In some forms of rheumatism it has done good, the pains being drawing and tearing, worse at night and from warmth, and felt in the ligaments and in the periosteum.

IGNATIA AMARA.

STRYCHNOS IGNATIA. FABA SANCTI IGNATII. ST. IGNATIUS' BEAN.

THE seed of a large tree, a native of the Philippine Islands. It contains strychnine, and in poisonous doses its effects are regarded as identical with those of Nux vomica.

The seeds are used in medicine. They are bruised and triturated.

By allopathic writers Ignatia is classed among the spinants, as acting exclusively upon the spinal cord. Containing strychnine, it is regarded as indentical in action with Nux vomica.

We shall see that, however great the similarity, there are yet great, and to us, as therapeutists, most valuable differences between these drugs. This is not the first instance in which a superficial use of chemistry has led to error.

GENERAL ANALYSIS.

Much of what was said of Nux vomica is certainly applicable also to Ignatia. Yet it appears that Ignatia acts less than Nux vomica upon the organic substance of the body, producing appreciable changes in the tissues, and much more exclusively upon the vital power.

Upon the vital power its action is not so much exalting or depressing, although in certain organs each of these varieties of action is distinguishable; but rather disturbing, destroying the harmony of action between different portions of the organism, perverting the co-ordination of functions. Thus, where we find heat of the body, and should anticipate such a condition of the nervous system as would make cool air agreeable, the contrary condition obtains; where we should, from the fever existing, except thirst, we find none, and *vice versa*. The great sensitiveness of the surface, instead of being aggravated by contact and by pressure, is relieved by it, etc., etc.

Now, it would seem as though such results from provings might be fanciful, were they not corroborated by too many witnesses to admit of the idea being entertained.

And yet, singular as this state of things is, it finds its analogy in the natural history of disease. For if you analyze the phenomena of hysteria, you will find this "perversion of the co-ordination of functions" to be the fundamental principle of the malady. And of all our remedies none so completely corresponds to hysteria, and so often cures it, as Ignatia.

In the words of Dr. Wurmb the whole character of Ignatia may be expressed in two words: "*Entgegengesetzte nebenbeschwerden.*" Accessory or concomitant phenomena which are contradictory to or inconsistent with each other.

SPECIAL ANALYSIS.

Head. The headache of Ignatia is aggravated by talking or listening or paying close attention to anything, but not by independent mental action. It is a sensation of heaviness, as if congested, relieved by stooping and leaning forward, not therefore a real congestion (here is a contradiction). There is sometimes a semi-lateral throbbing, sometimes a throbbing over the orbits.

The most characteristic pain is that as if a nail vere driven into the head. It is generally in the parietal or vertical region. Thuja has a similar pain in the occiput. This calls to mind the clavus hystericus, in which Ignatia is very useful.

Eyes. The affection of the conjunctiva is moderate. There is but little congestion. On the contrary, photophobia is sometimes intense, though capricious.

The vision is affected in this way: on one side of the axis of vision is observed a zigzag, white flickering.

Ears. Ringing and noises in the ears are observed.

Face. The muscles of the face and the lips often twitch and are convulsed.

Teeth. It is noted of the Ignatia toothache that though it consists chiefly in a soreness and tenderness of the teeth, it is felt more in the interval between meals than when eating. (Another contradiction.)

Throat. The sore throat of Ignatia, which is a sticking sensation, is felt more when swallowing than when the throat is at rest.

The digestive organs are much modified in action. The mouth is full of mucus. The taste is flat; food has a bitter, repulsive taste. There are fanciful aversions to special articles of food. There is sometimes craving for a particular article, and then, after a small portion has been taken with great enjoyment, a sudden and great aversion to it.

Frequent regurgitation of food and of a bitter liquid. Vomiting at night of food taken in the evening. Empty retching relieved by eating. (Contradiction.)

Distention of the abdomen after eating. Sour eructations. Salivation copious, frothy, sour. Hiccough.

In the region of the stomach great emptiness and qualmishness and weakness, with a flat taste in the mouth. Characteristic.

(The above three paragraphs are very important, applying to vomiting in pregnancy.)

There are sticking and soreness in the epigastrium, and moderate flatus, with cutting and griping.

The stool is but little affected. There is a tendency to frequent but scanty stool, as in Nux vomica; but Ignatia acts less on the substance of the rectum and more on its nerves. Thus in the rectum we have a distressing contraction and constriction of the sphincter, most painful after a stool, and when walking and standing, and relieved by sitting. (Contradiction.)

These are very important symptoms; violent stitches shooting from the rectum upward and forward into the abdomen. Along with these soreness, constriction and blind or bleeding hæmorrhoids, worse after a stool.

Besides these symptoms of hæmorrhoids and of proctalgia, itching and creeping at the anus indicate the presence of ascarides.

The chief symptoms of the urinary system are an incresed secretion of clear, lemon-colored urine. (Hysteria.)

Menstruation is too frequent and too copius, and for this state of things, other symptoms corresponding, Ignatia is a remedy.

Respiratory Organs. With regard to the respiratory organs, besides the itching of the nose and disposition to ulceration around the anterior nares, I call attention only to the cough.

This is characteristic of Ignatia. It arises from a feeling of constriction in the trachea or larynx, as if drawn together, then a tickling as if feather dust were in the throat; the cough is dry, violent, shattering; the shocks come in quick succession; the tickling irritation is not relieved by coughing. On the contrary, it becomes worse the longer the patient coughs, and is only relieved by a resolute suppression of the cough. (A marked contradiction, this!) The cough occurs chiefly in the evening, after lying down. This cough is unlike that of any other drug; the contradiction is the characteristic feature.

There is occasional spasmodic dyspnœa.

In the trunk various tearing pains, and lassitude.

There are jerking and twitchings in the extremities, especially after lying down at night, and startings when just falling asleep

Sleep is sometimes deep and irresistible, sometimes the patient is wakeful. It is disturbed by dreams.

The fever is partial in all its stages. The peculiarity of the chill is that it is relieved by external heat, and that it is accompanied by excessive thirst; whereas the fever, which is partial, is not attended by thirst. (Contradiction.)

The symptoms of the mind are most important. Anxiety, as though something terrible had happened; he cannot speak because of it, Hurry, fearfullness, terror, alternating with irresolution and inertness. Fixed ideas; the prover sits still and broods over thoughts and griefs.

PRACTICAL APPLICATION.

Ignatia is indicated:

1. When the bad effects of anger, of grief, and of sudden mental shocks produce still grief,

or a disposition to brood over sorrow instead of giving way. But when these emotions and shocks make the patient supercilious or crazy, given Platina; when boisterous and wild, Belladonna.

2. In convulsions. In epileptic attacks, with consciousness; in convulsions from grief; from dentition; from labor, when without fever or cerebral congestion; not, therefore, where Hyoscyamus or Belladonna is required.

3. In intermittent fever, when there is chill with thirst or fever without. Distinguished from Ipecacuanha, Eupatorium, Rhus toxicodendron.

4. In dyspepsia, for weakness in the epigastrium.

5. In proctalgia, after the stool; it is distinguished by stitches up into the abdomen; it is not indicated in fissure of the anus, which calls for Nitric acid and Plumbum.

6. For hæmorrhoids after labor.

7 For ascarides.

8. For the vomiting of pregnancy, if appetite, salivation, copious lemon-colored urine, etc., be present, and clavus hystericus.

9. In spasmodic cough. Note the sensation of constriction felt in the rectum and in the trachea.

Ignatia has a general correspondence to hysteria; to the form characterized by a mental character, which is mild, gentle, yielding though whimsical (else it were not hysteria), and introverted. There is another form represented by Platina, which drug will be the subject of the next lecture.

PLATINA.

THE physical and chemical properties and reactions of this metal are described from another chair.

It finds no place in the Pharmacopœia of England or the United States.

Trousseau and Pidoux cite a few vague and indecisive experiments upon animals and men with double Chloride of Platina and Sodium by Dr. Hœfer in 1840, and therapeutic experiments by the same physician, who proposed to substitute Platina for Gold and for Mercury in the treatment of secondary and of primary syphilis and syphilitic rheumatism.

Our knowledge of the action of Platina is derived exclusively from a proving by Stapf and Gross, two pupils of Hahnemann. It was first published in one of the earlier volumes of the "Archiv fur die Homœopathische Heilkunst."

For medical use, chemically pure Platina is dissolved in aqua regia. Into this solution a polished steel rod is plunged. The chloride is decomposed, and the resulting metallic Platina is precipitated in the form of a fine dust upon the surface of the rod. It is carefully washed to free it from the acid, and is then triturated according to the rules of the homœopathic pharmacy.

The action of Platina is exerted, in the most marked and peculiar manner, upon the mind and disposition; upon the second and third branches of the tri-facial nerve; and upon the sexual organs of women.

It acts, like Ignatia, much more upon the vital forces than upon the organic substance of the body.

It further resembles Ignatia in the fact that it interferes with and deranges the co-ordination of functions, destroying the harmony with which related functions are performed in the healthy body.

But the kind of perversion, and, in particular, the variety of mental perversion and disturbance produced by it, are altogether different from those produced by Ignatia, so that, if Ignatia correspond to one form of hysteria, Platina corresponds to a form altogether different.

The kind of pain characteristic of Platina is a cramp-like, squeezing pain,—a kind of crushing together. It is peculiarly characteristic of this pain that it begins gently, gradually increases in severity, and then gradually becomes less severe, until at last it ceases. In this respect Platina resembles Stannum.

Most of the Platina symptoms are worse when the patient sits or stands, and are ameliorated by

PLATINA.

walking. They generally occur, or are aggravated, at night.

It has been remarked as a peculiarity of the sleep of Platina, that however quiet the sleep may have been and however sound, the patient is always found, on awaking, to be lying on the back with the things drawn up upon the abdomen, with one or both hands above the head; and there is about or a little before the time of waking, a disposition to uncover the lower extremities. In connection with the form of hysteria to which Platina will be seen to correspond, and particularly with the nymphomania, which is a variety of this form of hysteria in which Platina has proved itself a most valuable remedy, these symptoms of the sleep have a great significance.

The action of Platina may be more particularly delineated as follows:

At first, the prover experience a distressing anxiety, a kind of deadly apprehensiveness, with a sensation of trembling throughout the body, a great disquiet of mind, which dose not admit of repose the prover believes death to be impending and has a great dread of it. (Like Aconite.)

Now, instead of grief, or despondency, or resignation under this state of things, there is great irritability, great susceptibility to anger and vexation; a trifling grievance produces a profound vexation, under the effects of which the prover remains a long time vexed, unfriendly, in fact "in the sulks."

Then, as the action of the drug becomes more profound, there is an alternation of this depression and this sulky despondency with an unnatural liveliness and gayety, so that the patient laughs violently, and this perversion of the natural functions (and of the co-ordination of the functions) of the sensorium goes so far that the prover laughs immoderately, even at the saddest objects.

Then finally there comes a state of mind, the outgrowth and development of that last described, in which the prover displays a most exalted and overweening self-esteem, overestimating herself beyond all reason, and entertaining a correspondingly low and contemptuous opinion of all surrounding objects and persons, even the most venerable and respectable; nay, this opinion is the more depreciating the nobler and more worthy the objects of it.

The extent to which this perversion of mind is sometimes carried, and the ludicrous scenes to which it gives rise, are among the curiosities of the materia medica. This is a characteristic action of Platina, and cases of disease in which something analogous does not appear, are rarely cured by Platina.

Headache also is produced. This presents the characteristics feature of Platina. A squeezing, constricting pain, as if a board were pressed against the forehead, as if the head were compressed, screwed together, etc., and at the same time a sensation of numbness in the head. Like other

Platina pains it begins gently, gradually increases in severity, and then gradually diminishes. Sometimes the cramping pain is in the temple, and then it is conjoined with similar pain in the zygoma and malar bone, constituting the temporo-facial neuralgia of Platina.

Besides these sensations, there is a variety of headache, consisting of a compression of the forehead and temples, as if everything would come out at the forehead; much worse from stooping forward, as well as from the slightest movement. It is preceded by anxiety, and by burning heat and redness of the face (a kind of "sick headache").

There are painful crampings and compression in the circumorbital regions, and particularly in the supraorbital and in these the globe of the eye sometimes participates, feeling sore.

The peculiar compressing, cramping pain is felt in the malar bone and zygoma, with a kind of uumbness and at the same time a burning pungent sensation, inducing one to rub or scratch the part.

This corresponds well to a certain form of facial neuralgia. It resembles most closely that of Verbascum thapsus.

It is distinguished from that of Arsenicum in this, that in the latter the pains are burning, and that they dart quickly, like red-hot needles, from place to place.

The pain of Verbascum is like a crushing with tongs. Platina has steady compression.

That of Spigelia is a shooting or piercing, and has its chief in the globe of the eye.

Chamomilla has aggravation by heat, and is further distinguished by the great impatience of pain exhibited by the patient. The neuralgia of Capsicum is provoked by external pressure, and is a fine line of pain coursing along the nerve. The constitutional symptoms still further aid us in distinguishing the indications for the several drugs which produce a form of prosopalgia.

Noises in the ears, of the greater variety, are produced in abundance by Platina. There is little evidence of any organic lesion. (This might lead to the selection of Platina for what is called "nervous deafness.")

There is little that is distinctive in the action of Platina on the digestive canal, except in so far as the stool is concerned.

This is retarded; the fæces are scanty, hard, evacuated with difficulty and almost dry. The evacuation requires great effort of the abdominal muscles; and this is followed by a peculiar sensation of weakness in the abdomen, or by a shuddering throughout the body.

In the rectum there are occasional sharp stitches, compelling one to cry out. In this Platina resembles Ignatia.

The menses appear much too early and are very copious. Moreover, there are uterine hæmorthages, copious and often recurring. As in most uterine hæmorrhages, the color and consistency of the blood furnish a valuable characteristic of the remedy. That of Platina is very dark, and without being coagulated in distinct masses, it is thick and tarry. It is accompanied by pains in the sacrum; but these sacral pains are only felt as a sequel to pains which have first been felt in the groins, causing a dragging and pressing downward in the entire pelvis, and have then passed to the sacrum; and, furthermore, there is always in connection with this metrorrhagia of Platina an unnatural sensibility and irritability of the genital organs.

It may be remarked of the pains of Belladonna that they pass through the pelvis either in its anterior-posterior or in its lateral axis; while the pains of Pulsatilla and Sepia pass around the pelvis from sacrum to groin, and are conjoined with scanty menstruation instead of profuse.

The labor like pains of Chamomilla are very severe, and the metrorrhagia is in paroxysms, the blood being thin and rather light, with firm coagula.

The flow of Secale cornutum is thin and painless, so is that of China.

Crocus has a dark flow, but it is not attended by a bearing-down pain, but rather by a sensation as of a living body moving in the abdomen.

Millefolium and Sabina both produce a light-colored, florid uterine hæmorrhage.

It is, thus, not difficult to distinguish the uterine flow of Platina from that of other drugs.

Attention should again be called to the hypersensitiveness and irritability of the genital organs.

These symptoms, together with those of the sleep already mentioned, have led to the use of Platina in cases of nymphomania; it has been of the greatest service, comparing with Hyoscyamus.

The organs of respiration are not especially affected.

In the trunk, we have first a weakness of the neck; the patient cannot hold up his head, and along with this, a kind of tensive numbness. There is pain in the spine and sacrum, as if they were broken, especially after a long walk or on bending backward.

In the extremities are felt cramp-like, pressing and compressing pains, such as are elsewhere experienced, conjoined with a kind of burning and numbness.

PRACTICAL APPLICATIONS.

Of the uses of Platina in treating disease, but little remains to be said.

The mental symptoms denote the forms of hysteria in which it is useful. Whereas Ignatia corresponds to cases in which there is a disposition to grieve, to brood in melancholy sadness over sorrows, whether real or imaginary, Platina, on the other hand, belongs to a variety in which the mind rises in defiant and distorted superiority over the causes of vexation or sorrow; becomes, first, demonstratively apprehensive, then alternately demonstratively lachrymose and boisterously merry, and at last absurdly supercilious,—a genuine representation of Mrs. Lofty. But, whatever the frame of mind may be, it is always demonstrative, and this is the character of Platina; the personality of the patient is obtruded on one's notice.

The character of Ignatia, on the other hand, is that it is undemonstrative; the sufferings and perversions are not obtruded on one's notice.

The peculiarities of the neuralgia and of the uterine hæmorrhage, which are marked Platina symptoms, have already been pointed out.

It remains only to call attention to the stool, and to say that in the constipation which is often so troublesome a concomitant of pregnancy, Platina is often a valuable remedy, standing in the same rank with Sepia, Alumina and Plumbum.

SEPIA.

SEPIÆ SUCCUS.

THE juice of the cuttle-fish; a blackish fluid contained in the abdomen of the animal, and from which the animal has the power of projecting the juice into the surrounding water.

For medicinal purposes the juice carefully dried, divested of its membranous envelope, and prepared by trituration according to the rules of the homœopathic pharmacy

Although Sepia has no place in the pharmacopœia of the old school, and is, indeed, so little known by them that one of their foremost writers has endeavored to fling ridicule on homœopathists by stating that they ascribe medicinal virtues to the cuttle-fish *bone,* which is mere carbonate of lime, it is a singular fact that Hippocrates set a high value on Sepia as a remedy in diseases of women and in dysmenorrhœa, and that Galen ascribes to it tonic and stomachic qualities; while Marcellus recommends it for gravel and for the removal of freckles. A very singular anticipation by the ancients of the exact deductions from the homœopathic law.

SEPIA.

Sepia is one of our most important remedies. Its action pervades almost the entire organism and is very enduring, the effects of a single dose often lasting for many weeks. Upon the vital force and the organic substance it acts with equal energy.

The sphere of action comprises, in particular, the sexual organs of women, the gastro-intestinal tract and its appendages, the skin and glands, and the nervous system of animal life.

The symptoms are most apt to occur or to be aggravated when the patient is at rest, sitting quietly, in the forenoon or evening; and to be relieved by vigorous exercise in the open air. In general, the aggravation occurs about the middle of the forenoon; especially the sense of "sinking at the pit of the stomach," which attends many uterine disorders.

Sepia induces a tendency to free and sudden perspiration from a nervous shock or from exertion, but it is noteworthy that this perspiration comes out after the exertion is over or the shock is past, and when one is sitting quietly. (Calcarea carbonica has sweat during the exertion.)

Sepia produces (and cures) what are well known as "hot flashes"—sudden accessions of heat, followed by a momentary sweat and weakness and disposition to syncope. These are frequent and very annoying incidents of the climacteric period in women. Lachesis resembles Sepia in this.

In many respects the symptoms of Sepia closely resemble those of Pulsatilla. As would be naturally inferred, these remedies often act as mutual antidotes; and so it happens frequently, when they are given in alternation, as the custom is of some physicians, no result is observed. In such cases, it is often sufficient to suspend the administration of one of them in order to get a prompt and satisfactory effect from the other.

The skin affections of Sepia are among its most important symptoms. We find itching of the skin, and itching vesicles and papules on the face, hands and feet; and also a vesiculo-pustular eruption in the hollow of the joints of the knee and elbow. After the Sepia eczema there is abundant desquamation.

While speaking of the skin, it should be mentioned that Sepia produces on the lower lip a swelling with a soreness, burning pain and a pricking as from a splinter of wood. This symptom, together with the constitutional symptoms, has led to the use of Sepia in the treatment of epithelial cancer of the lower lip, two cases of which, cured by Sepia^{800}, have come within my personal knowledge.

In like manner, the other skin symptoms have induced the successful use of Sepia in cases of Rhus poisoning.

The fever of Sepia is incomplete. Chilliness predominates, but, like the heat, is fugitive and transient. Perspiration is copious, especially at night, and is conjoined with great weakness.

SEPIA.

The disposition peculiar to Sepia is a depressed, anxious and fearful state of mind, with a sense of helplessness, and yet great susceptibility to excitement, and still more to terror, frequent attacks of weeping, and despair of life.

SPECIAL ANALYSIS.

Headache. Chiefly pressing and throbbing, with a kind of rush of blood to the face, which becomes red and hot, even to the ears. No general fever, however. General aggravation from motion. Itching of the scalp and falling out of the hair.

Eyes. The sense of vision is affected. There is photophobia by day, and a white flickering before the eyes, like a thousand suns or sparks or black specks; around the candle-flame there is a green halo. On attempting to read or white, the vision becomes obscured.

There are supra-orbital pains. The eyelids pain on awaking, as if too heavy, as if paralyzed, corresponding to ptosis—a malady in which Sepia has often been given successfully.

Then, conjunctivitis with biting and burning and itching, but very scanty secretion of mucus or pus.

The face is the seat of eruption already described. Moreover, on the forehead come irregular non-elevated brown spots, well known as "liver spots." The complexion becomes yellow and earthy. There are often, in connection with the headache or with uterine disorder, tearing pains in the facial bones and in the teeth. Finally, a characteristic symptom of Sepia is a brown discoloration extending across the bridge of the nose like a saddle.

In the mouth often form painful vesicles and ulcers —a form of stomatitis.

The gums swell and bleed easily. The teeth become loose. There is toothache, digging, tearing and gnawing pain, sometims in a single tooth, sometimes in a whole row, aggravated by warmth. The toothache is generally a sympathetic concomitant of uterine disorder or of pregnancy.

The tongue is often sore, as if scalded. Salivation occurs, the mouth filling with a saltish fluid, while at the same time the throat and fauces are so dry that the patient can hardly utter a sound. (This closely resembles the salivation of pregnancy.)

The taste in the mouth is offensive, slimy putrid like a bad egg, with eructations of the same character; or bitter, often bitter early in the morning, this ceasing after breakfast.

There are abundant eructations; hiccough after eating; nausea and vomiting of bile, or vomiting of bile early in the morning on rising, with, during the day, attacks of constriction in the hypochondria, and nausea.

There is no thirst. Appetitie fails; all food tastes alike. The stomach feels empty and weak with nausea at thought of food. A characteristic symptom is a peculiar faint sinking at the pit of the stomach, which is not necessarily painful to pressure. The faintness of Mercury is accompanied

SEPIA. 143

by tenderness; so is that of Calcarea carbonica. (Hydrastis.) Pressure and fullness are also sometimes felt. There are stitches in the region of the liver, which is sometimes sensitive to pressure. Also a fullness in the hepatic region and a pinching pain. It is peculiar to Sepia that the pains in the hypochondria are more tolerable when the patient lies on the painful side, while with Magnesia muriatica the opposite condition obtains. (Bœnninghausen.)

The abdomen is often distended with flatus. There are cutting pains horizontally across the abdomen, sometimes extending up into the chest.

In the rectum and anus a constricting pain which extends into the perinæum or the vagina, sometimes up into the abdomen. Sometimes a feeling of soreness and a kind of pressure outward, cutting burning and itching. Hæmorrhoidal tumors occur, which are painful and bleed. After stool, emptiness and weakness in the abdomen.

The stool is scanty and infrequent.

The evacuation of urine is preceded by pressure and tenesmus; it is frequent, painful, and often ineffectual until after long waiting and effort. At night frequent desire to pass water, which starts tardily, and flows slowly. Again, involuntary micturition at night.

On the sexual organs of women Sepia acts very distinctly. Along with cutting pains in the abdomen, a pressure is felt on the uterus downward, as if everything would fall out.

The menses come too early, but are scanty. They are preceded by violent aching in the abdomen, causing even faintness, and by chilliness and shuddering.

During the menses, restlessness, drawing pains in the limbs and abdomen. Palpitation and dyspnœa, with toothache and headache and epistaxis; with depression of mind.

At other times than the menstrual period, frequent stitches in the vagina in paroxysms, with or without a watery yet lavish leucorrhœa. The leucorrhœa is rarely acrid, whereas that of Kreosote is very acrid.

Sepia produces (and cures) a dry, fatiguing cough, provoked by a sensation in the region of the stomach, and seeming to come therefrom; or the cough comes, as it seems, from the abdomen. A symptom which I have often verified in practice.

Then again a cough with copious, saltish expectoration, white or grayish yellow: the cough being attended, as all the Sepia symptoms are, by accessory symptoms, such as stitches in the epigastrium or head, faintness, nausea, etc.

From these and other similar symptoms, we draw our indications for Sepia in pulmonary consumption.

It produces various forms of oppression of the chest, burning in the chest and palpitation.

In the sacro-lumbar region Sepia produces pain, which generally is relieved by sitting or lying, worse when standing or walking. The backache of Belladonna is worse when lying down; better when sitting. Sometimes the reverse.

It is a pressing, dragging pain over the sacrum and at the same time over the hips, and a burning pressure in the spine; also drawing pressure and burning pain across the dorsal region and under the scapula (often like that produced by sewing).

In the extremities, stitches and sticking, drawing pains, with lassitude, coldness of the feet, but sometimes only of the knees; sweat of the feet. The eruptions already described.

PRACTICAL APPLICATIONS.

Among the general affections for which Sepia has been found a useful remedy may be mentioned, first: Various forms of skin disease, and in particular those of a vesicular character, attended by much itching and followed by desquamation. The vesicular eruption is not attended by the erysipelatous inflammation of the contiguous skin, such as is characteristic of Rhus toxicodendron; and this serves in part to distinguish these drugs.

Sepia is especially successful in the treatment of herpes circinnatus or ringworm, when this occurs in isolated spots. Calcarea carbonica (or acetica) is also useful in this affection. The distinction is to be found in the constitutional symptom. When, however, the herpes circinnatus occurs, not in isolated patches, but over a great portion of the body in intersecting rings, and attended by heat, itching, fever and great constitutional disturbance, Tellurium seems to be indicated, as appears from a proving of that drug in the "American Homœopathic Review."

In connection with skin symptoms, may be mentioned again, the brown discolorations of the forehead and cheeks and of the skin across the bridge of the nose, known as "liver spots," and which are very frequently found conjoined with constitutional symptoms which indicate Sepia as a remedy, these symptoms being particularly those of the hepatic region and of the uterus and its appendages.

In paralysis of the upper eyelid—ptosis—Sepia often effects a cure; also in certain perversions of the function of vision.

The neuralgia, the toothache and the headache of Sepia, are almost always conjoined with some disorder of menstruation, with pregnancy, or with some disease of the sexual organs of women. And it is peculiar to Sepia that, along with its symptoms of disease in the sexual organs, there occurs a considerable number of sympathetic symptoms in distant organs, e.g.: the toothache, headache, salivation, neuralgia.

Attention has been called to the fact that two cases of epithelial cancer of the lower lip have been cured by Sepia. A third case of this disease is so interesting as to be worthy of narration.

SEPIA. 147

An epithelial cancer, far developed, had been excised. The wound healed kindly. After a few months the patient began to emaciate, and to exhibit every sign of cancer cachexy. The decline was alarmingly rapid. Eminent surgeons diagnosticated internal cancer. No hope of recovery was entertained. The complex of symptoms indicated Sepia, which was given, 200, and effected a complete and rapid restoration of health. The health remains good to this day (ten years).

In chronic or sub-acute hepatitis, Sepia does good. Its chief use, however, overshadowing all others, is in displacements and diseases of the uterus. In prolapsus it is the remedy, *par excellence*. Yet not to be used to the exclusion of Nux vomica, Pulsatilla, Belladonna and Podophyllum. The simultaneous irritability of the bladder and the presence of leucorrhœa, together with the hot flashes and the sympathetic affections of remote organs, serve especially to indicate it.

Sepia is rarely indicated by these symptoms but that there is present the peculiar "sinking and all-gone sensation" in the pit of the stomach, almost producing faintness, and relieved by lying down and by taking food or wine.

In amenorrhœa or retarded and scanty menstruation, it is often indicated.

Experience has shown its value in cases of ulceration and congestion of the os and cervix uteri. Its use in appropriate cases supersedes all local applications, which in the vast majority of cases are not simply unnecessary, but are very mischievous. The same may be said of mechanical contrivances in uterine displacements, especially pessaries and internal supporters of all kinds.

Sepia is also a remedy in functional derangements of the liver.

Medical practitioners, like other men, are apt to "run in grooves," and the grooves grow deeper by use. With regard to the materia medica, they are apt to remember of each remedy some one or two applications in which it is eminently useful, and to forget or ignore many others in which, though, perhaps, less frequently indicated, it is equally valuable.

Thus, every one has in mind the virtues of Silicea in suppurative inflammation of connective tissue, while comparatively few might think of it as a remedy in cerebro-meningitis, or in neuralgia, or in epilepsy.

Sepia, in like manner, suggests itself to every practitioner in cases of chronic uterine disease, and its value in such cases has caused it to be classed, in the medical mind, with remedies specially adapted to chronic cases. The remarks I purpose to make will show, I think, that it may also be a remedy for acute conditions. They will serve, likewise, to call attention to the re-proving of Sepia, made under the direction of the Bureau of Materia Medica of the American Institute of

Homœopathy, and published in the Transactions of that body for 1875. While this proving confirms in a remarkable manner, the Hahnemannian proving of Sepia, and may be said to have added little absolutely new to our knowledge of this drug, it certainly presents, in a definite form, symptoms that are somewhat shadowy in the original proving, and thereby furnishes evident indications, where formerly these were perceptible only to acute observers.

I propose to consider only the relations of Sepia to "functional derangements of the liver," taking from Murchison's recent work,* the symptoms of these derangements and placing under each of these symptoms the corresponding group of Sepia symptoms.

Before describing the symptoms of functional derangement of the liver, Dr. Murchison states that the functions of the healthy liver are—not simply nor chiefly the secretion of bile—but

"1. The formation of glycogen, which contributes to the maintenance of animal heat and to the nutrition of the blood and tissues, and the development of white blood corpuscles.

"2. The destructive metamorphosis of albuminoid matter, and the formation of urea and other nitrogenous products, which are subsequently eliminated by the kidneys, these chemical changes also contributing to the development of animal heat.

---

* "Functional Derangements of Lectures, etc., delivered in March, the Liver: being the Croonian 1874, etc., London."

"3. The secretion of bile, the greater part of which is re-absorbed, assisting in the assimilation of fat and peptones, and probably in those chemical changes which go on in the liver and portal circulation, while part is excrementitious, and in passing along the bowels stimulates peristalsis and arrests decomposition."

A "functional derangement" may be a modification or an arrest of any one or several of these healthy functions.

1. If the power to convert glucose into glycogen be impaired by functional derangement of the liver, glucose passes into the general circulation, is eliminated by the kidneys, and we have one of the several forms of glycosuria,—forms which agree in this one symptom (sugar in the urine), but differ profoundly in the pathological conditions on which this symptom depends, and in the indications for, and their amenability to, treatment. The form we have described is often transient, and always a mild and curable form of diabetes; or, this glycogenetic function may be modified in another way, and we may have a more serious form of glycosuria by an increased conversion of glycogen into sugar, from hyperæmia of the liver depending on paralysis of the vaso-motor nerves, resulting from irritation of the roots of the pneumo-gastric nerves, injuries of the spinal cord, poisoning by curare, etc.

2. When the function by which the liver disintegrates and eliminates albuminoid matter is imperfectly performed, the disintegration stops short of

the formation of urea which is soluble; and products more sparingly soluble, and which are less completely oxidized, than urea, are formed, viz., uric acid, etc.; or products still less oxidized, such as leucin and tyrosin, which we find in acute atrophy of the liver when this function of that viscus is almost abolished. Where, under this functional derangement, uric acid is formed instead of urea, we find in the urine deposits of uric acid, of urates, and abnormal pigment.

Such is a brief statement of Murchison's views of the functions of healthy liver, and the results of some of their derangements. I shall restrict my remarks upon Sepia to the second form of derangement above described, viz., that of the function by which albuminoid matter is disintegrated and eliminated, and the derangement of which is manifested, among other symptoms, by excess of uric acid and urates in the urine.

Murchison gives the following names of diseased conditions resulting from this derangement:

1. Atonic dyspepsia, of which the symptoms will presently by given in detail.

2. Gout—anomalous or regular; urates in the blood, and deposited in or near the joints.

3. Urinary or biliary calculi.

4. Granular degeneration of the kidneys, from their constant work in eliminating urates. (Dr. Geo. Johnson.)

The symptoms of the atonic dyspepsia are given more particularly by Murchison, as follows:

After each group I cite, from the new or from Hahnemann's proving, the corresponding Sepia symptom:

1. Tongue: that of atonic dyspepsia, large, pale, flabby, indented. Sepia: tongue coated brown or yellow (148, 149); tongue feels too large. (155.)

2. Appetite good, but suddenly satisfied; loathing of fat. Sepia: sudden craving, sudden satiety· (185, 184); good appetite, but loathing of meat. (Hahn., 510, 522.)

3. Bitter or coppery taste; worse in the morning. Sepia: putrid, insipid taste (177, 178); bitter, repulsive taste in the morning. (Hahn., 499.)

4. Flatulence (from lack of bile?). Sepia: obdomen very much distended after the least bit of food. (207, 215.)

5. Constipation, from lack of normal stimulus to the excretion, and with great depression of spirits; or there may be pale or dark offensive diarrhœa. Sepia: constipation; seems to have lost power (243, 241); constipation, with bleeding and weight and pain in the rectum (236); only small, hard lumps passed (241); hard stools; fæces covered with mucus, followed by slimy, bilious or catarrhal stools. (255, 256.)

6. Intestinal hæmorrhage; hæmorrhoids. Sepia: considerable bleeding from the rectum and intense bearing down at the anus. (261, 262.)

7. Hepatic pains; weight, fullness, tightness; worse when lying on the left side. Sepia: as if the abdomen were full and bloated across the epi-

gastric region (214, 215); as if a load rested on the epigastrium (217); soreness around the umbilical region on pressure, especially on the right side (221); Bœnninghausen names Sepia under the rubric "worse from lying on the left side."

8. Jaundice (?). Sepia: yellow face and whites of eyes. (Hahn., 325.)

9. Aching of the limbs and lassitude. Sepia: weakness and aching of the thighs and legs (419-421); general weariness and prostration in the joints. (422.)

10. Pain in the right shoulder and about the scapula. Sepia: long-continued pain under the right shoulder. (410, 413.)

11. Hepatic neuralgia, with great depression of spirits. Sepia: stitches in the hypochondria, across the abdomen, making her cry out (Hahn., 626); frequent stitches under the right ribs. (Hahn., 627, 629, and 624, 625.)

12. Cramps in the legs. Sepia: cramps in the calves at night. (Hahn., 1310-1314.)

13. Dull headache in the forehead and occiput in th morning on waking, lasting part of a day, or several days, with constipation and pain in the right hypochondrium. Sepia: dull, stupid headache, with great mental depression (40-43); dull pain over both eyes (55); dull headache through the temples and forehead (59); waked with dull headache in the back of the head (74).

14. Vertigo and dim vision. Sepia: dizziness (35 Hahn., 87-100); obscured vision. (Hahn., 258, 259.)

15. Noises in the ears. Sepia: both ears feel stopped (111); ringing, singing, roaring, etc. (Hahn., 293-304.)

16. Sleeplessness. Sepia: restless nights; tired mornings (504); disturbed sleep. (508, 509, 511, 512.)

17. Depression of spirits; irritability of temper. Sepia: mental depression; very low spirited, with headache (2-5); very irritable; very cross. (5, 6, 10, 12.)

18. Palpitations and fluttering of the heart. Sepia: palpitation, very nervous (360, 365); seemed as if the heart occupied all the cavities of the body (359); pulsation with soreness in the stomach (199.)

19. Irregularities of pulse; intermission (which is always due rather to hepatic indigestion than to cardiac disease; intermission of pulse. (Hahn., 1098, 1099.)

20. Feeble circulation; anæmia. Sepia: pale, sickly aspect. (Hahn., 324.)

21. Angina pectoris, Sepia (?).

22. Pulsations in various parts of the body, especially in the epigastrium. Sepia: pulsations felt in the body, in the head and extremities, day and night, especially in the night. (Hahn., 1409, 1410.)

23. Urine heavier than normal; it deposits uric acid and urates. Sepia: every prover noticed marked diminution in the quantity and increase in the specific gravity of the urine, which deposited uric acid and urates. This was reported by

SEPIA. 155

provers of both sexes, and from various potencies of Sepia.

24. Chronic catarrh of the fauces. Sepia: feeling of rawness in the posterior fauces, etc. (165, 167).

25. Chronic bonchitis. Sepia: coughing spells in the morning, with either difficult expectoration, or copious sputa, easily raised; harsh dry cough. (342,344.)

26. Spasmodic asthma. Sepia: tightness and constrictive sensation in the chest. (346).

27. Eczema, lepra, psoriasis, lichen, urticaria, boils, pigment spots, pruritus. Sepia: vesicular, papular and pustular eruptions (484-495); itching (484); yellow spots on the face and a yellow patch over the dorsum of the nose. (Hahn., 326.)

In an excellent physiological study of Hahnemann's proving of Sepia, Dr. V. Meyer of Leipzig, in 1853, used the following language: "This remedy operates especially on the portal system, by retarding the circulation, and causing an overloading of the vascular system with venous blood, or with blood more or less resembling venous. A plethora venosa, as it is called, gives rise to most of the various symptoms. The pathological process is also marked by a state of depression. * * All further morbid conditions are but secondary." * * "All disorders of the portal system must first affect the neighboring organ, the liver." ("Homœopathische Vierteljahrschrift," iv., 2. Translation in "British Journal of Homœopathy," xiii., pp. 635, 636.)

Cases illustrating the use of Sepia in acute dissease, connected with functional derangement of the liver.

Case 1. August, 1875. A lad, seven years old, was brought home from the country, said to be suffering from remittent fever; he had been ill three weeks, and presented the following symptoms: febrile condition persistent, very weak, keeping his bed, extreme depression of spirits and irritability of temper, occipital headache, sudden, excessive desire for food, but eats only a small quantity. Two or three stools daily and one or two at night, of normal consistency; but clay-colored and offensive. Successive outbreaks of furuncles on the nates; on the right side of the abdomen, just below the arch of the ribs, a very tender spot which is the seat of constant pain; the whole right hypochondrium is tender and heavy; aching in the right shoulder, restless sleep; the urine has a pink deposit, stains every thing it touches red and stains the vessel; heavy sweats at night. He is reported to have had Podophyllum, China, Bryonia, etc., etc., without perceptible effect.

I gave Sepia^{30} trituration, in solution, a dose every four hours during the day. In two days a vast improvement was manifest; and in a weak he was perfectly well, and has so continued to the present. Improvement was noticed first in his fever, spirits and temper, then in his appetite and

SEPIA. 157

digestion; then the pain and soreness vanished; then the stools and sleep became normal; last of all, the urine became normal

Case 2. A lady, aged thirty, has been ill nine or ten days; is in a remittent febrile condition with evening exacerbations, no chills, pulse at eleven A. M., ninety-six. Aching weight and soreness in the right hypochondrium, and distress and aching in right shoulder and scapula; cheeks flushed, the forehead and conjunctivæ yellow; irregular yellow patches on the forehead, lassitude; the limbs and back ache, obstinate constipation and occipital headache; anorexia, she loathes fat and milk; thirst, tongue flabby and indented, great flatulence after food, restless sleep, dry hot skin, urine scanty and loaded with urates. Her disease is said to have been pronounced remittent fever and prescribe for as such. She has taken Podophyllum and she knows not what else.

I gave Sepit^{30} trituration, in solution, a dose every four hours. In twelve hours the fever had gone and did not return, the side was better, the bowels had moved; in a week she was entirely well.

MUREX PURPUREA.

A VISCOUS juice, found in a small sack between the heart and liver of the mollusks of the genus purpura, of the family buccinidæ, and also of the muricidæ. A similar sack and juice are found in several conchiferæ belonging to the family limacidæ.

When brought into contact with the atmosphere, this juice becomes successively yellow, green, blue, and finally, a reddish purple. It is insoluble in water, alcohol or ether; consequently for homœopathic use the attenuations are prepared by trituration.

The proving which we possess was made chiefly under the observations of the late Dr. Petroz of Paris. Some additional ovservations have been collected by Dr. Hering; and a résumé of our knowledge to the present date was published in the "American Homœopathic Review," vol. iv., 1864.

In its origin, Murex is very closely akin to Sepia; and it will be perceived that its pathogenesis closely resembles that of Sepia, especially in its relations to the female genital organs. What its analogies or contrasts may be, with reference to other organs or apparatus, we can hardly venture to conjecture, for our proving of Murex is fragmentary, and the number of provers was very small.

Head. Upon the sensorium, Murex produces a depressing effect. There is confusion of ideas and diminished intellectual activity.

The pains are heaviness and pressure in various parts of the head, chiefly in the forehead, or, in one or the other temple. Heaviness or tightness in the head, relieved by bending the head backward.

Stomach. A peculiar and distressing sensation of "sinking" or faintness or vacuity in the epigastrium. The patients call it an "all-gone" feeling, something like the sensation produced by excessive hunger. Sepia has the same symptom, but in a less degree.

Abdomen. An acute sensation like a sharp point in the left side of the abdomen, which extends, and is felt in different isolated spots. The left side of the abdomen remained painful.

Tension (painful) in the right hypochondrium. Uneasiness in the abdomen like that which is caused by the approach of the menses; which, however, are retarded.

Stool. Constipation, lasting several days.

Anus. Pressure upon the anus like painful points.

Genital Organs. Our symptoms relate only to those of women.

In the right side of the uterus, acute pain, which crosses the body, and ascends to the left mamma. Pain in the uterus as if wounded by a cutting instrument. In the evening, two violent lancinations in an upward direction on the left side of the abdomen. Throbbings in the uterus.

Vagina. Heaviness in the vagina during the pains in the adbomen.

Pudenda. Sensation of weight and of dilatation in the labia majora.

Functional Symtoms. Excitement; sexual instinct so violent as to fatigue the reason.

Platina has similar excitement. Hyoscyamus also, but with disturbance and perversion of the intelligence and moral sense, constituting nymphomania.

Venereal desire, increased or renewed by the slightest touch.

Discharge. The menses are delayed. After flowing a few days the menses cease, and after twelve hours re-appear. Sepia has a similar symptom. Kreasote the same, together with irritation of the bladder, and a very acrid discharge from the vagina, causing the pudenda and thighs to swell and become raw, burning and itching.

Thick and greenish, or watery, leucorrhœ.

Urinary Organs. In quantity the urine is diminished, but the calls to pass urine are more frequent and urgent than in the normal state, especially during the night.

The urine is fetid, or has an odor like that of valerian. It has a white sediment, and its evacuation is followed by a discharge of blood or bloody mucus. (These symptoms occur in females, and probably this discharge is from the vagina.)

Trunk. Pains in the loins, burning or excoriating. Pains in the hips and loins when lying down, and especially in bed. Here we have a contrast to Sepia, the lumber and coxal pains of which are relieved by lying down; and a point of resemblance to Belladonna.

Pains around the pelvis.

Extremities. Pains and aching in the arms and legs. Feebleness, the limbs give way. Lassitude and fatigue; disposition to lie down. On rising, acute pain in the middle anterior portion of the right thigh. It will not bear to be touched.

Sleep. Drowsiness in the evening. But the sleep is disturbed by troublous dreams, by pains like menstrual pains, and by an urgent necessity to rise and urinate.

These are in substance the symptoms ascribed to Murex. We gather from them and from clinical experience, that Murex acts peculiarly upon the sexual system of women; although the pains in the right hypochondrium and the constipation point to an action on the liver similar to that of Sepia.

Murex produces general lassitude and feebleness in the body and limbs, as well as in the sensorium; but the feeling of prostration is most marked in the sinking, "all-gone" sensation in the epigastrium, which is very characteristic of Murex, and which is so frequent a concomitant of uterine disease, especially of prolapsus uteri.

In the loins and hips and around the pelvis, aching, drawing or burning pains, and pains and tenderness in the anterior part of the thighs,—such as often coincide with uterine disease,—are marked symptoms of Murex.

Again, the irritation of the bladder, which does not tolerate a large accumulation of urine in it,—the desire to evacuate being sudden and urgent,—points rather to uterine than to vesical disease.

Most peculiar to Murex, however, are the sensations ascribed to the uterus itself. First among these is a sensation described by one of Dr. Hering's provers as a "consciousness of the womb." Patients sometimes describe it thus: "I feel that I have a womb, and it is uncomfortable; whereas when I am well I am not conscious of the organ." More positive symptoms are the lancination, cuttings and throbbings felt in the uterus, and chiefly on the left side. Finally the sensation of sharp pain passing upward on the right side of the uterus, then crossing the body and extending to the left mamma.

There is leucorrhœa, thick or watery.

It is noteworthy that the sexual instinct is very active, and the susceptibility greatly increased, so as to annoy the subject. In this aspect Murex resembles Platina (and perhaps Phosphorus) and differs from Sepia.

The applications of Murex follow directly upon this statement. In the "American Homœopathic

Review," *loc. cit.*, cases are given of its successful use in treating prolapsus uteri and other uterine affections.

I have in my records a case of a large cyst, supposed to be connected with the left ovary, which occupied the space between the rectum and uterus and vagina, so as to obliterate the posterior cul de sac and almost occlude the vagina. In addition, it somewhat distended the abdomen. The patient had been confined to her room and bed for more than a year. The subjective symptoms so clearly indicated Murex that I gave the sixth. Whether it were mere coincidence or not I cannot say, but it is certain that within three weeks the tumor discharged a limpid fluid per vagina, and the local as well as general symptoms completely vanished, so that in a month thereafter the patient could walk freely and look after her housekeeping; nor has she since (for five years) been disabled or ailing.

KREASOTUM.

THIS remedy, of which a proving was published by Dr. Wahle in the "Archiv," and which, in Dr. Bœnninghausen's opinion, has not received from practitioners the attention which it merits, I mention here, because of the analogy of its action on the female sexual organs to that of Sepia and Murex. And for the reason that Kreasotum has been but little used in practice, and few of its symptoms have been verified by clinical experienc, I shall not attempt a systematic statement or analysis of the pathogenesis, but proceed at once to symptoms.

The Head. Dull feeling in the head, and as if a board were pressed against the forehead. Headache, as if the head were too full, and would burst out forward. In various parts of the head, pressing from within outward. Jerking, tearing and stitching pains in the anterior part of the head, semi-lateral, and extending to the cheeks, jaws, teeth and neck. Kreasote has proved curative in neuralgia, where the sensations were burning, and where the paroxysms were induced by talking, moving or sitting up or lying on the side not affected; and attended by great excitability and nervous irritability.

In the digestive apparatus, Kreasote produces, among other symptoms: rising of tasteless air after a meal, or of frothy saliva. Nausea and vomiting before breakfast, with tightness across the epigastrium, and yet an inability to bear tight clothing. It is useful in the vomiting of pregnancy.

Various pains in the abdomen, which constipation.

Urinary Organs. The secretion of urine is reported as both diminished and increased. But whichever be the case, there is also a disposition to evacuate it more frequently than in health, especially at night, there being much pressure upon the bladder. Bœnninghausen calls attention to the value of Kreasote as a remedy in cases of incontinentia urinæ nocturna, where the patient dreams he is urinating *comme il faut.* Sepia has incontinence during the first sleep. The desire is very sudden and imperative; and, in women, the evacuation is attended and followed by much smarting and burning of the pudenda. The urine is often turbid and offensive, depositing a reddish sediment. This is similar to Sepia, of which a characteristic symptom is "deposit of red sediment which adheres to the chamber and is removed with difficulty." Lycopodium has also a red deposit, but it is granular like sand. The deposit of Cantharides is granular but is grayish white, looking like fragments of old mortar. (Of course it is to be remembered that besides these deposits, both Lycopodium and Cantharides, as well as Dulcamara and Cannabis and Hepar may present—and be indicated where there exist—deposits of mucus, pus and blood.)

In women, Kreasote has a discharge of bland, yellow leucorrhœa preceding each urination, with frequent desire to urinate.

Female Sexual Organs. Much excitement is produce. There are pains in the pudenda; stitches in the vagina proceeding from the abdomen. Intolerable itching in the vagina; the labia swell and become excoriated; and in this condition smart exceedingly during and after urination, which is frequent. The leucorrhœal discharge is very acrid, excoriating the parts which it touches. The menses come too soon and are too copious, the flow being dark and thick. It is followed by leucorrhœa and by the local symptoms just described. The menses are accompanied by many accessory symptoms, *e. g.,* nausea, deafness, and abdominal colics. The menstrual flow often ceases on the third or fourth day, and after a few hours, or a day, re-appears. In this respect Kreasote resembles Sepia, but the flow of Sepia is scanty and retarded, while that of Kreasote is abundant and anticipates; and the local symptoms and general condition of Sepia are less pronounced, or decidedly different.

KREASOTUM.

The menses are followed by leucorrhœa, which is at first very acrid and dark brown in color, and quite offensive. Nitric acid has a dark flesh-colored discharge after the menses, but it is thin and watery, looking like the washings of meat, and it is not offensive.

In a day or two the leucorrhœa of Kreasote becomes deep yellow, and has a peculiar odor, like that of fresh green corn when it has just been husked.

Along with the leucorrhœa there is much pain in the back, a dragging pain from above downward, a pain as if something would come out, or as after long stooping. This pain is relieved by motion and is worse during rest; just the opposite of the backache of Sepia and Nux vomica, and similar to that of Belladonna.

These series of symptoms have led to the use of Kreasote in prolapsus uteri, in which it has proved of great value. Along with Sepia, Pulsatilla, Stannum, Nux vomica, Belladonna and Podophyllum, it enables us to avoid altogether the use of those miserable make-shifts, pessaries and supporters, which, affording temporary relief, entail so great miseries on those who use them.

The Kreasote cough is noteworthy. It is spasmodic and fatiguing and wheezing, excited by a sensation of a crawling below the larynx, or as from mucus in the bronchi which cannot be dislodged.

There is a copious expectoration of thick, yellow mucus. Along with the cough heaviness upon the chest with dyspnœa, as though the chest were bruised on inhalation. Pain as though the sternum would be crushed in, with stitches here and there. These symptoms have led to the successful use of Kreasote in "nervous asthma."

Lassitude in the limbs, and numbness of the fingers.

The present general use of carbolic acid may give us new symptoms.

SECALE CORNUTUM.

ERGOT.   SPURRED RYE.   MUTTERKORN.

"A METAMORPHOSIS of rye, or other grain, by which it is converted, wholly or in part, into a curved, purplish-black, cylindrical, tapering and grooved excrescence, from one to three lines in diameter, and usually from six to ten lines long. When dry it is firm and brittle, but when moist is soft and flexible. It gives out a sickening, heavy smell. Its color externally is purplish black. Internally it is pinkish white. It has a nauseous and slightly acrid taste."

It is said to be more active if gathered while the grain is still standing, about harvest time, than if collected after harvest.

It appears from the popular German name of this substance that it has been in domestic use as a parturifacient from early ages. So it certainly was in France. Indeed, its use as such in France was interdicted in 1774.

Still, it was ignored by physicians until Dr. Stearns of Waterford, N. Y., introduced it in 1807 as "a substance which he had used for several years to expedite lingering labors when the pains had subsided, and were incompetent to expel the fœtus." Since that time it has been more or less generally used in lingering labors. It is well understood that its power to cause violent contractions of the muscular fibres of the uterus, is so great that it should never be given when the os uteri is not fully dilated, nor unless there be satisfactory evidence that no mechanical obstacle interferes with the completion of the labor; otherwise, there is great danger of death of the fœtus from violent compression, or of rupture of the uterus from the same cause.

It is justly regarded as unfortunate if the labor do not come to an end soon after the administration of the Ergot, since if it be delayed there is reason to believe that the child will be poisoned by it.

Ergot is used in the forms of infusion, tincture, wine, trituration, and watery extract.

Its effects on the lower animals are as follows: The pulse is lessened, the action of the heart becomes irregular, the breathing slow and deep, appetite and flesh fail; tremulousness, staggering and dulness come on. Hæmorrhage of black blood from the nostrils, bowels or vagina occurs, then diarrhœa and death ensue. Moreover, it acts uniformly in a greater or less degree upon the gravid uterus, causing abortion or premature delivery, and, not infrequently, death of the fœtus.

On man, in small doses, not often repeated, it is said to have produced colic, nausea and vomiting, salivation and diarrhœa. Depression of the pulse always results from its use.

These poisonous effects are said to be due to the oil of the Ergot, which if given alone to a parturient woman, does not cause contraction of the uterus, but does poison the fœtus. Whereas, on the other hand, the Ergot, deprived of its oil, acts on the uterus, but does not poison the fœtus.

These statements should be taken *cum grano salis*.

In certain districts and throughout some countries, Poland in particular, the grain has at certain periods been so completely ergoted that the nutriment of the entire population has been more or less contaminated with this poison. Hence have arisen epidemics of a malady called ergotism. One of the earliest dates 1096. Ergotism is of two kinds, spasmodic and gangrenous.

The spasmodic is ushered in by a general feeling of illness. Then follow formication of the whole skin, cramps and numbness of the extremities, and pains in the head and back. After a few weeks occur heart-burn, vertigo, syncope, deafness, paroxysmal or permanent curvature (flexure) of the joints, and equally violent extension and opisthotonos, twitching of the facial muscles, sometimes violent delirium with cold skin, intense internal heat, and fœtid sweat. These attacks last several hours.

After a while the convulsive aspect of the disease ceases. It is following by exhaustion, debility, oppression, heart-burn, and a ravenous appetite, which it is dangerous to gratify. Sometimes strabismus or loss of sight succeeds, with general insensibility of the skin. After death the stomach and bowels are found inflamed and the parenchymatous organs congested. It generally proves fatal in three or four weeks. It is very fatal.

The gangrenous form is very different. It commences with dull pain and weariness of the limbs, with heaviness and stupidity of the face. The skin acquires an earthy or jaundiced hue. The extremity about to be affected (sometimes it is the nose) becomes cold, and the skin over it gets dusky red. Then gangrene begins in the inside of the end of an extremity (or of the nose) and extends outward to the skin. It also extends upward toward the trunk. The parts affected shrivel, dry up, become black and harden until they look like those of a mummy. They separate from the living flesh without hæmorrhage and by a clean line of division Death is sometimes preceded by diarrhœa. Beside weakness, there is not much general disturbance. The cases run their course in about three weeks, and are almost always fatal.

ANALYSIS.

To describe more particularly the more characteristic symptoms of Secale, we may mention :

1. General numbness and formication over the whole body.

2. The disposition is exceedingly melancholy, and depressed, with apprehension and dread of death. There is also violent mania.

3. Vertigo and stupefaction; dull headache.

4. Dilatation of the pupils, the eyes stare. There is double vision, squinting, obscuration of the sight.

5. Humming and roaring in the ears.

6. The face is pale and sunken. The complexion is earthy and sallow.

7. The voice becomes feeble. Speech is slow and difficult and inarticulate. There is tingling in the tip of the tongue, which is stiff.

8. Bleeding from the nose; dark blood is discharged.

9. Appetite gone.

10. Eructations, heart-burn, vomiting. Constant retching and oppression. Burning in the stomach.

11. Coldness in the back and abdomen. Burning in the abdomen.

12. Painful diarrhœa, with great prostration. Involuntary diarrhœa; putrid, watery, fetid, brown, profuse diarrhœa, with great exhaustion; a sudden change of the expression of the face, sinking of the eyes, etc., etc., as in cholera; suppression of the urine, etc.

13. Diminution and suppression of the urine.

14. The menses too profuse and too soon. Metrorrhagia, the blood being very liquid, but dark and attended by formication. Labor-like pains.

15. Weakness of the extremities. Formication. Convulsions. Rigidity. Gangrene.

PRACTICAL USES.

1. In lingering labors, where no obstruction exists, it is in common use. The infusion is preferred. Two drachms of pulv. Ergoti in eight ounces of water. The dose is two drachms every five minutes. The objections are its bad effects on the child. Hence the rule not to use it except where labor may be expected to end within a short time after giving it.

I prefer the Dublin mode of using the forceps early. In homœpathic practice, Ergot is generally superseded by Pulsatilla or Nux vomica.

2. In uterine hæmorrhage, whether as a sequel of abortion or labour, or an independent occurrence, or a concomitant of cancer, etc. It is characterized by the blood being dark and liquid, and by the general symptoms, especially the formication. It is used by allopaths to bring on abortion, provoking hæmorrhage; yet Gardner recommends it to arrest abortion begun from other causes!

In Asiatic cholera, Ergot has been used with success.

In diarrhœa, fetid, brown, watery, passing involuntarily, or nearly so, it is a most valuable remedy.

In cancer uteri it arrests hæmorrhage and relieves the terrible burning pains at night which torment the patient. This it does in small doses, even the 200th.

In paralysis, and particularly in paraplegia, as well as in dry gangrene, Secale should receive greater attention than is generally accorded to it.

JUNIPERUS SABINA.

SAVINE.

AN evergreen shrub of South Europe. The leaves and tops are used in medicine. Their properties depend on an essential oil, which dissolves in alcohol.

It was used by the ancients to stimulate indolent ulcers, to hasten the menses, and to cure chronic gout and rheumatism. Also to induce abortion.

It is described by allopathic writers as the most powerful emmenagogue of the materia medica, and also (!) as the best remedy for unduly abundant menstruation and threatened abortion! M. Aran says: "Strange as it may appear, this powerful emmenagogue has the power of suspending uterine hæmorrhage!"

Time fails me to enter upon a more minute analysis of Sabina than that of the uterine system.

It produces copious and early menstruation. Likewise metrorrhagia, and it is characteristic that the flow is paroxysmal and of a very bright color. It is always attended by pains in the joints,

It produces leucorrhœa, with itching irritation.

Besides cases of uterine hæmorrhage characterized thus, cases of threatened abortion have been cured by Sabina.

It is used (symptoms corresponding) in protracted uterine hæmorrhages at the "change of life."

ACHILLÆA MILLEFOLIUM.

MILLEFOIL. YARROW

THIS wayside drug produces hæmorrhage from all the mucous surface. The hæmorrhage is painless, and the blood very light coloured and fluid.

In painless drainings from the uterus (or nose or lungs) after lobor, after abortion, or when an abortion threatens, if the blood be bright and there are no pains in the joints, Millefolium does good.

So sometimes it checks too profuse menstruation.

ARSENICUM ALBUM.

METALLUM ALBUM. ARSENIOUS ACID.

THIS substance is generally prepared by sublimation from the ores of cobalt, and is often found adulterating the ores of zinc. It is a white powder, completely soluble in boiling water. It has neither taste nor smell but leaves a somewhat acrid sensation of the fauces; and when fused and thereby deoxidized, it emits the odor of garlic which characterizes the heated metal.

In medicine, the forms of Arsenicum chiefly used are the arsenious acid and the solution of the arsenite of potassa known as "Fowler's solution," or the "tasteless ague drop." The latter is prepared by dissolving equal parts of arsenious acid and carbonate of potassa in boiling distilled water. A very little compound spirit of lavender is added to give color and flavor. It contains four grains of arsenious acid to the fluid ounce.

Dose: Five to twenty drops; it may be repeated several times daily.

Arsenious acid has been known since the eighth century. In the fourteenth century, it was used as a medicine in the treatment of diseases of cattle. In the seventeenth and eighteenth centuries, it was used as a caustic application to malignant ulcers, but its use was condemned by regular physicians. Irregular practitioners, however, had learned its value in the treatment of skin diseases and of intermittent fever. How they found this out is more than we can say.

The same has been true of nearly every drug of the materia medica. It is certain howrver, that while in irregular and domestic practice intermittents and skin diseases were being cured by Arsenicum every day, its use was condemned by the faculty; and Goeffroy said, "Though it may be a good remedy for the present, it will afterward prove a poison and bring on very dismal symptoms. Arsenic, therefore, is, in my opinion, worse than the fever!"

Not so, however, thought the patients who were glad to get rid of their fevers, and to run the risk of the dismal symptoms. The popularity of the remedy, and its extensive use, unsanctioned by the faculty, at length converted learned doctors; and Arsenic was received into the orthodox pharmacopœia, and became forthwith "a safe remedy," and much better "than a fever itself."

Arsenic is a poison to plants as well as to animals.

Upon animals it acts in its well-known peculiar way, however it be introduced into the system, whether by the stomach or by the rectum, or through the external surface of the body by the endermic method. Cases of fatal poisoning are on record in which the arsenic was introduced in a wash applied to cutaneous eruptions or to ulcers.

The fumes of arsenious acid act very sensibly on the system. It is recorded that persons have been poisoned by inhaling the air of a room in which had been burned candles the wicks of which had been saturated with a solution of arsenious acid. The same result has followed the use of arsenious acid in candles to harden them. Clay tobacco pipes are glazed with a preparation of arsenious acid,—at least those having a superior finish, and designed for the use of the aristocracy. At the first smoking this glazing is volatilized, and the smoker inhales a dose of arsenic. Every new pipe involves a new dose. Some persons scorn to use any but a new pipe. Fatal poisonings have resulted from this fastidious extravagance.

A beautiful green wall-paper gets its color from the arsenite of copper, a pigment known as Scheele's green. The exhalations from this paper have caused illnesses and death. The same pigment is used in almost every form of ornamentation of dress and furniture and condiments, from the artificial flowers of the fine lady's head-dress, which give her the mysterious arsenical neuralgic headache, to the green candy toy of her spoiled child, which, when eaten, gives the child the equally mysterious arsenical stomachache.

ARSENICUM ALBUM. 181

The effects of small doses of arsenic frequently repeated, producing chronic arsenical poisoning, are thus described:

"Loss of appetite, nausea, deranged digestion, diarrhœa, thirst, salivation, tenesmus, colic and intestinal cramps; respiration labored and painful; a sense of oppression with pain in the breast; cough; extreme wasting of the flesh, and hectic fever; the limbs grow tremulous, and not unfrequently are paralyzed, especially the lower extremities; pains in the whole body, but particularly in the hands and feet; stiffness and contraction of the extensor muscles succeed; numbness invades the extremities, and the mental faculties subside into insensibility and torpor; œdema of the face and extremities, and even general anasarca are not unusual; the hair falls out; epidermis scales off; pustular and other eruptions, ending in ulceration, attack the skin, which acquires a lifeless, earthy hue; the countenance, if not œdematous, is sunken; the conjunctiva is strongly injected, and a reddish circle surrounds the eyes."

The symptoms of acute poisoning are as follows:

"Immediately after the poison is swallowed a metallic taste is perceived, with constriction of the fauces. A violent burning pain, which soon becomes excruciating, is felt in the stomach, and gradually extends itself over the whole abdomen, steadily increasing in severity until it becomes intolerable. Retching and vomiting and cramps of the bowels ensue, with spasms of the œsophagus and chest, which resemble those of hydrophobia. The thirst is insatiable, but even the mildest drinks cannot be retained. The tongue is generally fissured, hard and dry, although occasionally there is profuse salivation, and the voice is hoarse. There is also tenesmus, with bloody and offensive stools and retraction of the abdomen. The irritation extends to the urinary organs, producing strangury. Sometimes the urine is completely suppressed, and sometimes it is mixed with blood. Christison says that in women there is burning in the vagina and excoriation of the labia, but this does not happen unless life is prolonged beyond three days. Bachman had previously noticed the pain above alluded to, and also profuse menorrhagia among the symptoms in women.

"The pulse is irregular, rapid and intermittent; the muscles are spasmodically affected; the skin presents a livid eruption, as already described. The sense of anguish is unutterable, and sometimes there is delirium. The breathing is oppressed. A consuming fire seems to prey upon the vitals, while the whole body is pale, cold, shivery and clammy. The features are sunken and sharp; if vomiting occurs it is convulsive and affords no relief. Exhaustion and mind and body; prostration and despair, with anxious restlessness, generally attend this stage of the attack. On the approach of death, spasm yields to general exhaustion, the pulse grows slow and feeble, and urine and fæces are passed involuntarily, but sensibility and consciousness are lost only in the last moments of life.

"The duration of the symptoms is variable, and may be stated, in general, as from six to twelve hours, but occasionally they last several days.

"But even when recovery from the acute symptoms takes place it is rarely complete. For months or even years, the joints remain stiff and swollen, rendering walking difficult and painful; the digestive organs continue irritable and feeble, and all the functions of the nervous system are impaired. In some cases paralysis of the upper or lower extremities occurs, and gangrenous ulcers attack the legs."

"The quantity of arsenious acid sufficient to cause death will depend," says Œsterlein, "on the condition of the stomach at the time the arsenic is swallowed. If the stomach be full of food at the time a large quantity may produce only a slight effect." Thus Œsterlein reports a case in which just after a hearty meal a man swallowed a quarter of an ounce. Emetics were given immediately and no evil followed.

On the other hand, very small doses may produce very violent and fatal symptoms.

Four, three, and even two grains of arsenious acid have destroyed life.

A summary review of the effects of Arsenic leads us to conclude:

1. From the fact that, after death from poisoning by it, it is found in almost every tissue and secretion of the body, that it is universally

diffused throughout the body and acts upon every part.

2. From the fact that its action and diffusion are uniform, however it be introduced into the body, whether through the skin or by the alimentary canal, that its action is specific and not local.

3. From its effects in chronic poisoning, producing anæmia, exhaustion, emacination, etc., that it acts upon the blood composition, as well as directly on the tissues and on the nervous system.

We consider now the more intimate specific effects as gathered from provings on the healthy body, made by Hahnemann and his pupils.

A few words from Hahnemann's introduction to his proving may not be amiss, and especially since the use of Arsenic as a remedy has been denounced on the ground of its frequent abuse as a poison.

"When I utter the name Arsenic, powerful recollections possess my soul.

"In creating Iron, the All-Merciful left it free to His children to transform it at their pleasure, either into the murderous dagger or the blessed ploughshare, and to use it either for destruction or preservation.   *   *   *   *   *

"It is not the fault of Him who loves us all that we abuse powerful medicinal agents, giving them either in too large doses or in cases for which they are not suitable, being merely guided by the caprice of miserable authorities, and without having taken the trouble to investigate the inherent curative virtues of the drug, and to make our selection depend on the knowledge thus obtained."

GENERAL ANALYSIS.

1. Arsenic exhausts the vital power of certain organs or systems or of the entire organism, produces symptoms of impeded activity in the functions of organs; indeed, in some cases, positive paralysis.

This asthenic condition characterizes the entire symptomatology of Arsenic. For this reason, the sensations of prostration, lessitude, weakness, etc., sinking of the forces, etc., are highly characteristic indications for Arsenic. They are so peculiar to Arsenic that Hahnemann says: "Even circumstances that are in themselves not very important and would otherwise produce but little effect, occasion in the Arsenic patient a sudden and complete sinking of the forces." This is a vital phenomenon and not a result of chemical or physical destruction of vital organs, as the stomach or intestine; for this sinking occurs when there is no such destruction.

2. The organic substance of the body is acted upon throughout. A cachectic dyscrasia and colliquative destruction of tissues is indicated by symptoms of the complexion, excretions, ulcers, eruption, and the skin generally.

Hence the use of Arsenic in persons of a cachectic habit, in leucophlegmatic persons.

3. The sphere of action embraces almost all the organs and systems of the body, but it acts especially on the mucous membranes and the external skin.

4. It is one of the most eminent periodics of our materia medica.

5. As characteristic peculiarities may be mentioned:

That the symptoms of Arsenic are almost always accompanied by great restlessness and anxiety, indeed sometimes by frantic desperation.

That they are sometimes relieved for a time by external warmth.

That they occur and are aggravated during repose, but are ameliorated by standing and by moving.

That the symptoms are almost always attended by concomitant symptoms; that is, by symptoms which stand in no pathological relation to the former.

That as regards the time of day at which the symptoms occur or are aggravated there is a great variety. Most of them occur at night after lying down, or about two A. M.; some on rising, and after dinner.

SPECIAL ANALYSIS.

The action on the head is not very striking.

Pressing pain and semi-lateral headaches are mentioned by provers, but not graphically. It is probable that the general symptoms alone will suffice to guide the prescriber in selecting Arsenic for headache.

Eyes. Upon the eyes and their appendages Arsenic produces: itching, drawing and pressure around the eyes, swelling of the lids, pains on moving the eyelids, as if they were dry and rubbed against the eyeball; agglutination of the lids; increased lachrymation; drawing and pressure, but especially tickling, itching and *burning* (the characteristic sensation produced by Arsenic.) The conjunctiva is reddened, there is photophobia, the pupils are contracted; in fact there is very symptom of inflammation. As regards vision itself, it is obscured and weakened.

With regard to the ears, no symptom seems characteristic, except that, almost all the paroxysms of pain, wherever located, begin with roaring in the ears. But when it is remembered that great debility and exhaustion attend the pains of Arsenic, and that these in turn are apt to be attended by roaring in the ears, this symptom will not be regarded as indicative of a special affection of the ear.

Let me, however, caution you against supposing that because Arsenic has hitherto produced no definite ear affection it cannot nevertheless cure one. I shall have occasion to relate to you a severe case of otalgia, cured in a very short time by a single dose of Arsenic; which was indicated by the *general* constitutional symptoms of the case.

The face is altered in complexion, which assumes a sunken, yellow, ghastly aspect; the skin around the mouth is livid, the face is cold and sunken.

Swelling and inflammation of the lips, bleeding of the lips, painful tumor in the lip, an ulcer, phagedenic, with a tearing, biting, burning pain, aggravated by touch, and in the air, and especially at night. These symptoms must be remembered in connection with the well-known and long-known use of Arsenic in ill-conditioned ulcers of the lip, lupus, and epithelial cancer.

The toothache of Arsenic is a pressing, tearing, jerking, not infrequently conjoined with swelling of the cheek, relieved by sitting up in bed, and by external warmth. Many other remedies produce the same effects. The indication for Arsenic must, therefore, be drawn rather from the constitutional than from the local symptoms.

Arsenic produces great dryness of the mouth and excessive thirst, yet at the same time the prover drinks but little at a time. The saliva is sometimes bloody. The tongue is dry as if burnt, deprived of sensibility, stitching pains in the root of the tongue, burning pain in the tongue.

The tongue is excoriated at the tip, which has a biting or burning pain.

In the throat, dryness and burning, a scraped, ulcerative sensation. Constrictive feeling in the œsophagus and throat. Gangrenous inflammation of the throat.

Action on the fauces is eminently exerted by Arsenic, however it be introduced into the system.

ARSENICUM ALBUM.

The same may be said of its action upon the entire alimentary canal.

Arsenic alters the normal taste; sometimes this is extinguished. Again, the taste is bitter, sour, or putrid. Appetite is abnormal; there are cravings for acids, for coffee, etc., but especially loss of appetite; there is nausea at the idea of food.

The nausea which Arsenic produces is conjoined with a sensation of the greatest weakness, with anxiety; it recurs periodically. It is often conjoined with symptoms that seem to have no pathological connection with it; is worse during repose, and is aggravated by motion.

Actual vomiting occurs, with great anxiety, with diarrhœa, with severe griping and burning pains in the stomach and obdomen.

The vomiting requires great effort; is scanty in quantity, as are all the excretions of Arsenic; and it is followed by extreme prostration.

The matters vomited may be first water, then thick, glairy or grass-green mucus, and then blood. The stomach becomes at times so irritable that it will not tolerate food.

Hahnemann says, Arsenic provokes in the stomach rather an irregular convulsive action than an ordinary peristaltic or anti-peristaltic motion; rather an anxious, fruitless retching than a copious vomiting.

In the stomach itself, pressing, gnawing, *burning,* and a feeling as though the stomach were distended.

The burning pains are the most constant. With them come violent thirst, lamentation, anguish.

They may be continuous or periodic. If the latter, they occur most frequently at two A. M., or after eating.

Intestines. All the varieties of pains analogous to that which is so characteristic of Arsenic., viz.: burning, may be confined to single parts of the abdomen, or may be general,—generally in the hypogastric region,—accompanied by thirst, restlessness and the other conditions of Arsenic.

Stool. Most important symptoms.

Arsenic produces diarrhœa; it is our most important remedy for diarrhœa. As all the excretions of Arsenic are scanty, so is the stool. The irritation is disproportionately great. The stool is preceded by restlessness, anguish, and pain in the abdomen. It is accompanied by vomiting, excessive pain in the abdomen, burning in the rectum, tenesmus. It is followed by burning in the anus, palpitation, trembling of the limbs, great weakness—out of all proportion to the amount of stool.

It is of great importance to note the concomitant symptoms that precede, accompany and follow the stool. They often indicate the remedy. Thus Nux vomica, Mercury, Aloes, Capsicum, Podophyllum, Veratrum and Phosphorus are distinguished.

The stool, as regards its character, is diarrhœic. It consists of a pappy (not often watery), yellow, bloody or greenish, or more frequently a blackish, very offensive substance.

The characteristics may be said to be small quantity, dark color, offensive odor; great prostration following it.

ARSENICUM ALBUM.

No other drug combines all these characteristics. Phosphorus has some; but Phosphorus is never indicated where the loss of power, the prostration, is a striking symptom.

Veratrum has some, but the quantity of the excretion is as remarkably large, as, under Arsenic, it is notably small.

Secale cornutum has some, but the stool is watery, putrid, dark brown; and there is not the restless anguish of Arsenic.

Graphites has some, but the stool is pasty, of a light brown color, and a most atrocious odor, with scarcely any pain, and no restlessness, nor weakness, etc., etc.

There is burning in the bladder and in the urethra. The urine is scanty. Three cases of chronic poisoning,—recorded in the "Edinburgh Medical and Surgical Journal,"—one from which the patient recovered, two in which death occured, present us perfect pictures of Bright's disease, even to the pathological anatomy of the disease.

Arsenic produces a yellow, acrid leucorrhœa, and increases the menstrual flow.

During the menses, sharp sticking in the rectum, extending to the anus and pubes; cutting pains in the abdomen, with the conditions characteristic of Arsenic.

The menses are often followed by a discharge of bloody mucus.

It should be added, that, in cases of chronic poisoning, profuse metrorrhagia has occurred; and this fact has led to the successful use of Arsenic in such cases, where the constitutional symptoms correspond.

Arsenic seems to produce in the mucous membrane of the respiratory organs a hyperæmic and inflammatory condition, the symptoms of which vary according to the locality.

Thus, in the nasal membrane, the irritation is shown by frequent sneezing, by obstruction alternating with fluent coryza, with hoarseness and drowsiness; the nares burn, and the discharge is watery and very acrid.

On the larynx, the action is not marked. But we have constant tickling in the entire trachea, which provokes a cough, a feeling of rawness, soreness and burning in the chest; scanty, tenacious mucus in the chest, hard to dislodge; and when dislodged it is blood-streaked.

The cough is dry, and very fatiguing. It is paroxysmal, worse at night; and is sometimes so violent that it seems as though suffocation would ensue. It is aggravated by drinking, by movements of the body, and by the open air.

But the cough symptoms, etc., are by no means so violent, nor indeed so significant, as those of several other remedies. On the other hand, Arsenic produces a series of chest symptoms very peculiar and significant, viz., the asthmatic series.

Constriction of the chest (here we meet the characteristic constriction, as in the œsophagus, the rectum and the bladder), dyspnœa, asthma, whistling respiration—indeed all degrees of difficult

ARSENICUM ALBUM. 193

respiration, dyspnœa, orthopnœa, apnœa. They may be paroxysmal, intermittent, periodically recurring, worse at night.

Burning in the chest.

The heart is especially affected by Arsenic, and it is probable that some of the dyspnœa is thus explained.

We find anguish in the præcordia, stitching and sore pain there on coughing; pain under the præcordia restricting respiration; palpitation; at night, about three A. M., an irregular but very violent palpitation, which seems to him audible, with great anguish; palpitation much worse when he lies on the back.

Pathologico-anatomical investigations show the heart to be "lax, not over-filled with blood, the muscular substance infiltrated with blood. The pericardium contains serum." It would appear that Arsenic affects the muscular substance of the heart.

In the trunk, Arsenic produces various pains of stiffness, lassitude and powerlessness.

Autopsies show that the spinal marrow is always affected, especially the lower part of it.

In the upper extremities (as might be supposed) the symptoms are few, chiefly those of loss of power.

In the lower extremities they are numerous, but may be reduced to three varieties: pain, spasm, paralysis.

The pains are stitching, boring and tearing. The spasms are generally tonic contractions. The paralysis occurs, generally, in fatal cases, not long before death, and is hardly a specific effect of Arsenic, but rather a forerunner of dissolution.

The skin is one of those organs on which the action of Arsenic is most powerfully exerted.

Thus Arsenic produces: 1. Pains, itching, biting, gnawing; but above all, burning.

2. Watery swellings; from puffiness of the feet or the face to general anasarca.

3. Eruptions. Inflamed spots on the face, head and neck; nettle-rash, yellow spots.

Whitish papules or elevated spots, itching and burning, like lepra, red pimples, pustules.

4. Soreness between the arms and trunk. Ulcers already existing and hitherto painful become very sensitive, as if red-hot coals were laid upon them; the margins become elevated, and they bleed, discharging black blood; the ulcers become offensive.

The sleep is disturbed; sleeplessness alternates with restlessness and tossing, twitching and jerking. There are vivid, anxious dreams. Sleep does not refresh.

The fever may be continued, or remitting, or distinctly intermittent; quotidian, or quartan.

The paroxysm is not complete. One stage is generally wanting.

The fever is most apt to occur at night.

The sweat occurs only at the end of the fever, or only at the beginning of sleep.

The pulse is small; quick, but weak.

ARSENICUM ALBUM.

Thirst never accompanies the chill, but comes after it. It does not accompany the night fever, but is very violent during the sweat.

The disposition is:
  a. Depressed, melancholy, despairing, indifferent.
  b. Fearful, restless, anxious, full of anguish.
  c. Irritable, sensitive, peevish.

PRACTICAL APPLICATIONS.

Masked ague. Otalgia. Neuralgia. Bright's disease. Dyspepsia. Diarrhœa. Metrorrhagia. Skin diseases (psoriasis). Intermittent. Coryza. Asthma. Chorea. Heart disease. Ulcers.

The fact cannot be too often called to mind, nor too strongly insisted upon, that our most characteristic indications for the use of a drug which presents well-defined general symptoms, as Arsenic does, and indeed as every well-proved drug does, are derived not from its local action upon any organ or system, not from a knowledge of the particular tissues it may affect, and how it affects them, but upon the general constitutional symptoms and their conditions and concomitants. If this were not so, in the presence of how many maladies, of the intimate nature of which we are wholly ignorant and which nevertheless we cure, should we be utterly powerless for good.

I mention and urge this, because the opposite is strongly presented by an author whose voluminous productions are evidence in themselves of the notorious fact that his life has been that of a student and compiler; that he entirely lacks the practical experience in the treatment of the sick, which serves as the test and corrective of any theoretical opinions we may form of the mode of selecting drugs, and of their mode of action.

A few cases will illustrate what I mean.

A lady of middle age suffered from intense pain in the inner ear. There were no indications of external inflammation. The pain had lasted several days. No remedy had given any relief. Morphine had only temporarily assuaged the pain, which afterward became worse again. Here was the case. What organ was affected? Doubtful. What tissues? Who could say? Could Arsenic be the remedy? Certainly Arsenic produces no such symptoms. What were the constitutional symptoms and the conditions? Did the patient endure the pain patiently? On the contrary, the pain was intolerable. Her whole demeanor indicated positive anguish. She could not retain one position for more than a few seconds, but tossed and moved about, and was constantly changing her posture. Then, the pain was not constant.

It intermitted, the intervals varying from ten to ninety minutes.

As regards character, the pain was described as a fine, burning pain.

The effects of the pain were very remarkable. Whereas during its continuance the patient's vio-

ARSENICUM ALBUM.   197

lent movements indicated the possession of no inconsiderable muscular vigor, no sooner had the paroxysm passed over than she fell into a state of really pitiable exhaustion and weakness. Moreover, she had burning thirst, though she cared to drink but little at a time.

Here, then, we have, though none of the local symptoms corresponded to Arsenic, yet a complete picture of the general or constitutional action of that drug. We have burning pain, intolerable paroxysmal pain, followed by disproportionate exhaustion, and attended by burning thirst, in which, however often the patient drinks, she takes but little at a time. A single dose of Arsenic^{30}, given at the commencement of a paroxysm of pain, caused the disappearance of the pain in the space of five minutes. The patient fell asleep. There was never any return of the pain. She was well.

A second case will serve to illustrate not merely this point but also another, viz.: the detection and treatment of what is sometimes called "masked intermittent;" by which is meant a disease clearly resulting from marsh-malaria, and which nevertheless does not manifest itself by the customary paroxysm of chill, heat and perspiration, which constitute intermittent fever.

A precocious child in Dutchess County, twelve years old, had complained for more than eighteen months of a severe pain in the left ear. She was brought to my office for treatment, with the statement that for this affection she had been treated, both locally and constitutionally, for an inflammation of the middle ear, by some of the most distinguished surgeons of the city of New-York, but with no good result. I could discover no distinct signs of local lesion, but nevertheless supposed it to be a case of otalgia, and from a very close correspondence of the case, as described to me, with the symptoms of Chammomilla, gave that drug.

She got no better. I then learned that she had been under the care of a good homœopathic physician, who, if it had been simple otalgia, would surely have cured her. This fact induced me to scrutinize the case very carefully before I prescribed again. Visiting the patient repeatedly at her residence, at different times in the day, I found that the attacks of pain were regularly and distinctly paroxysmal; that they were attended by the peculiar thirst so characteristic of Arsenic, and by the restlessness and anguish, and followed by the prostration, equally characteristic. Furthermore, concomitant symptoms in the shape of an Arsenic gastralgia and an Arsenic diarrhœa were also present. It then occurred to me that this was probably a case of masked intermittent. The situation of the house, and the topography of the neighborhood favored the idea. On the strength of the symptoms recited, I gave Arsenicum^{200}. Within fiive days the pains had ceased to appear, but in their stead came a regular paroxysm of chill, fever and sweat, indicating the existence of quotidian intermittent fever. These paroxysms recurred for four days, gradually, diminishing in intensity. They then ceased, leaving the patient well.

Instances almost without number might be adduced in corroboration of this statement, that cures are to be made in a multitude of instances which present local symptoms and lesions of tissue, to which the symptomatology of the drug presents no analogy; provided always the general and constitutional symptoms correspond closely to those which characterize the drug. And it may be added that perhaps no other drug is so often useful and available in this way as Arsenic, for the reason that hardly any other drug produces general symptoms so strongly marked, and so easily detected; I may add, so frequently met with in patients. Whatever, then, may be the local nature of the disease before, whatever pathological name it may bear, if the general symptoms correspond to those of Arsenic in the way that I have pointed out, do not hesitate a moment to give that drug. (How otherwise could we cure lupus, cancer, ulcers; for these do not occur in provings!)

The eminent periodic character of the action of Arsenic upon the healthy subject, would mark it at once as a drug likely to be very useful in the cure of intermittent fever. But long before systematic provings on the healthy body had made known to us this peculiarity, popular experience had discovered the value of Arsenic in such cases. It was found to be the sole ingredient of a nostrum, very famous in the last century under the name of "the tasteless ague-drop."

During the wars consequent on the French Revolution, and the Napoleonic wars on the continent of Europe, while England held control of the ocean and effectually blockaded the European seaports, thereby preventing the importation of foreign products, and among them of Peruvian bark, the recognized specific for intermittent fever (for, whatever opinion the English may now entertain of the barbarity of our withholding medicines from our enemies, they had then no doubt of the propriety of withholding them from theirs):—at this time attention was turned to the practicability of using Arsenic as a substitute for bark in treating intermittent; and large rewards were offered for an effectual method of so using it, or for any efficient substitute for bark. It is amazing that this idea of using one specific as a substitute for another specific could ever be entertained; since the virtues of a specific reside in its peculiar, individual properties, which are never common to two different substances. Nevertheless, even at the present day and in our latest words on materia medica, we find the subject of the substitution of Arsenic for Quinine gravely discussed and statistics referred to to show, as the case may be, its inferiority or superiority to Quinine. As might be supposed, the testimony of different physicians differs widely on this point. Some affirm that almost all the cases treated by them during a certain period, were promptly cured by Arsenic, while they proved rebellious to Quinine. Others succeeded with Arsenic in a smaller proportion of cases, and in a larger with Quinine; while others, again, found Arsenic of comparatively little use, Quinine curing nearly every case. Finally, others again failed with Arsenic and Quinine alike, but succeeded with other drugs less often used, as Ipecacuanha, or Eupatorium, or Nux vomica.

Now, it is a wonderful thing that medical men should still argue, in the face of these statistics, upon a question of the relative value of certain drugs in the treatment of a disease, regarded not in the light of the individuals affected by it, but solely with reference to its great pathological features. It seems to me the only sound deductions from these testimonies are these: That there are diversities in the form in which intermittent fever appears in different persons and in different epidemics; that these forms require different remedies, and that thus there is a form which is capable of being cured by Arsenic, and by nothing else; a form capable of being cured by Quinine, and by nothing else; and so of other drugs. In this view, when a case of intermittent fever presents itself, the question can never be: Is Arsenic a better remedy for this disease than Quinine is? Does it offer greater chances of a cure? There can be no better or worse. The question is between right and wrong; suitable and not suitable. The question would be always: Which remedy corresponds to this particular case, and is, therefore, indicated in it?

Attention should again be called to the fact which has been previously mentioned (see Bryonia), that in different epidemics the indications, though uniform, are aften quite different; and that in the endemic fevers of certain malarious districts, the indications for remedies are often very uniform, and yet different for each locality. Thus it has been found, by experience, that the intermittents which are endemic near Rome (Italy), require Quinine or China; those of the head of the Adriatic require Arsenic; those of the Maremma, along the Tuscan gulf, require Bryonia; those of Salonica, in Turkey, yield to Ammonium muriaticum; while those of the Dobrutscha require Rhus toxicodendron.

The special indications for Arsenic in intermittent are thus admirably stated by Dr. Wurmb ("Homœopathische Clinische Studien," i., 179):

"Arsenic is one of those few drugs whose action is distinguished not alone by its intensity, but equally by its extent; it involves the entire organism. Every system, every organ of the body, every nervous filament, is so subjected to its powerful influence that we are not able to say which of its symptoms are primary, and which are secondary, and where the focus of its action chiefly lies.

"We see the entire nerve-life attacked in all directions, from the slightest excitement to the most violent irritation; from the more sensation of weakness to actual paralysis; and then we see, likewise, another series of disturbances arise from its action, which advance in regular gradation from the most inconsiderable acceleration of the circulation to the most violent febrile storm; from the slightest irregularity in the vegetative sphere to a cachectic dyscrasia, yes, even to decomposition and destruction of the organic substance.

"In addition, we remark the striking similarity between the symptoms of chronic, arsenical poisoning and those of the intermittent cachexy; as well as the fact that Arsenic has the property of causing the periodical recurrence of symptoms in so high a degree as to surpass in this respect all other drugs; in a word, no other drug known to us has such a power of affecting so intimately and so variously those organs that are especially affected in intermittent fever; and none corresponds so well as Arsenic does to all the requirements of a remedy for intermittent.   *   *   *   *

"'Arsenic in indicated in cases which are distinguished not only by weakness in the vital power and deterioration of the organic substance, but also and at the same time by symptoms of excitation of the circulation, or of the nervous system alone, or of both together.

"Again, it seems to be the more especially indicated the more malignant the influence from which the disease has sprung. Marsh-miasm is the chief of these influences; in this originate the most serious and most dangerous cases of fever; and in these, Arsenic is often the only remedy that will rescue the patient.

ARSENICUM ALBUM.

"Again, the longer the disease has lasted, the more is Arsenic generally indicated; because the more deeply have the organs and tissues been affected, the more nearly has the patient's condition approached that known as the intermittent cachexia, and which so nearly resembles the arsenical cachexia. Especially is this the case when the liver and the spleen have become swollen.

"The intermittents which find this homœopathic remedy in Arsenic present in their paroxysms the following peculiarities: the paroxysms are general, violent, and of long duration; the stages are either distinctly developed, and equally proportioned to each other, or else, as is most frequently the case, the one or the other stage is absent, or is very feebly present; if the latter be the case, it is genearlly the cold stage which fails, and the hot stage, is all the more violent. The more intense the heat, the longer it continues, the higher the degree of development of the accompanying excitement in the vascular system, and the more burning and insatiable the thirst, the better is Arsenic indicated. The sweating stage may be altogether wanting; or the perspiration may be very copious; it breaks out generally several hours after the end of the hot stage, and lasts a long time.

"With the paroxysms are associated many distressing accessory symptoms, which are connected, some with the disturbances in the nervous system, some with those of the vascular system, *e. g.*, spasms, pains, delirium, paralyses,

ARSENICUM ALBUM. 205

and the anguish and restlessness that are so characteristic of Arsenic.

"The apyrexia is not pure, but is disturbed by symptoms of the most various kinds; restlessness, sleeplessness, spasms, digestive disorders, feeling of weakness and general prostration; and it is especially characteristic for Arsenic, that, after every paroxysm, there is a notable increase of prostration."

Much of what has been said will serve to point out the indications for Arsenic in continued fever as well as in intermittent. A careful analysis of the symptoms of Arsenic shows them to be a mixture of prostration and of destruction in the vegetative system, with erethism and excitement in the animal system and in the circulation. In this respect it is related to Rhus toxicodendron, being more active and more penetrating in each respect than Rhus. As representing torpor and collapse without erethism, we have already (following Wurmb) mentioned Phosphoric acid as the less powerful and Carbo vegetabilis as the more powerful drug,—correlatives respectively or Rhus toxicodendron and Arsenic.

Wurmb thus describes the typhoid fever in which Arsenic is indicated:

"The patients are very restless and anxious, and generally so weak that they move only the hands, feet and head, and not the trunk; and hence do not voluntarily change their posture in bed. The pulse is very frequent, small and irregular;

the temperature greatly elevated, the cheeks burning hot and red, the thirst insatiable. With these symptoms of excitement those of decomposition of the blood hold equal pace, as is shown by the exanthema and ecchymoses, the often profuse hæmorrhages from various organs, the character of the blood thus excreted, and the destruction of the tissues in the parts on which the patient lies.

"The sensorial functions are withdrawn from the influence of the will; the delirium is always full of anguish and distress, and is sometimes violent, but more frequently is muttering. There are sudden startings and jerkings of muscles in the face and trunk.

"The patients often perceive nothing, and complain of nothing; the excretions pass involuntarily, but the urine is frequently retained, and the bladder is often so distended as to threaten a rupture, which indeed really takes place if the urine be not drawn off. The lips and tongue are dry, the latter often hard and either clean and dark red, or else thickly coated, the coat being a dark-brown fur, which also covers lips and teeth; speech is aften impossible.

"The stool bears the marks of colliquation; the stools are frequent, watery and bloody; the flatulent distention of the abdomen is enormous. There is rattling in the lungs. Emaciation is very rapid and very great. In such cases perforation of the intestine is a common occurrence."

ARSENICUM ALBUM. 207

The indications for Arsenic in neuralgia, in affections of the eyes and teeth, must be drawn from the character of the pain and from the general symptoms. In cholera morbus, in diarrhœa, and in malignant dysentery, it may be indicated, as the symptoms, both general and local, already described, clearly show.

HYDRARGYRUM.

A METAL, known to the ancients.

It was used medicinally by the Arabs, from whom the Europeans derived a knowledge of it through the Moors of Spain. Its general introduction into medical use is ascribed (perhaps wrongly) to Paracelsus (died 1541).

At ordinary temperatures, Hydrargyrum is liquid, hence its name liquid silver, or quick, that is, living silver. It freezes at 39.4° Fahr. and boils at 66_2° Fahr. It is very important to know that it gives off vapor at ordinary temperatures, and that from the inhalation of these vapors serious poisonings have resulted.

No drug, not even Opium, is in so constant and universal use among medical practitioners of the old school as Mercury. No drug has wrought so much mischief upon the human race through its abuse. Like every other drug, it has its proper place in the treatment of disease. This place cannot be supplied by any other drug. When used in this proper place, and used in a proper manner, it is a most powerful instrument for good. These considerations require that the subject of

HYDRARGYRUM.

the properties and uses of Mercury should be carefully and fully treated.

Mercury has been and is used in various forms:

1. Metallic Mercury, Hydrargyrum.

Mercurius vivus of Hahnemann, prepared for use by homœopathicians, by triturating Hydrargyrum with Milk Sugar, according to the rules of the Homœopathic Pharmacy, until the required attenuation is reached.

2. Hydrargyrum cum creta. Mercury with chalk. Trituration 3 oz. H. to 5 oz.

3. Pillulæ Hydrargyriæ. Blue pill. Blue mass.

Mercury 1 oz., confection of roses 1½ oz., powdered liquorice root ½ oz.

Then there are combinations of metallic Mercury with fats, for external use.

4. Unguentum Hydrargyri. Mercury 2 lbs., lard 23 oz., suet 1 oz.

5. Black oxide, protoxide; the precipitate in black wash.

6. The Hydrargyri oxydum rubrum.

Red deutoxide. Red precipitate, used chiefly in the red precipitate ointment.

7. Black sulphuret, or Ethiop's mineral.

8. Red sulphuret, bisulphuret; cinnabar.

9. Dichloride, Subchloride; Hydrargyri Chloridum mite; mild chloride of Mercury; Calomelanos; calomel; prepared by treating a sulphate of the protoxide of Mercury with chloride of Sodium,—two atoms of Mercury and one of chlorine.

Its English name, calomel, with signifies "beautiful black," is said to have been given it by Sir Theodore Mayerne, in compliment to a negro who assisted him in preparing it.

The officinal compound cathartic pill contains calomel, with compound extract of colocynth, extract jalap and gamboge.

10. Hydrargyri chloridum corrosivum; "bichloride of Mercury"; corrossive sublimate. Generally regarded as a bichloride, but really a chloride. An acrid poison of great activity, forming a scarlet precipitate with iodide of potassum, and insoluble compounds with albumen and fibrine.

11. Hydrargyrum ammoniatum. Ammonio-chloride of Mercury. White precipitate, precipitated by ammonia from a solution of corrosive sublimate.

12. Hydrargyrum iodidum.

13. Hydrargyrum biniodidum.

14. Hydrargyrum oxydulatum nigrum. Nitras ammoniacus cum oxydo hydrargyroso. Mercurius solubilis Hahnemanni. Ammonio-nitrate of Mercury. Soluble Mercury of Hahnemann.

Three parts of pure quicksilver are treated with four parts of concentrated nitric acid until about two parts of the quicksilver are dissolved. To the hot solution are then added twelve parts of distilled water; it is filtered, and to it is added a mixture of one and a half parts of strong aqua ammonia, sp. gr. 95, and eight parts of distilled water. A black precipitate is formed, which is the soluble Mercury of Hahnemann.

HYDRARGYRUM.

It is a tasteless, black powder, volatile in heat.

This preparation was introduced by Hahnemann into medicine, long before he had made any of those discoveries and observations which afterward became known as homœopathy. It was extensively used as a mercurial preparation, more certain and less severe in its action than calomel or corrosive sublimate, and is still highly esteemed and much used in Europe, especially in Paris, at the hospital St. Louis.

Hahnemann's excellent proving of Mercury was made chiefly with this preparation.

In treating of the action of Mercury on the organism, I propose to follow Hahnemann's proving of mercurius solubilis; speaking afterward of differences in the action of other preparations.

GENERAL ANALYSIS.

The action of Mercury is most profound and extensive. It affects the entire organism. The sensorium, the nerves of reflex function, and those which preside over vegetative life, are all modified in action. The substance of every tissue is more or less altered.

But, in considering the action of Mercury on the vital force, we distinguish at once that its action on the sensorium, on the nerves of animal life, is subordinate to that on the nerves of vegetation.

Here is a distinction at once between Mercury and the narcotics or cerebrants.

The nutrition is depressed by Mercury in a wonderful degree. Yet this depression is conjoined with a high degree of erethism, so great as often to mask the depression. Here is an analogy with Arsenic, and a distinction from Lachesis and Carbo vegetabilis.

On the organic substance, Mercury works eminent destruction in every tissue. The skin is the seat of destructive ulceration, so is the mucous membrane, so are the lymphatic glands, so are the bones, especially the alveoli. The periosteum is likewise destructively affected. Even newly organized deposits, the result of disease, are unquestionably absorbed and removed by Mercury.

The secretions, especially from the glandular surface (salivary and pancreas) are increased and altered. These and those from the intestines betoken destructive changes in the blood composition. The sweat is increased. The color of the blood becomes depraved,—witness the sallow complexion and the pale and flabby tongue. The albuminous constituent of the blood passes away through the kidney,—whether from change in the composition of the blood, or from change in the kidney, or from both, pathology has not yet taught us,—and we have albuminuria.

The subjective symptoms corroborate this view. The exhaustion consequent on the action of Mercury can hardly be expressed. It is sickening and death-like.

HYDRARGYRUM. 213

The all-pervading character of Mercury is a subject of ocular demonstration. Metallic Mercury has been found in every tissue of the body of those who have taken it as a medicine. Its persistence is likewise demonstrable. Once introduced into the system, it remains. Some remarkable instances of this are on record.

In cats that had been rubbed with Mercurial ointment, Œsterlen found globules of Mercury in the pancreas, liver, spleen, lungs, heart, mesenteric glands, kidneys, etc., and also in the bile, milk, urine and saliva. Van Hasselt has proved that metallic Mercury itself, and not merely the oxide, is absorbed.

It is notorious that nurses and internes in hospital wards become salivated from inhaling the mercurial atmosphere of these wards. (Colson, in "La Pitié," 1821-24; and Goulard, Van Swieten, "Comments," 1726.)

In 1810, Bruckmann published an account of a lady who, a year after being salivated, having become violently heated by dancing, had dark stains appear upon her breast, and metallic Mercury was found upon her linen. Here a year had elapsed since she had taken Mercury.

Jourda gathered a quantity of metallic Mercury from the urine of a syphilitic patient who was taking Mercury.

Elk and Buchner found it in the blood of a person who had been salivated. Colson found that a brass plate, which had lain for some time in the blood of a person treated by Mercury, became covered with a coating of Mercury. Biett, by a prolonged use of the warm bath, got Mercury from the axillary glands of a mercurialized syphilitic patient. Gmelin detected Mercury in the saliva of a person who had been salivated by mercurial inunction. So did Œsterlen and Andouard and Lehmann.

In this connection Melseus reminds us it would be improper to overlook the fact, that when Mercury has been taken so as to produce its constitutional effects, and these have entirely disappeared, they may long afterward be re-excited by the action of medicines, which, becoming decomposed in the system, form soluble compounds with Mercury. One of these is the iodide of potassium. Therefore, iodide of potassium has been recommended as a cure for symptoms which depend on Mercury retained in the economy (Melseus), and it is held by many that iodide of potassium is useful only in those cases of constitutional syphilis in which the body has been impregnated with Mercury; the action of which it certainly has the power of re-awakening.

These facts show the permanence of the action of Mercury; how it makes itself at home in the organism and "will not out."

A few more facts may be cited to show its diffusibility, and its penetrability into the tissue.

A quantity of metallic Mercury escaped from the bags, in which it was being conveyed, into the hold of a vessel. Not only were all the vermin on board killed, but the crew were all salivated.

In Idria, where the ores of Mercury are smelted, the whole population is affected. The mortality is one in forty. Premature births and abortions are very common. Even the cows are salivated and cachectic, and abort.

The chronic diseases, and especially the mercurial trembling, produced on gilders, are well known.

Even the secretion of milk in nursing women is altered; and infants who take it become mercurialized. This fact has been made use of therapeutically; and nurses have been mercurialized in order that their milk might be the vehicle for administering Mercury to infantile victims of congenital syphilis; and this has been successful, too. (Bouchut: "Maladies des Enfans.")

I cannot forbear interrupting the methodical treatment of this subject to call attention to the facts that:

1. Mercury is shown by the above evidence to permeate the tissues, reaching every part of the body. This leaves no room for doubting that it acts on the tissues by virtue of its presence in them. When we desire the action of Mercury, therefore, upon the tissues, the indication is to minutely subdivide it, so as to facilitate its introduction into the tissues.

2. Mercury acts energetically on the system when presented to it in inconceivably small quantities, in a most attenuated form.

It is difficult to estimate the quantity of Mercury that can be contained in the exhalations from the bodies and from the saliva of persons labouring under mercurial salivation. How much more difficult is it to express the infinitesimal smallness of the dose of Mercury which salivates an infant, given in the milk of a mercurialized nurse. Two grains of calomel judiciously used will salivate an adult. Let the average weight of the nurse be 125 pounds, equal to 720,000 grains. Considering the nurse as the non-medicinal vehicle in which those two grains of calomel are distributed, you have here about what homœopathicians would call the third centesimal dilution of calomel. But remember that the tissues of the nurse are constantly undergoing change, that she is constantly secreting fluids, in which Mercury can be detected by chemical re-agents. It appears at once that the dose is equivalent to a much higher dilution. Then consider that the effect is violent salivation, much more powerful than is needed for a cure.

When all these things are duly weighed, is it not amazing that physicians who testify to and accept all these marvelous facts, will accord neither merit nor credence to homœopathicians, who divide the drug very minutely, in order that it may easily penetrate the tissues; and who give exceedingly small doses, even smaller than those given by Bouchut, through the intervention of the nurse.

Peculiarities. It may be mentioned as a peculiarity of Mercury, that the symptoms are aggravated just after getting warm in bed, and that they are attended by a disposition to sweat.

Periodicity is not strongly marked in the action of Mercury, though salivation has been known to recur regularly at certain seasons for years. (Stillé.) The first appreciable effect of a moderate dose of Mercury is an increased activity of the secretions, particularly of the intestinal canal; the discharge becoming liquid and bilious. The mucous membrane of the respiratory apparatus, and sometimes also of the urino-genital, displays a similarly augmented secretion. Then the appetite fails, digestion is impaired, the secretions become still thinner and more copious, the firmness of the tissues diminishes, recently healed wounds open afresh; the muscles waste, the skin becomes earthy-pale, the eyelids and ankles becomes œdematous, and even general dropsy may ensue. These symptoms seem to depend on a radical change which the blood has undergone by losing a large proportion and its normal, solid constituents, and perhaps a portion of that vitality on which its coagulability in part depends. The unwonted fluidity of the blood predisposes to hæmorrhages, which may become dangerous.

Salivation takes place. It is often preceded by an erethism of the system, in which, beside the increased secretions already noticed, the patient loses appetite, but has a quick and frequent pulse, and manifests great nervous excitability. If the salivation is profuse, this state is strongly marked.

HYDRARGYRUM.

As the system is becoming mercurialized, there is a coppery, metallic taste in the mouth, and the teeth are sore when struck together. The breath acquires a characteristic fetor. The gums become puffed, with a red line along the attachment to the lower teeth. This redness gradually extends to the whole buccal, mucous surface. The tongue is coated with white slime, has a sodden, dough-like look, and bears on its margin the imprint of the teeth.

The salivary glands become swollen and tender, the saliva is increased in quantity, it is ropy, alkaline, and has a penetrating taste and smell. The daily discharge sometimes amounts to several pints. In bad cases it is very distressing. The mouth and tongue swell, the patient cannot speak or eat; extensive ulcers, sometimes coated with false membrane, appear on the gums, cheeks and fauces; and in healing, these sometimes cause adhesions of adjacent parts; œdema glottidis may occur, the breath is horribly fetid, the teeth loosen and fall out; and caries attacks the residue and the maxillæ.

The digestive apparatus is affected, appetite impaired, tongue coated; there is nausea, with oppression, and sometimes pain and tenderness at the epigastrium; the bowels are loose, and the stools often contain blood. Œsterlen found metallic Mercury in the intestine of a person who had used the medicine only by inunction.

It used to be thought to increase the discharge

of bile, though how it does so is disputed. But it does not.

It certainly produces enlargement of the liver. Dr. Cheyne says it actually produces jaundice. (The homœopathicians know from daily experience that it cures some forms of jaundice.) It produces green stools. (Green stools are not always bilious.)

It produces great depression, great sensibility to cold, pain in the limbs, irritability.

It causes menorrhagia.

It causes albuminuria (and cures it).

In persons long exposed to its vapor it causes a singular quasi-paralysis, the "mercurial trembling." This is gradual in its approach, beginning with formication of the hands and sometimes of the feet, and with more or less pain of the thumbs, elbows, knees and feet, which also renders the movement of these parts imperfect. After a time the hands begin to tremble, and then the arms and lower limbs, the muscles of the lower jaw and tongue, and indeed all the muscles of animal life. The muscular contractions takes place rapidly, but by starts, so that the patient feeds himself with difficulty. Walking is difficult from the same cause. So are articulation and mastication. It resembles chorea, being worse from mental emotion and relieved by alcohol. Sometimes single groups of muscles are absolutely paralyzed.

Mercury produces also an irritative fever. The patient is weary and chilly. The pulse is frequent (not full nor hard), tongue coated, great tendency to perspire, skin very sensitive to cold, often relieved by salivation.

Mercury produces a skin affection, which may be a rash, closely resembling measles ; or a miliary eruption, or an erysipelatous inflammation, or a gangrene.

Ulcers appear on the gums, on the inside of the cheeks, and on the tongue, attended with salivation. These ulcers usually advance from within outward, raising and then casting off the epithelium, and exposing a red, irritable surface, which secretes an acrid fluid. They are irregular in shape, without defined edges; they bleed readily, have a dirty, whitish surface, are surrounded with a dark halo, and are apt to run together.

Let me call attention to the difference between these and syphilitic ulcers of this membrane. The latter are "circular, attack the posterior parts of the mouth, have well-defined edges ; the surrounding membrane has a coppery hue, and they do not extend from their primary seat." I may remark that these ulcers find their remedy more often in Nitric acid than in Mercury.

Hæmorrhage may occur from these mercurial ulcers, or they may prove fatal by gangrene.

The destructive action of mercury on the glands (lymphatic) is unquestionable. Ulceration of both the inguinal and exillary glands occurs.

The bones are the seat of destructive inflammation. Periosteal nodes appear, which ulcerate, and then ulceration progresses from without inward into the bone. Canstatt says "it is most frequent in the spongy bones at the base of the cranium, and in the ends of the long bones."

To these details of the general action of Mercury on the human organism I shall append the finer and more exact data which resulted from Hahnmann's proving on the healthy subject :

1. As regards the action on the skin, the eruptions itch ; the discharge from them is acrid, excoriating adjacent surfaces. Indeed, this is a general characteristic of the secretion under Mercury, from the discharge in ophthalmia to the intestinal evacuations. They cause smarting and excoriation. Intertrigo s common.

Further, there is a general itching about the joints and over the body in the evening and at night.

2. *Limbs.* Tearing and drawing pains, wrose at night; the limbs twitch. There are lassitude and soreness; all the bones ache.

Jaundice ; the perspiration stains the linen yellow.

Great disposition to perspire on slight excercise.

As a general thing the symptoms are aggravated in the evening, and during repose, when lying or sitting. Great restlessness in the limbs in the evening; cannot remain anywhere quiet nor in any position; must constantly change posture.

Great weakness and prostration, yet orgasm of the blood; erethism.

Sleepiness by day, not relieved by long sleep. Difficult falling asleep in the evening, because of restlessness, anxiety, etc. Sleep at night disturbed by frequent wakings, and dreams which terrify.

The fever, which is irritative, is attended with decided thirst. Very marked is the disposition to sweat, which occurs during sleep. The heat is attended by great anxiety, and by the peculiar gastric symptoms of Mercurius.

The disposition is restless, anxious, irritable, and yet despondent.

Vertigo with nausea, distracted thoughts, momentary loss of vision.

Headache. Tearing, burning in the temples; semi-lateral tearing in the head at night, as if the head would burst, along with soreness and a tired aching in the nape of the neck. Sensation as if the head were bound around with a hoop.

Eyes. The margins of the lids are ulcerated and scabby. Ophthalmia and intolerance of firelight. Great lachrymation. Pain as from a cutting body under the eyelids. Biting and burning in the eyes, especially in the open air. Black spots before the eyes. Photophobia.

Ears. Earache, with tearing or stitching pain. Ulceration of the concha. Discharge of blood and offensive pus from the ears. Fungous growths in the meatus. Swelling of the parotids. Deafnesh, relieved by blowing the nose. Noises in the ears.

Nose. Red, shining swelling of the nose. Epistaxis. Earthy, yellow complexion. Dirty yel-

HYDRARGYRUM.

low scabs in the face, which bleed when scratched. Swelling of the submaxillary and cervical glands.

The *Gums* swell and burn, and are sore, worse at night, worse by touch and by eating. Ulceration. Teeth are loose.

Toothache, tearing at night, excited by cold air, by eating, and by both cold and warm drinks. Worst in the evening and at night; intolerable when warm in the bed.

Offensive smell from the mouth. Burning ulcers or aphthæ. Swelling of the soft palate and fauces. Burning and ulceration of the fauces. Constant disposition to swallow. When swallowing, sticking pain in the throat and in the tonsils. Copious, offensive saliva. Swelling of the tongue. Induration and ulceration of the tongue. Cannot talk. Voice hoarse and rough.

Canine hunger. Aversion to food.

Insatiable, burning thirst.

Flat, putrid or metallic taste.

Nausea, with sweetish taste.

Weak digestion, with constant hunger, oppression of the stomach, and feeling as if the stomach were dragged down after each meal.

Inflammation and hardening of the liver, with stitching pains.

Abdomen distended, with soreness; cutting and pinching pains.

Stool. Frequent desire for stool, ineffectual, especially at night. Dysenteric diarrhœa, with tenesmus. Tenesmus continues after stool. Stools acrid, of bloody mucus. Sour-smelling, green, acrid stools.

Prolapsus ani, when straining at stool and after stool.

Frequent, rapid urination, with scanty discharge, often followed by discharge of mucus. Urine dark red, offensive, or it may be very abundant and light.

Menses too copious, with anxiety and abdominal cramps. Leucorrhœa purulent and acrid.

Violent fluent coryza, with an acrid watery discharge, making the nose and lip red, and very sore.

Dyspnœa on rapid motion.

Dry fatiguing cough—as if the head and chest would burst—from tickling in the larynx. Hemoptysis.

Burning in the chest; palpitation.

Secretion of the mammary gland repulsive to the infant.

Upper Extremities. At night, tearing in the shoulder and arms. Hot, red swellings in the forearm. The fingers crack. Paronychia.

Lower Extremities. Tearing in the legs at night. Dropsical swelling of the feet and legs. Painful swellings on the bones of the feet and legs.

The warmth of the bed increases all the symptoms until they become intolerable.

The practical applications of Mercury are very diverse.

PRACTICAL APPLICATION.

The discussion of the practical application of any remedy in the treatment of diseased persons should always be opened by the reminder that each diseased state is to be regarded as a new case, distinct from all others, and different from every other; and that a remedy must be selected for it in accordance with the similarity which the symptoms produced by the remedy in the healthy subject bear to the symptoms of the sick person for whom it is selected. This cannot be too often repeated, nor too strongly insisted on.

This being premised, I may call attention to a few cases in which Mercurius is more especially likely to be required and useful.

And first, of general diseases.

That in which Mercury was first employed, and in the treatment of which it has acquired the dignity of a specific, is syphilis.

Touching this disease I desire to say, that in so far as my experience in the treatment of it is concerned, I have not found it less amenable to treatment than other constitutional maladies. The patient, otherwise in vigorous health, who presents himself for treatment, without having previously saturated his system with drugs, and without having undertaken to eradicate the morbific poison by caustic applications to its primary local manifestation, the chancre—such a patient, if Mercury be indicated by his symptoms, will be cured as readily and by as small doses as though his disease were something of a totally different character. (A prejudice to the contrary exists.) And my professional experience satisfies me, that in these, as in other cases, the high potencies, and infrequent doses, produce a more speedy and a more effectual cure than low potencies and frequent doses do. But inasmuch as I do not regard the chancre as the "fons et origo mali," but rather as the blossom and product of a constitutional infection which already pervades the system, I am not in so great haste as some are to destroy the chancre, well satisfied if, under internal treatment, I perceive it gradually heal by healthy granulations, no other symptoms meanwhile appearing. Above all, I dread the local treatment by caustic, the much-vaunted method of Ricord. For observation has satisfied me that even a majority of his patients, discharged as cured through the local cauterization, present, after the lapse of from one to eight weeks, all the signs of secondary syphilis, and become candidates for, and victims of, the "constitutional treatment."

It is not every case, however, of so-called chancre, for which Mercury is indicated.

That which is now denominated chancroid, and which, being a shallow and flat-bottomed ulceration, shows a disposition to spread irregularly and indefinitely, having never well-defined outlines nor a lardaceous bottom; but exuding a thin, serous discharge, and which is probably not at all syphilitic in its origin, does not call for Mercury, and is not benefited by it; indeed is rather aggravated. I have found the totality of the symptoms to indicate Nux vomica more frequently than any other drug, and under this a speedy cure to follow.

The form of chancre in which Mercurius is indicated is the regular indurated Hunterian chancre, with the lardaceous base.

In continued or remittent fevers, particularly those which are complicated with enlargement or subacute inflammation of the liver, Mercurius may be indicated by the symptoms.

The peculiar headache of Mercurius—dullness in the forehead, stitches through the temples, a band around the head, and aching, and weariness in the posterior cervical muscles, from the occipital ridge downward—is often found conjoined with gastric symptoms and a state of the tongue which clearly call for Mercury.

A catarrhal or superficial otitis often exists, which is promptly relieved by Chamomilla or Pulsatilla, according as the characteristic indications for one or the other may be present. But there is another form, in which the inflammation is deeper seated, affecting the sub-mucous and sub-cutaneous cellular tissue, extending to the parotid gland, which becomes swollen and tender, and accompanied by throbbing pain, worse at night on getting warm in bed; accompanied, too, by the tongue and gastric symptoms peculiar to Mercury; in which Mercury is the proper remedy.

The throat affection that calls for Mercury is a parenchymatous tonsillitis, in which the pain is throbbing, the tonsil and fauces yellowish red, often covered with a thin, false membrane; the breath fetid, the tongue pale, flabby, and indented by the teeth; the pain on deglutition much greater than on empty swallowing. Salivation increased; the throat sore externally when pressed. The difference from the sore throat of Belladonna is evident. From that of Lachesis it will be differentiated in the lecture on Lachesis. It closely resembles that of Hepar sulphuris, which, however, has the sharp, sticking pain in the tonsil, as from a splinter.

The stomatitis has been described.

I may mention that qualmishness and a peculiar sense of weakness and tenderness at the pit of the stomach, are very characteristic symptoms of Mercury.

To be distinguished, however, from Calcarea carbonica, which has soreness and intolerance of pressure from the hand or by clothing; and from Sepia and Murex purpurea, which have a "sinking", an "all-gone feeling", and a faintness and die-away sensation at the pit of the stomach.

The stool of Mercury is a symptom of great importance.

In large doses, Calomel produces copious semi-fluid, pasty evacuations of dark green or greeenish brown fæces, with great weakness and prostration at the epigastrium, griping and soreness in the abdomen, moderate tenesmus and burning in the rectum, with exhaustion after the evacuation. If the administration be continued, the discharges become frequent but small in quantity; consist of mucus and blood mixed together, and often containing shreddy substance, like strips of mucous membrane; and are attended by tenesmus, which is not relieved by the evacuation of stool, but continues almost without interruption; also with burning and soreness in the rectum and anus, as if the secretions were acrid.

This describes a form of dysentery of which every year furnishes examples in practice. The chief point is to distinguish such cases from those which correspond better to Nux vomica or Podophyllum or Sulphur than to Mercurius.

Under Mercurius the desire for stool is not relieved by the evacuation; the patient would glodly sit and strain for an indefinite period. Under Nux vomica the tenesmus is relieved by stool; and the patient enjoys a respite from suffering.

Under Sulphur, likewise, the tenesmus is relieved by stool, and the Sulphur stools have the peculiarity that the blood is not uniformly mixed through the mucus, but occurs in thready streaks.

It is needless, I hope, to remark that to those who are capable of looking at the entire condition of the patient, and of keeping their attention from being engrossed by the one group of symptoms made prominent by the patient's complaints, the general symptoms furnish an unfailing guide. For excellent distinctions between remedies for dysentery, I refer to Dr. Well's articles in the "American Homœopathic Review," iii.

Homœopathic preparations are: Mercurius solubilis; Mercurius vivus; Mercurius corrosivus sublimatus; Mercurius protiodide and biniodide; Cinnibaris.

Proto iodatus. *Throat symptoms.*

Tongue thickly coated, yellowish white at the back part, the front and edges being clean and red.

Empty deglutition; is painful. Desire to swallow; sense as of a lump in the throat.

Posterior wall of the pharynx red and irritated, and dotted with patches of mucus and spots which look ulcerated.

Patches on the tonsils and soft palate, easily detached. Worse on the right side. Great thirst.

CUCUMIS COLOCYNTHIS.

SQUIRTING CUCUMBER: BITTER APPLE.

WE use in medicine the pulp of the fruit, an exceedingly bitter and nauseous production.

It was known to the early Greeks, and a great regard for its medicinal virtues is expressed by all the ancient writers. Among moderns it has fallen into disuse and some discredit, except as an ingredient of the officinal and other compound cathartic pills.

It was classed as a drastic or as a hydragogue cathartic along with scammony and gamboge. And in modern times, under the sway of the physiological school, which denied to drugs the possession of any individual specific properties peculiar to each, according them only certain general properties which were common to them and other members of a group, it was thought that for Colocynth might be advantageously substituted some less powerful, perhaps, and less distressing, purgative. But we shall see that Colocynth has certain properties which no other drug possesses.

I may remark, in passing, that it seems remarkable that physicians who dreaded the too powerful action of Colocynth, should yet so often,—in seeking to blend with it a drug or a complex of drugs which should moderate and correct its vigorous action,—have selected for this purpose other powerful drastic cathartics, such as scammony, gamboge, veratrum, black hellebore, ect. Nay, Dodonæus even says that violent purges are the best corrigentia of Colocynth. It can hardly be but that, under the law *"Similia similibus curantur"*, these violent drugs, to a great extent, neutralize and antidote each other. Of the fact of this neutralizing effect there can be no question. It is universally admitted. Why may it not be accounted for by the same law which accounts for the subsidence of morbid symptoms through the action of the similar remedy?

But what a discovery was that of Hahnemann, so laughably simple, yet so unsuspected, that the too powerful action of a drug may be moderated by just diminishing the dose, and by going on to diminish it until the dose acts as gently as you wish.

Another Columbus with another egg!

The action of Colocynth in large doses is shown forth by the following cases:

"A woman, aged forty years, had a chronic rheumatic pain in the left thigh and left shoulder. A kind friend advised her to infuse half a pound of Colocynth in a half pint of red wine, and to drink the fluid before going to bed. By good fortune she took only one-half part of the infusion.

Scarcely had she swallowed this, when she was seized with fearful pains in the region of the stomach, great anxiety, vertigo, faintness and cramps. She vomited several times without relief; then evacuated copious stools, at first watery and feculent, then consisting of pure blood, with distressing tenesmus; along with these came large pieces of the inner membrane of the intestine. The pain then concentrated in the stomach and in the lower part of the rectum; the abdomen because collapsed; at last the tenesmus ceased, and the patient gradually fell asleep. Great exhaustion followed, but she finally recovered."

In another case of the kind, which proved fatal, the autopsy revealed that the intestines were red, with black spots, glued together by false membrane. A white fluid had exuded into the cavity of the abdomen, and in it white flocculi were floating. On the coat of the stomach here and there an ulcerated spot could be seen. There was no trace of inflammation in liver, kidney or bladder.

Hahnemann and six of his pupils proved Colocynth, but the result was quite meagre. It was reserved for the Austrain Proving Society to show us a full picture of the pathogenesis of this drug.

These provings, viewed collectively, show us, what indeed we knew before, that the effect of Colocynth upon the alimentary canal is immediate and profound, that it produces vomiting and purging of watery matters, and then of mucus and blood; great flatulent distention of the abdomen;

and cruel, griping, flatulent colic. They give finer shades of delineation, however, than cases of poisoning could.

Furthermore, they reveal to us an action of Colocynth that was heretofore masked under its violent action on the alimentary canal. I mean its power to produce neuralgia, affecting; 1, the trifacial nerve; 2, the solar plexus; 3, the lumbar and femoral nerves and their branches. Yet this knowledge has enable us to effect some most brilliant cures, and to grope our way toward others, which could never be clearly indicated by any proving. Furthermore, a power to affect the ovaries is shadowed in the proving of Colocynth.

SPECIAL ANALYSIS.

Upon the mind Colocynth exerts no deep action. It produces impatience, vexation, excitement, followed of course by prostration and dejection.

Sensorium. Dullness of the head, vertigo, confusion.

Violent headache, as if brought on by exposure to a current of air. Aching pain along the sagittal suture, increased by exercise and by stooping.

Pressing and drawing pain in the left side of the forehead. Drawing in the forehead as if it would be pressed out. Digging in the left temple. Pulsation in the left temple, which afterward changes to lancinations, the same being felt simultaneously in the left shoulder.

Tearing and tension in the left side of the face, extending to the ear and head. Cramp-like sensation in the left malar bone, extending into the left eye. Feeling of pressure in the orbits near the root of the nose, with confusion in the head and chilliness.

Scraping and burning in the mouth and throat. Eructations. Nausea. Vomiting of food and vomiting of greenish fluid. Vomiting with diarrhœa.

Pain in the stomach after eating. Fullness in the epigastrium. Squeezing and wringing pain in the stomach.

Colic and diarrhœa after taking the least nourishment.

Flying pains in the hepatic region.

Constricting pain in the centre of the abdomen, recurring at short intervals, and passing into a sharp griping.

Griping in the abdomen, especially about the umbilicus, like a cutting or squeezing; relieved by bending forward or on evacuating the bowels.

Pain in the whole abdomen, as if the bowels were squeezed between stones.

Rumbling and commotion in the hypogastrium.

The colic comes on every fifteen or twenty minutes, and is relieved by pressure and by bending forward.

Diarrhœa, with nausea. Stool semi-liquid, brownish yellow, retained with difficulty; preceded by colic; some tenesmus. Liquid frothy stool; saffron yellow, and of a musty odor; watery-mucous and bloody stools. Sensation of weakness in the rectum.

Abundant urine. Frequent desire to pass water, with burning in the bladder and stitches in the bladder; alternating with stitches in the rectum.

Menses early and more abundant.

Under Dr. Frohlich, Colocynth was proved by two young women, who both experienced, beside the symptoms of the abdomen and bowels, deep stitches in the ovaries on both sides, but worse on the left.

The respiratory organs are not markedly affected.

Drawing, lancinating pain in the left shoulder, extending thither from the left side of the face over the neck. Drawing pain and stiffness in the muscles of the left side of the neck. Generally this pain is relieved by motion.

In the upper part of the nape of the neck, close to the occiput, a sensation as if a heavy weight were there. Rawness in the right scapula, a feeling as if the nerves and blood-vessels were stretched. Severe contusive pain from the right side of the neck down to the scapula.

(It is to be remarked that with all these symptoms there is no fever, no sensitiveness, no heat; motion generally relieves.)

Drawing and paralytic pain in the arms.

The lower limbs are weak and heavy.

Tension in the right groin, Pressure at the left sacro-iliac articulation, with tingling at the sole of the foot.

Drawing in the right thigh down to the knee. Pain darting from the tuber ischii to the knee. Drawing, darting and obscure pulsation in the left hip. Tingling in the left foot, with simultaneous pressure about the sacro-iliac articulation. Pulsation in the left gluteal region. Drawing in the right thigh down to the knee.

Only during motion pain in the right thigh, as if the psoas muscle were too short; better on ceasing to walk; recurring on moving again.

Cramp-like drawing in the internal femoral region. Stiffness of the knee, as if bound around with a cord.

Tearing, drawing and pressure throughout the limb.

Dr. Watzke of Vienna says:

"The hemicraniæ and prosopalgiæ which Colocynth will cure, are, in all cases, purely functional derangements of the filaments of the trifacial nerve.

"In the prosopalgiæ of Colocynth there are no twitchings of the muscles, nor any palsied feelings in the affected side; the pain follows the course of the nerve, is periodical, and accompanied by toothache." Colocynth is related to Belladonna, Capsicum and Verbascum.

Colocynth is adapted to what Romberg describes as neuralgia hypogastrica, and which is often described and regarded in women as menstrual colic;

and in men as hæmorrhoidal colic; attended by pains and aching in the thighs.

"The intestinal affection indicating Colocynth is hardly inflammatory (and yet the autopsy shows it)"

"The ischialgiæ are not due to strumous diathesis or to organic changes."

And yet unless many skillful physicians have been greatly deceived, Colocynth has arrested and cured, in its early stages, morbus coxarius.

It is not easy nor safe to undertake to distinguish, in early stages, functional and organic affections, and to set apart remedies for the one and for the other on pathological grounds. Experience gives the lie to our hypothesis.

The presumptive action of Colocynth on the ovaries deserves attention and experimental research.

PODOPHYLLUM PELTATUM.

THIS remedy has been flippantly called the *"Vegetable Mercury."* It resembles it no more than the "greenback" or paper dollar is like the precious metal which, by a financial fiction, it purports to represent

Podophyllum is a remedy of great value, and possessing a distinct individuality. It can neither be used as a succedaneum for, nor be replaced by, any other remedy.

It was proved under the auspices of Dr. Williamson of Philadelphia. A very extended easy upon it is contained in Hale's "New Materia Medica."

I propose to notice, in a cursory way, some of its best established relations to the organism.

And first, upon the digestive apparatus.

The secretion of saliva is increased, the breath is offensive, tongue coated white, with a foul taste; worse in the morning.

Sore throat, beginning on the right side and going to the left. Dryness of the throat. Soreness extending to the ears. This is the reverse of Lachesis and the same as Lycopodium.

Regurgitation of food; increased appetite; satiety from a small quantity of food, followed by nausea and vomiting; thirst; putrid taste.

This satiety resembles Lycopodium and Nux vomica, but Lycopodium has also great flatulence; flatus being incarcerated under the false ribs.

Acidity of the stomach, nausea and vomiting, heart-burn, heat and throbbing in the stomach, followed by diarrhœa. The vomiting is forcible, and the matter vomited is dark green.

Much pain in the abdomen, as in the transverse colon, occurring or worse about three A. M., and followed by diarrhœa. The colic is relieved by warmth and by bending forward while lying on the side. In this it resembles Colocynth colic.

It is at first accompanied by general coldness, which soon gives place to heat and perspiration.

Feeling of fullness; weight and dragging in the hypochondria, especially in the right, with stitches, twisting pain, and heat.

The stool is increased in frequency and altered in character. Diarrhœa occurs; frequent pappy yellow stools. Diarrhœa immediately after eating or drinking. Similar to Colocynth and China. Watery yellow stools without pain from three A. M. till nine A. M., followed by a natural stool toward evening. These forms of diarrhœa stool are followed by a sensation of great weakness in the abdomen, and especially in the rectum. This sensation of weakness in the rectum is characteristic of Podophyllum.

Besides this modification of stool, Podophyllum produces chalky evacuations, which are very offensive.

Likewise, stools yellow, green or brownish and watery; mucus streaked with blood; and these attended by heat in the rectum, by flashes of heat running up the back, by painful tenesmus, and by a descent of the rectum. Hence a valuable remedy in dysentery, especially when the patient complains of a sensation of weakness in the rectum.

This prolapsus is to be distinguished from that of Ignatia, Carbo vegetabilis and Hamamelis, in that it occurs before the evacuation of fæces and not after it. The anus is extremely sore.

From these symptoms we might gather that Podophyllum would be a valuable remedy in prolapsus ani following dysentery, in hæmorrhoids, in dysentery, and in certain watery diarrhœas,—an inference abundantly confirmed by experience. The time of occurrence and the concomitant symptoms furnish the distinctive indications. The diarrhœa generally occurs or is worse in the morning, and the stool is followed by a sensation of extreme weakness in the abdomen, or only in the rectum.

From the green, watery diarrhœa and the evident hepatic condition associated with it, one might think of Podophyllum in cases of diarrhœa during dentition; and Drs. Williamson and Bell have used it successfully in dentition-diarrhœa where there was present also cerebral irritation, as shown by the following symptoms:

Grinding the teeth at night, "rolling the head."

It is to be noted also that in the symptomatology, the diarrhœa (yellow, watery) alternates with a morning headache—a heavy, dull headache in the forehead, with soreness of the forehead and eyes. Such an alternation is observed in many hepatic affections. It reminds one of Aloes.

The urine is increased.

Menstruation is retarded. There is much bearing down in the hypogastric and sacral regions, increased by motion and relieved by lying down. Like Sepia.

Much pain in the region of the right ovary.

Leucorrhœa thick and transparent, with bearing down in the genital organs, and constipation.

Dr. Williamson and others have found Podophyllum a valuable remedy in prolapsus uteri, following parturition, especially when there was also a numb, aching pain in the region of the ovaries, particularly the left.

I shall speak further only of the febrile symptoms of Podophyllum. Dr. Williamson gives the following indications: Chilliness in the evening or morning early, preceded by backache, accompanied by pressing in the hypochondria and aching in the joints of the extremities. Heat comes on before the chilliness disappears. Heat with delirium, loquacity, violent headache, and great thirst with loss of appetite.

Sweat, during which the patient sleeps.

Podophyllum has been used successfully where indicated, in intermittent, remittent and typhoid fevers.

LACHESIS.

THE very excellent and convincing article on Lachesis by Dr. Lippe in the last number of the "Review,"* calls to mind the fact that this remedy, so highly prized by many practioners—I might say by all who make any use of it whatever—is, by a large number of homœopathists, regarded as of no account at all.

Those who do not use Lachesis in their practice give various reasons for their course. Some express the views laid down by Dr. Lippe. These are theoretical and *a priori* objections, and they cannot stand one moment against the testimony of experience and *a posteriori* demonstration.

Others hesitate to use Lachesis because they cannot procure it in the "mother tincture," or the "first decimal preparations," or in any dilution below the sixth. Inasmuch as, by both faith and practice, they are committed against "infinitesimals," they cannot employ Lachesis in any case, since they could not use it in any but an infinitesimal

---

* "Lachesis," by Ad. Lippe, M. D. "American Homœopathic Review," June, 1863, p. 552.

dose. No doubt many are sincere in this objection. A few, it must be feared, gladly avail themselves of so fair a pretext for avoiding the study of the long list of symptoms which Lachesis presents. It is a pity that this whole class of objectors could not bring themselves to the point of fairly testing, by clinical experiment, the virtues of Lachesis. The result would be happy in a double sense. It would enlighten them respecting a most valuable remedy, and at the same time it would be a satisfactory demonstration of the action of infinitesimal doses.

A third class of objectors throw discredit on the proving of Lachesis, and on very singular grounds. Because it is fragmentary? Scanty? Has but few symptoms? Is carelessly arranged? Criticisms like these have been made with more or less justice upon many provings in our materia medica. No! the objection made to the proving of Lachesis is that it is too rich; there are "too many symptoms;" it is too thoroughly elaborated! "What!" it is asked, "can one remedy produce so many symptoms?" The answer comes readily to hand,—"No!" The inference is at its elbow,—"Some symptoms, then, must be false." Then come the conclusions,—"Some are false; we cannot tell which they are; we will therefore reject all, and the remedy along with them!"

One of the oldest and most widely known homœopathic practioners in America said to the writer: "In the American 'Jahr's New Manual,' thirty pages are devoted to Lachesis. If all were reduced to a concise statement of verified, unquestionable Lachesis symptoms, even Dr. Hering would admit that there would not be matter for more than three such pages. I therefore reject the whole proving and never give the remedy."

To this objection I could not help replying: "In yonder wheat-field, I doubt not the proportion of chaff, straw and stubble to good wheat is as ten to one. And yet the farmer willingly submits to the labor of harvesting, threshing and winnowing for the sake of the ten per cent, of wheat; he would not think of abandoning the grain in his field because of the tenfold preponderance of chaff. And if there be, as you admit, in those thirty pages, the equivalent of three pages, or even of one page, of verified and trustworthy symptoms, how can you, as a conscientious prescriber, deliberately refuse to make yourself master of them and to use in your practice the remedy which produced them?"

This question, which received at that time no conclusive answer, addresses itself to all who stand in the position of that practitioner.

If, of the three thousand and more symptoms ascribed to Lachesis, there be thrity, if there be three, symptoms that are trustworthy and that are peculiar to Lachesis, a case of disease may occur presenting those symptoms and no others, and which, therefore, Lachesis, and no other remedy, will cure. How can those gentlemen who determine beforehand that they will have nothing to do with Lachesis because of the two thousand and seventy or the two thousand and ninety-seven symptoms which they discredit—how can these gentlemen, with a clear conscience, run the risk of meeting such a case and of losing it from the want of knowledge of the characteristics of Lachesis?

The objection to the length and complexity of the treatise on Lachesis comes from those who have cursorily turned over the leaves of the Manual, and not from those who have made an earnest study of the symptomatology. The latter class of students make no such complaint. They find, indeed, no great difficulty in getting a clear idea of the relations of Lachesis to morbid conditions. And the facility with which they can do this is due chiefly to the care with which Dr. Hering has elaborated the proving, to the immense labor he has devoted to the collation of the symptoms, to his caution in avoiding any sundering of pathogenetic groups, and to his faithful repetition of each group under every rubric to which it has any pertinence. All these points of excellence, while they have made the original proving of Lachesis a model for fullness and clearness of arrangement, have made its length a bugbear to the timid reader.

But it is not to be supposed that either *a priori* doubts of the efficacy of a remedy, or any practical difficulties in the mastery of symptomatology, would deter physicians from studying and using it, when the testimony of those who have employed it successfully shall have been placed before them.

In 1850, while assisting in the autopsy of a woman who had died of puerperal peritonitis, the writer received a dissecting would in the index finger of the left hand. Within a week, the finger had quadrupled in size, the hand and forearm were much swollen and œdematous, a hard, red line extended from the wrist to the axilla. The axillary glands were swollen. The arm and hand were intensely painful; the whole left side was partially paralyzed. The constitutional symptoms were: extreme prostration,—causing the disease to be at first mistaken for a typhus,—low muttering delirium at night, marked aggravation of suffering and prostration on awaking from sleep. The general condition grew steadily worse, abscesses forming under the deep fibrous tissues of the finger and hand. No homœopathic practitioner was in the neighborhood. The allopathic surgeons in attendance advised calomel and opium, but gave a very discouraging prognosis. The patient refused to take any drugs, determining to trust the issue of the case to Lachesis. The first dose (of the twelfth) was taken on the third day of the illness, and a dose was taken thrice daily for five days, at the end of which period the constitutional symptoms had substantially vanished. The recovery of the finger was slow but complete. The effect of the Lachesis could not be mistaken by the patient.

FROM MY CLINICAL RECORD.

April 9th, 1860. Josephine Birmingham, aged nine years, well grown, had, last winter, scarlatina very severely. It left her delicate and deaf. Nine days ago she was exposed to the measles. The rash appeared on the 6th inst., along with a copious discharge from the ears. Yesterday (8th) this discharge suddenly ceased and the rash disappeared. She immediately became very feeble and prostrate; was seized with wild, muttering delirium. She had great thirst, drinking, however, but little at a time. There was a singularly biting heat of the skin.

I saw her first at eleven A.M., on the 9th inst. She had lain in alternate delirium and stupor for twenty-four hours; was irrational; had low muttering dilirium; the pulse was soft, wavy, hardly to be counted; there was calor mordax; the respiration was attended by moaning; it was very rapid, whistling; there was an occasional single cough, with a moan following each cough, and a grasping at the throat, as if to tear away the clothing from it. The pupils were widely dilated; there had been no stool for two days; the urine was scanty and seldom passed; I could not secure any for analysis. The expression of the countenance was cadaverous; the odor of the breath putrescent. I ordered Lachesis[30], six globules in water, a tea-spoonful every two hours. Also strong beef tea every two hours.

At six P.M. I found her sitting supported in an arm-chair, playing with some toys; rational; the skin of a pleasant temperature; the pulse eighty, regular and soft. The attendants reported that after the second dose she had slept quietly, had had no more delirium and no thirst. I found the eyes normal, the cough infrequent and not painful I ordered Saccharum lactis.

The rash did not re-appear. The patient convalesced from this point, and I gave no other remedy and did not repeat the Lachesis.

This change from apparent impending death to established convalescence within the space of seven hours was very impressive and even startling.

In the year 1853 there prevailed, quite extensively, in Brooklyn, an epidemic of what was called "malignant pustule." A furuncular formation appeared, generally upon the lower lip, attended with severe pain, and frequently surrounded by an erysipelatous areola. The most marked constitutional symptom was a very rapid and excessive loss of strength, the patient being reduced from vigor to absolute prostration within the space of from twenty-four to thirty-six hours. Allopathic physicians at first resorted to the local application of nitrate of silver to the pustule. In those cases, thus treated, which came under my personal observation, death followed cauterization within twenty-four hours.

In eight cases treated by myself, Lachesis was the only remedy used. It relieved the pain within a few hours after the first dose was given, and the patients all recovered very speedily.

I have three times been called to cases of chronic ulcers of the lower extremities (probably of syphilitic origin), in which the discharge had ceased; the extremity had become œdematous, and a hard, slightly red swelling extending up along the course of the principal veins, together with a great and sudden prostration of strength, low muttering delirium and general typhoid symptoms, gave good reason for supposing that the secondary phlebitis had occurred. In these cases a careful study of the symptoms induced me to give Lachesis. The effect was all that could be desired, the patients rallying promptly, all symptoms of phlebitis speedily disappearing.

During the prevalence of diphtheria on the banks of the Hudson in 1858-60, many cases occurred in which the severity of the constitutional symptoms was very much greater than the local manifestations of disease in the pharynx would have led one to anticipate. In some cases in which the tumefaction in the throat was slight, and the redness of the mucous membrane hardly noticeable, and in which the diphtheritic deposits consisted merely of two or three little patches hardly larger than a pin's head, the prostration of strength was quite alarming; the pulse became, in a very short time, slow, feeble and compressed, a cold, clammy sweat frequently covered the forehead and extremities, the breath was fetid, the appetite entirely destroyed,—indeed, the patient passed with alarming rapidity into a completely asthenic condition. Not infrequently the prostration had become quite considerable even before any local evidences of disease could be detected.

In these cases,—in all in which the constitutional symptoms thus predominated over the local symptoms,—Lachesis produced prompt and lasting improvement, so that very rarely was any other medicine given subsequently.

Several cases of carbuncle have come under my notice, in which the progress of the inflammation was very slow, the skin over the dead cellular tissue showed little disposition to ulcerate, and when, finally, it became perforated in three or four places, there was but a scanty discharge of thin, sometimes bloody, sanies. Meanwhile the constitutional symptoms denoted very great prostration, *not* preceded nor attended by the nervous and vascular erethism which are sometimes observed in similar cases. Lachesis is the remedy on which experience has taught me to rely in the treatment of such affections, provided the symptoms do not conclusively indicate some other remedy. In the cases to which I refer, the symptoms corresponded very closely to those of Lachesis.

About a year ago, I was called to take charge of a patient who had suffered for several years from a succession of carbuncles and indolent boils. During the four months preceding my visit to him, he had had four successive carbuncles, none of which ran a complete course. After the skin covering the dead cellular tissue had become perforated, a slight discharge of sanies had taken place, and the perforations had closed again, without any discharge of slough, leaving an indurated mass, with a dull, burning pain and considerable tenderness, but scarcely any discoloration. After each of these carbuncles, a marked deterioration in the patient's health was observed, until, after the last, he was so much reduced as to be confined to his bed, with well-marked hectic fever.

Pretty soon, a severe pain in and below the right groin and along the inner aspect of the femur, gave indication of trouble in that region. An abscess was discovered deep in the adductor muscles of the thigh. An opening was made by a distinguished professor of surgery in New-York upon the anterior surface of the thigh (as the patient was confined to the bed and lay on his back, this was the superior aspect of the thigh), and nearly a quart of pus was discharged. The formation and discharge of pus continued to be profuse for fifteen days, the patient all the time becoming rapidly more feeble, with severe hectic, total loss of appetite, and great local suffering, when the case was placed under my charge. I found that the evacuation of the pus was a very difficult matter, the aperture being at the highest point of the abscess. The attending surgeon had been compelled to withdraw the pus by means of an exhausting pump, attached to the free end of a gum catheter which he previously introduced into the abscess. I continued this method until the abscess closed. The patient, his family, and the physicians in attendance had abandoned all hope of his recovery.

In view of the copious formation of pus, one's first thought would naturally be that Silicea would be the appropriate remedy. This remedy, however, had been given in every variety of potency. It had never failed to aggravate the whole condition of the patient, without any subsequent benefit.

Considering, now, the history of the patient—the long succession of boils and carbuncles, the four aborting carbuncles, each followed by a marked deterioration of health, and each leaving a painful induration which might be supposed to be a portion of dead cellular membrane retained in contact with the living tissues, and that the present abscess had followed immediately upon the last of this series of abortive carbuncles, very much as a secondary abscess follows the absorption of pus in pyæmia—I resolved to trust the case to the action of Lachesis. At the same time, I informed the patient that, in my judgment, after the healing of the abscess, the indurated remnants of the four aborted carbuncles would inflame again and be discharged, and that this process must precede the re-establishment of his health.

I gave a dose of Lachesis^{200} every morning, noon and night. The progress of the case was tedious, but uniform and prosperous. In twelve days the hectic had ceased, the appetite was restored, and the formation of pus had decidedly diminished. In six weeks the abscess had healed. In seven weeks the patient walked on crutches. But now, when he seemed almost well, fever came on again and he was prostrated. After twenty-four hours of fever, the indurated remnant of the last carbuncle became inflamed, an abscess formed and a slough was discharged. The same thing occurred in the locality of the three remaining indurations, and, singularly enough, in the inverse order of their original appearance. After the last of these abscesses had healed, the patient rapidly gained health and strength, and has since been perfectly well. In this case no remedy was given save Lachesis[200] When the treatment was begun, the patient was in a most deplorable condition, and his recovery was hardly hoped for by his attendants. Improvement began as soon as he began to take Lachesis, and continued, with scarcely an interruption, until he was completely restored.

Now, let us suppose that to a man in perfect health there be administered daily a dose of a drug, which, a person familiar for some years with its properties predicts, will cause the man to exhibit a definite series of symptoms and finally to die. As soon as the administration of the drug is begun, the man begins to exhibit the predicted symptoms, and finally, as was foretold, he dies. What jury, with these facts before it, would hesitate to say that the man was deliberately poisoned, and to convict the one who gave the drug of murder? Now, shall not such evidence as would convince a jury of citizens that a man has been poisoned by a drug, convince a body of physicians that a patient has been cured by Lachesis? Shall not testimony that would hang a malefactor convert a skeptic?

The diseases which I have cited as those in which Lachesis has been of unquestionable service in my hands, present, in name at least, a considerable variety. Pyæmia, repercussed measles, malignant pustule, diphtheria, phlebitis, carbuncle, have not necessarily a great deal in common. A close examination, however, of the cases as I have described them, will show, notwithstanding the diversity in name, a considerable approach to identity in morbid condition. In all there was great prostration, as manifested by loss of muscular power, slowness and softness of pulse, stupid delirium, etc. In this respect the cases resembled those in which Arsenicum is indicated and has so often proved curative. These cases, however, did not present that vascular and nervous erethism conjoined with prostration, which is so characteristic of Arsenicum. Nor, on the other hand, was the asthenia so complete as to call for Carbo vegetabilis. Lachesis may perhaps be held, in so far as the symptoms of asthenia are concerned, to occupy an intermediate position between Arsenicum and Carbo vegetabilis. This statement would at once suggest its usefulness in typhoid fevers; and those who have made themselves familiar with Lachesis have learned from clinical experience to place great dependence upon it in treating certain forms of these diseases.

LYCOPODIUM CLAVATUM.

SENSORIUM. Vertigo, occurring particularly in the forenoon, and in a hot room; accompanied by nausea; it seems as though everything were turning around.

The perceptive faculties are singularly affected. One cannot read, because the meaning of certain letters is not clear; errs in speaking, because he cannot get the right words; this when talking about every-day matters; whereas when the subject is very important, so as to call forth the most energy, the words are correctly chosen. Analogous to the state of mind in certain typhoid conditions.

Generally it is difficult to collect and hold the thoughts.

Head. Confused; heaviness.

Headache; often semi-lateral. A shattered or concussed sensation at every step. China; Rhus.

Often a semi-lateral headache, especially at evening much aggravated by reading or writing.

Pain over and between the eyes, early in the morning.

There are also pressing and throbbing pains in various parts of the head. The most frequent is an aching pressure in the occiput, or ever the eyes.

The head easily becomes cold, which results in a cutting soreness of the scalp. The hair becomes gray, and falls out. Consider, in this relation, the eruptions of Lycopodium.

Complexion. Pale, sallow; sunken eyes and blue rings around them.

Eyes. Dazed by light, and painful as if bruised.

They present many symptoms of inflammation, as redness and swelling of the eyelids, with aching pains, ulceration and nocturnal agglutination; itching in the canthi and much lachrymation.

In the eyes themselves, redness, aching and burning and stitching pains.

Vision is affected; in artificial light all objects tremble; a constant flickering, or black spots before the eyes; vision obscured; letters run together or are indistinct; one must vary the distance of the book from the eye.

Ears. Tearing or stitching pains in the meatus, with the sensation that it is too narrow. The open air provokes a kind of earache.

Itching in the ear, and discharge from the meatus.

Roaring, buzzing, etc., in the ears.

Deafness: sometimes over-sensibility to noise, while walking.

Nose. Externally, pressure and aching. Internally, soreness.

Frequent epistaxis.

Sense of smell keen; sometimes perverted.

Mouth. Gums swollen, hot and tender. Jumping toothache, relieved by warm drinks. (Relieved by cold water indicates Coffea. Hahnemann.) Sometimes the toothache comes on from the slightest touch to the teeth or from the shock of coughing. Sometimes only at night, and causing great nervousness.

Tongue. Sore; ulcers under it, paining when speaking and eating. Dryness in the mouth and throat, with and without thirst.

Throat. Diseases of the throat that begin on the right side and go to the left. (Lippe.) Lachesis has the reverse. Tearing and aching in the throat. The uvula is swollen. The glands are swollen, and are the seat of stitching pains.

Digestive Apparatus. The mouth is dry; bitter taste, in the morning or all day; but food had its natural flavor. Sometimes a sweet or even a sour taste.

Heart-burn, A burning sensation comes up from stomach to throat, with a sour taste in the mouth; sometimes so violent as to take away the breath. Or a kind of incomplete burning eruption which comes as far as the pharynx and leaves a burning in the throat.

Empty, sour eructations, especially after each meal; with gulping up of digested food.

Water gathers in the mouth, with nausea.

These are the symptoms of slow and enfeebled digestion.

LYCOPODIUM CLAVATUM.

Every morning, on rising, nausea, and water-brash, with oppression of the chest, heat in the abdomen, and cold face.

Appetite fails. No thirst. (Constant sense of satiety.)

After eating, oppression of the stomach and bitter taste. The abdomen is in a ferment. Also, after eating only a very small quantity, a sudden feeling of satiety and even of fullness in the epigastrium, with flatulent rumbling in the bowels. This is characteristic of Lycopodium. Sepia alone has the same symptom. Acidity and heart-burn with constant sleepiness after dinner.

Stomach and other digestive organs. After eating and after slight cold, violent stomach pains with chilliness, the fingers becoming waxy white, as if dead. The gastralgia is like a constriction, or a gnawing, and the patient cannot bear anything tight around the epigastrium.

In the liver region, frequent pains and tenderness to pressure.

The chief sensation under Lycopodium is aching pressure, and we find this produced in stomach, epigastrium and liver, with pain on pressure and deep respiration.

I have found in a case of chronic duodenitis, relieved by Lycopodium, always present this symptom: pressure on the hypochondrium produced tender pains in the epigastrium, and *vice versa*.

Especially often the aching pressure in the

region of the liver, like a dull and tensive aching and pressure, on respiration, on bending the body, or on pressure with the hand. Sometimes this extends to the left side of the abdomen, and sometimes down to the hip.

In the abdomen, squeezing pressure, so severe one cannot walk erect, but must go bent over or lie down; it produces dyspnœa.

Tensive, tearing and cutting pains.

The great characteristic of Lycopodium is the production of flatus in the intestines.

The abdomen is distended thereby; flatus becomes incarcerated in the abdomen, producing pain, finally relieved by eructations. Tension and rumbling in various parts of the abdomen. It appears that most of the abdominal pains of Lycopodium are due to flatus.

Pains in the region of the abdominal ring, outward pressing; and the old hernia protrudes. Swelling of the inguinal glands, which pain as though suppurating.

About the anus, itching and a moist, tender eruption. Aching and pressure in the rectum, especially at night. Stitching and burning at stool, even when the fæces are not hard. Hæmorrhoids swell and protrude and bleed, even when there is no constipation.

Inclination to stool, but at stool a spasmodic pain or constriction of the anus, which makes the evacuation difficult. It is scanty, infrequent and difficult. After stool, much rumbling in the bowels and either flatulent distention of the abdomen or uterine cramps, or great lassitude.

Urinary Organs. Secretion diminished. Urine dark, with a yellow or reddish deposit. "Red sand in the urine. Terrific pain in the back before every urination, relieved by urinating." (G.)

Smarting and burning, when passing water, in the female urethra; and stitches or drawing or cutting pains through the urethra and toward the abdomen. Painless discharge of blood through the urethra.

Sexual desire and power diminished markedly in males.

The menses anticipate a little and are too profuse; preceded by flatulent distention of the abdomen; great heaviness of the legs; chill and heat at night; ill humor and disposition to weep.

During the menses, acid taste, headache, severe backache; swelling of the feet, nausea and a kind of faintness.

Leucorrhœa in spells; of a blood-red color; "with cutting pains going across the body from right to left." (G).

Respiratory Organs. Fan-like motion of the alæ nasi (Dr. D. Wilson's indication in severe pneumonia). Catarrhal conditions. Frequent sneezing. Coryza, both dry and fluent. When dry, oppressing respiration, with burning headache. When fluent, with swelling of the nose and copious acrid and offensive discharge.

The cough is provoked by a tickling irritation in the larynx, as if from vapor of sulphur. Sometimes dry; and, when so, very fatiguing, producing pain in the head, stomach and abdomen; sometimes loose, the sputa being a thick gray, grayish yellow, or yellow, or mixed with blood and having a saltish taste. These and other symptoms have led to the successful use of Lycopodium in consumption, etc.

In the chest, a sensation as if the lungs were full of mucus, with a whistling sound in the trachea on inspiration; a fullness and appression in the open air and after eating.

Aching, with or without soreness, producing some dyspnœa and much mental depression. Tearing and tension under the clavicles, and stitch on deep inspiration.

Externally, stitches and burning pains in the nipples and discharge from them of blood and water; hence Lycopodium in sore nipples, etc.

Back. Backache so severe that it makes it impossible to sit, and the pain even extends, as a constrictive sensation, to the chest.

Tearing in the sacrum, kidneys and back, especially near the spine. Drawing and aching between the scapulæ.

The aching in the kidneys is increased before, and diminished after, urinating.

In the extremities we find tearing and aching pains; and more frequently during repose than motion. Pains, tearing, etc., from the neck to the shoulder and elbow, especially at night and during repose; also in the whole arm to the wrist; in the hand and fingers while they are in bed, but ceasing when they are taken out of bed. Tearing and aching in the joints and ends of the fingers, with burning and sometimes itching of the palm. Consider these symptoms in connection with the red deposit in the urine. (Rheumatic gout?)

In the lower extremities the same pains about the hips, in the nates; down the thigh and legs; under the heel and in the toes.

A paralytic weakness is often left in the arms; as though they would fall by the side; yet they are strong enough in work.

The same sensation in the limbs.

The limbs go to sleep easily.

Every four days a pain in the leg from the hip to the foot, causing limping. (Verified.)

Intertrigo. The finger joints are red, inflamed, swollen; and burn and pain.

Swelling of the feet and limbs. (Dropsical.)

Feet cold, with cold sweat, which makes them sore.

Sleep. Fruitless efforts to yawn (like chloroform). Great day sleepiness, but late sleeping at night. Restless; wakes often with vivacious, troublesome dreams. Starting on falling asleep. Tired on waking in the morning.

Fever. Chill predominates; comes more in the evening; not much heat, nor sweat; generally every second day, often affecting only one side of the body.

Sometimes the sweat follows the chill without intervening heat; or the chill and heat are mixed up.

Sweat mostly on the chest and trunk; at night or early in the morning.

Lippe says: "Night sweats cold, clammy, sour, fetid, bloody, smelling like onions."

Disposition. Great anxiety; timidity; fears to be alone.

Also indifference to external influences. Depression; sadness; inclined to weep. "Great fear of being left alone."

Weakness: bodily; mental; moral.

Skin. Red, itching and burning, or painless spots of eruption.

Eczematous, suppurating eruption on the head, with swollen cervical glands.

Dark red spots and blotches on the face, suppurating. Fine eruption about the mouth and on the chin. Warts on the fingers and hands. Intertrigo; especially between the thighs and on the scrotum; also, under the arms.

Compare Carbo animalis and Calcarea sulphuris.

Stiffness in the limbs and joints, and great weakness.

Generalities. The pains are aching,—pressive, drawing and burning.

Restlessness, and excited circulation in the evening, producing a feeling of trembling.

Ulcers that are present bleed when bandaged, and have a stitching pain.

The symptoms are worse from four to eight P. M., and recur regularly; as do those of Sabadilla.

Lycopodium affects the mucous membranes of the respiratory, digestive, and genito-urinary organs; makes digestive processes slow; hence wind, water and acidity.

Produces lithic acid deposit in quantities; hence pains in the kidneys and bladder, etc; and hence indirectly the pains in the limbs and joints. Produces catarrhal condition, and muco-purulent sputa.

Nervous action weakened; a great remedy for overworked brains and where brain trouble, for *e. g.*, softening, threatens from overwork or from metastasis of ulcers suddenly healed; see the torpor; the use of wrong words; failure to collect and command the thoughts, etc.

NATRUM MURIATICUM.

THIS remedy cannot often, in chronic cases, be repeated without an intercurrent.

Head. Vertigo; when walking, everything goes round in a circle; when sitting quietly with a downward pressure of the head; when rising from the bed.

Sensorium. Absence of mind; incapacity; confusion of ideas; does not know what to say; slow in coming to a resolution; indecision.

Memory much weakened; forgets what he would write; cannot remember what happened yesterday.

Head. Confusion, as after much mental exertion.

Headache produced by quick movements of the head, sudden turning, etc.

Heavy aching (pressure) in the forehead, with pressure outward in the eyes. Pressure inward on both temples, as if the head were in a vise; or a fullness, as though the head would brust, increased by reading or writing; often accompanied by nausea; worse in the afternoon.

But such a headache succeeds the chill of febrile

paroxysm, and then comes in the morning. Throbbing also during the fever.

The scalp is cold, and chills run over it.

Itching. The hair falls out when touched or combed (common in nursing women, and Natrum muriaticum stops this).

Complexion. Sallow, earthy, yellow, with pain in the abdomen (torpid chlorosis).

Eruptions. Miliary eruption on the forehead, perceptible to the touch only. Papules on the cheeks and chin.

Aching around the eyes, in the malar bones and zygomatic arch. The eyelids quiver and twitch, are ulcerated and red, with soreness and agglutination. Hordeola are frequent.

The eyes itch, especially in the inner canthus; or ache. Conjunctiva reddened, and burns on slight exposure to the wind, with acrid lachrymation.

Vision obscured, as if the eyes were covered with mucus or a thin veil. Half vision; one side of the object is distinct, the other side looks dark (Lithium). Also, accommodation is modified, myopic or presbyopic. Fiery points before the eyes. Aggravation from using the eyes in reading, etc.

Ears. Heat of the external ear; swelling of the meatus and discharge of matter; much itching, both internally and externally. Drawing and stitching pains from the ear down the neck to the shoulder; or from the teeth up to the ear. Noises in the ear; rushing and ringing. Deafness.

Nose. White papules at the root of the nose. Alæ nasi inflamed, with redness, heat and swelling, and great soreness. One-half of the nose becomes insensible and as if dead. Epistaxis from stooping, but especially on coughing and at night, with soreness in all the limbs.

Lips. Swelling, with vesicles; also vesicles on the tongue, which burn and smart and, finally, have a scab on them. The lips crack. Pain in the submaxillary glands, as if swollen or compressed; and on coughing.

Gums. They bleed easily, are sensitive to cold and warmth, and to pressure with tongue.

Teeth. Very sensitive; toothache on drawing the air against the teeth, and on pressure of the tongue and of food. They become loose.

Drawing pain from the teeth, extending to the ear; extending throughout all the teeth. The pain extends into the malar bones.

Tongue. Heavy and clumsy, as if paralyzed. Can only speak with much effort. One-half of the tongue seems numb and stiff.

Burning and sore vesicles on the tongue; also on the gums; very sensitive to contact of food.

In the throat, some stitching sensation behind the tonsil, and a sense of constriction.

Digestion. Sense of taste blunted or annihilated; sticky or bitter taste; water-brash. Nausea frequent, especially early in the morning, with prostration after eating or drinking even agreeable things; first food, then bile.

NATRUM MURIATICUM.

Abdomen. Stitches in the right hypochondrium and stomach; also in the left hypochondrium on deep inspiration and on bending to the left side, which also produces a sence of stiffness in the liver. Tension in both hypochondria.

Pinching in the hypochondria. Cannot lie on the sound side; also in the umbilical region and thence into the sacral region, and into the rectum and anus. Distention of the abdomen, and much flatus. Herniæ protrude.

Stool. Insufficient; frequent, ineffectual efforts; great exertion is necessary to evacuation; often blood follows.

Tenesmus in the rectum with discharge of flatus and slime. The rectum seems constricted, and it is only after great effort that some little hard fæces pass, which tear the anus so that it bleeds and smarts; and then comes some dirty water. Stool preceded by pressure in the region of the bladder; soreness in the abdomen, accompanied by labor-like pains in the abdomen; pressing-down pain, followed by tenesmus; vain efforts, and sensation as though diarrhœa would ensue; burning and smarting soreness in the anus.

Beside this, stitches in the rectum and anus; violent pains in the bladder and anus; prolapsus ani, with bloody mucus and water; and burning, preventing sleep at night.

Urinary Organs. Urination almost involuntary after violent tenesmus. Pressure on the bladder, and stitching pain. Cutting and burning after urination; and discharge of thin mucus, leaving translucent spots on the linen. Urine clear; deposits of urates, white or red, or red sand.

Sexual Organs. Male. Frequent pollution, followed by cold exterior and lassitude. Sexual desire increased. Gonorrhœa.

Female. Menses retarded and less in quantity, or delayed and weak two or three days, and then a copious flow. Preceded by anxiety and disposition to faint, or nausea, with sweet taste and bloody sputa; accompanied by constipation, or tearing toothache; followed by dull headache. Leucorrhœa copious, with bearing down as if the menses were coming.

Respiratory Organs. Dry catarrh of the larynx and trachea. Voice hoarse.

Sneezing. Coryza, although dry and somewhat loose, impedes respiration very much.

Cough, provoked by tickling in the epigastrium, day and night; increased at night or early in the morning. Generally dry, with wheezing and vomiting and headache and soreness in the larynx and trachea. Vague pains in the thorax. The heart's action is affected. Palpitation, forcible and anxious, with aching as if a pressure came from the abdomen and compressed the heart; increased by lying on the left side and on every motion; palpitation and fluttering.

Back. In the sacro-lumbar region, pulsation and stitches; a paralytic soreness, increased in the morning on rising; cannot stand erect nor walk;

diminished when lying down. Soreness in the loins, as if beaten; also in the back and between the scapulæ. In the back, tension and stiffness. Tearing. Burning in the scapulæ, as from hot water.

In the extremities, a marked feeling of lassitude and weakness; cannot raise the arms or lift anything; can hardly move them.

The same in the lower extremities.

Sleep. By day sleepiness. Sleeplessness at night; restlessness. Dyspnœa.

Fever. A full and powerful paroxysm complete, occurring early in the morning; a severe chill, then frontal headache, red face and high fever; sweat in the evening.

Professor Guernsey says:

"Thirst for large quantities of water before the chill; this thirst continues through the paroxysm. Violent chill with headache, and after the chill the headache increases greatly; feels as if the brain were being beaten with thousands of little hammers. After the fever, sweat, and the patient wishes to lie a long time. If the disease lasts long, the corners of the mouth become sore, and finally the lips."

Disposition. Impatient and hasty. Easily angered. Then melancholy; sadness; anxiety.

VERATRUM ALBUM.

WHITE HELLEBORE.

THE root of the plant is used in medicine. It may be prepared by trituration, or used in the form of a tincture.

It was known to the ancients, and was used by them to cure insanity and various spasmodic affections; and it is recorded of Hippocrates that he cured with it a case much resembling Asiatic cholera, as follows:

"A young Athenian, affected with cholera, evacuated upward and downward with much suffering; nothing could arrest the vomiting or alvine evacuations. His voice failed; he could not stir from bed; his eyes were lustreless and sunken; he had convulsions of the lower extremities from the abdomen downward; he had hiccough, and the alvine dejections were more copious than the vomitings. He took Veratrum in lentil-juice and recovered." This was a most excellent homœopathic prescription.

The action of Veratrum on the vital force is but moderate in so far as the sensorium and the nerves of animal life are concerned, but in so far as the system of nutrition is concerned it is most profound. The entire system of vegetation is affected in such a way, and to such a degree, that it seems as though the body were in a great measure withdrawn from the control of the vital forces, and given over to the action of mechanical and chemical laws.

The blood tends to separate into its proximate constituents, as it would do if suddenly withdrawn from the body; the liquid constituents seem to filtrate in a half-mechanical manner through the tissues, and thus we have a copious cold, clammy sweat; copious serous vomitings and diarrhœas; evacuations that are astounding from their quantity and from the mechanical manner of their ejection; the stomach seeming to become completely filled, and to be emptied by a sudden convulsive effort provoked by its complete distention.

This, then, is the key to the pathological character of the Veratrum disease—torpor of the vegetative system, with comparatively slight affection of the system of animal life.

As might be inferred from the above, the fever of Veratrum is characterized by predominant and sometimes exclusive coldness. The sweat is cold and clammy, and it is notably characteristic that almost every important symptom of Veratrum, wherever produced, is accompanied by cold sweat of the forehead.

As a matter of course, among the symptoms of Veratrum great weakness occurs. It is to be observed, however, as distinguishing Veratrum from Arsenic, that this weakness is not disproportioned to the other symptoms, is not unexpectedly great, and is not more than might be expected from the symptoms of diarrhœa, vomiting, or general disturbance which mark the case. Neither are the symptoms attended by the restlessness, anguish and intolerance of pain which are so characteristic of Arsenic; nor indeed do the symptoms involve a great amount of pain. That which is felt is philosophically endured. The patient is quite.

It must not be inferred from what has been said that Veratrum exerts no action whatever upon the sensorium. On the contrary, it produces a kind of mania; and Hahnemann affirms that it is a most precious and indispensable remedy in the treatment of various forms of mania and insanity. Moreover, he found it an indication for Veratrum if various kinds of pain were accompanied, now and then, by a kind of temporary or transient delirium or mania.

The affection of the mind and disposition is as follows: A kind of busy restlessness, a hurried and driven feeling that induces one to undertake a great variety of labor, which, however, he has no heart to finish. Still more common, however, is a gentle melancholy, a disposition to weep, and an inconsolable grief over an imaginary mishap, which cause the patient to sit weeping and not to be comforted, or else to run crying and howling about the apartment. This condition ends in a

VERATRUM ALBUM. 275

raving mania, with cursing and scolding, endeavors to escape, biting and tearing everything and everybody that offer opposition; accompanied by foolish imaginings.

Veratrum produces vertigo.

The headache is a pressure upon the vertex, generally attended by pain in the stomach. It is noteworthy that this pressing pain of the vertex is relieved by pressing on the vertex with the hand. I know but one other remedy of which the pressing headache in the vertex is thus relieved, viz.: Menyanthes trifoliata. The headache of Menyanthes is accompanied by icy coldness of the hands and feet.

The pupils contract. The sight becomes weak. Double vision is observed; and black spots and sparks appear before the eyes.

The eyelids are dry; the upper lid seems paralyzed, the patient cannot raise it; ptosis occurs, and has been cured by Veratrum (like Sepia).

The face is cold, the features are distorted, the complexion is cyanotic. The face is covered, particularly the forehead, with a cold, clammy sweat, during the symptoms of the stomach, bowels and chest.

The digestive organs are eminently affected by Veratrum.

We notice first an aversion to warm drinks, and a longing for fruit and for acids. The taste is diminished, or there is a feeling of coolness in the mouth, such as peppermint produces.

Nausea occurs, often with a taste of bile in the mouth; sometimes it is felt after breakfast and ceases after taking dinner.

The matters vomited are food or green bile, and tenacious mucus; the vomiting is preceded by a general shudder, and the nausea continues during the intervals between the Vomitings. The vomiting prostrates the patient, but not more than the quantity and violence would lead one to expect.

Pressure in the epigastrium, extending to the sternal and hypochondriac regions, and down to the os ileum. Pinching, tensive, cutting pains, as if the intestines were cut with knives, and with this pain diarrhœa is associated.

In the inguinal regions, frequently, a sensation as though a hernia would protrude; and when coughing, a sticking pain along the inguinal canal. These symptoms have caused a successful use of Veratrum in hernia.

As regards stool, we find two different conditions:

1. Constipation, characterized by a disposition to stool in the upper part of the intestinal canal, but an indisposition, sluggishness or apparent inactivity of the rectum and lower intestine. It is a most useful remedy in obstinate constipation when Nux vomica has failed to relieve, and especially in the constipation of infants.

2. Diarrhœa, watery, light-colored. Sometimes colorless, very copious.

It is characteristic of the vomiting and diar-

VERATRUM ALBUM. 277

rhœa of Veratrum, but particularly of the vomiting, that they are provoked by taking liquid into the stomach, which is no sooner taken than rejected. This is equally true of cold and warm drinks. Phosphorus, on the other hand, has nausea, relieved by cold drinks : which, however, are vomited as soon as they become warm in the stomach. The gastric symptoms of Veratrum are aggravated by motion.

The vomiting of Tabacum is relieved by eating or drinking.

The vomiting and diarrhœa of Veratrum being sudden and copious, are accompanied by exhaustion, cold sweat, a pinched, shriveled and livid aspect of the face and hands, and loss of voice; but by no great mental or sensorial disturbance, no great depression of spirits or anxiety.

The menses are hastened and increased.

Veratrum produces a catarrhal condition of the nasal membrane, with incessant sneezing and a tickling in the trachea, which extends thence through the bronchi to their extremities. The cough is generally dry, and if so, it is induced by the least motion of the body, or by going from a cold into a warm atmosphere. The opposite of Rumex crispus.

Sometimes the cough is loose and it is then accompanied by constriction of the chest.

Sometimes the slightest bodily exertion produces dyspnœa and palpitation.

Pains, stiffness and lassitude in the trunk and back.

In the extremities, lassitude; and in the lower extremities a kind of paralysis, as from too long a walk. Besides this, tonic cramps in the calves and thighs.

PRACTICAL APPLICATIONS.

It is useful in intermittent fever, when coldness predominates. The symptoms which call for it are, especially, great weakness and prostration; actual sinking of the forces; very slow pulse, and the impulse of the heart very weak, during the apyrexia as well as during the paroxysm, but especially during the latter; cramps in the limbs, and especially in the stomach and abdomen; paralytic sensations; syncope; watery diarrhœa, or obstinate constipation depending on inactivity of the rectum; collapse ; cyanosis.

The cold stage always predominates, and indeed often overshadows and extinguishes the hot stage. The changes of temperature are most marked in the extremities.

The hot stage often fails entirely, and it never reaches a high grade; generally it consists rather in a subjective sensation of warmth while the objective temperature is hardly elevated, nay, is sometimes diminished. The pulse is but slightly accelerated; it becomes somewhat more frequent, but not fuller nor harder.

The thirst is proportioned to the amount of the excretions.

The sweat is cold and clammy. It comes even before the paroxysm ; lasts untill the next. The results of the abuse of Quinine often require Veratrum.

The same general characteristics indicate Veratrum in typhoid and typhus fevers.

The use of Veratrum in cholera, in diarrhœa, in hernia, in constipation, and in bronchitis, has been alluded to and the indication have been noticed.

HEPAR SULPHURIS CALCAREUM.

LIVER OF SULPHUR.   IMPURE CALCIC SULPHIDE.

THE "liver of sulphur" of the shops and of the British and United States pharmacopœias, is a sulphuret of potassium, or a potassic sulphide, being prepared with potash and not with lime. It should never be used to prepare the drug known in the homœpathic pharmacopœia as Hepar sulphuris. It was discovered, in the course of experiments, that it produces solubility of sulphur. It is prepared by fusion; sulphur one part and carbonate of potash four parts. It is used to resolve exudations, as in swollen glands, etc.; it is also used in obstinate skin diseases, and in the preparation of sulphur baths. (Balneum sulphuratum of Raye.) Care must be taken if an acid is added, because then sulphuretted hydrogen is evolved, and there is danger of asphyxia.

Dupuytren added glue to the bath, and made the Balneum sulphuratum et gelatinosum.

Hahnemann prepared Hepar sulphuris as follows:

"Equal weights of the interior of the oyster-shell and pure sulphur flowers which have been well

HEPAR SULPHURIS CALCAREUM. 281

washed and dried; mix well, and place in a well-heated porcelain crucible; cover and keep at a white heat for ten minutes. When cold, open the crucible and preserve in well-stoppered bottles."

It is prepared for use by trituration up to the third centesimal or higher.

Some physicians use the third only of Hepar sulphuris who use higher potencies of other drugs.

SPECIAL ANALYSIS.

Sensorium. Vertigo when shaking the head or from jarring, as, for example, from driving in a wagon, so that on getting out one cannot stand alone. Sometimes faintness accompanies it.

Head. The pains are aching, boring, and soreness as if beaten.

As regards locality, the pain is in the temples, forehead and sides of the head, and is sometimes confind to one side of the head,—a kind of megrim.

As regards the time of day, the early morning and the forenoon are the favorite times of headache.

As regards conditions, motion and rising from a stooping posture produce or increase the pains; also moving the eyes increases the boring pain at the root of the nose.

To recapitulate, we find :

Aching pain in the temples and in one-half of

the head, a sensation as if a nail were driven into the brain; the clavus hystericus. (Ignatia, Thuja.)

Then, on rising from stoping or on moving, and especially after walking in the open air, a stitching pain; likewise on coughing.

Boring pains in the temples and a boring aching at the root of the nose, worse from moving the eyes. The forehead and scalp are sore and tender. (Bryonia, Eupatorium, China.)

The hair falls out in spots, leaving them bald. Papules and pustules form on the scalp and nape and are sore to the touch. Also on the forehead; worse in warmth; better in cold air.

Eyes. Eyes and lids inflamed. Lids swollen, red and aching, worse on being touched. Nocturnal agglutination; much muco-pus; obscured vision. Eruption on the eyelids and below them on the cheek.

It is a valuable remedy in strumous opthalmia and ulcer of the cornea, occurring with milk crust, etc., etc.

Complexion. Yellowish, with blue rings around the eyes. Red cheeks by day, without heat or thirst; but in the afternoon and night, heat. Sometimes erysipelatous swelling and redness of the cheeks.

Ears. External: hot, red and itching. Stitching in the inner ear on blowing the nose.

Roaring and noises, worse P. M.

Nose. Boring aching at the root of the nose from seven to twelve A. M. Dorsum sore to the touch. Frequent epistaxis. Loss of smell.

Mouth. Corner of the lips ulcerated and eruption on the lips, with heat; also vesicles, etc., on the chin and neck, very sore to the touch.

Gums. Swollen, and aching of the molar teeth as if pressed out; painful on biting. Toothache occurs when eating; drawing pain, worse in a warm room; and on biting it becomes a jumping toothache.

Throat. Very important symptoms. Stitching, as if a sliver of wood or a fish-bone were in the throat, occurring on swallowing, yawning, on taking a deep inspiration, and on turning the head, extending into the ear. Even also in the exterior parts of the throat, as in the cervical muscles. Feeling of internal swelling and pressure, as if a plug of mucus or some other body had stuck in the throat and could be swallowed away. Scratching, scraped feeling in the throat, increased when swallowing solid food. Constant desire to hawk out mucus, and much saliva from the mouth, like water-brash.

Digestive tract. Bitter or earthy taste in the mouth and throat, yet food has its natural taste.

Appetite fair. Longing for sour or strongly flavored food. More thirst than hunger. Burning eructations. Nausea when sitting or walking, A. M. Sour vomiting. Pressure, aching and hardness in the epigastrium after eating.

Distention of the abdomen and much flatus, which accumulates in the epigastric zone. Tearing and grasping in the umbilical region, with nausea and heat of the face. Soreness of the abdomen where flatus moves.

The inguinal glands are swollen and sore, and ulcerate.

Stool. The character of the stool and urine is sluggish evacuation. Then, though the fæces are soft, they are discharged with difficulty and slowly and with much tenesmus.

Sometimes diarrhœa and bloody slime, or greenish and clay-colored diarrhœa.

Green, slimy diarrhœa, of a sour smell. (See Hering.)

Urine. Sluggish stream; must wait long before it starts. It burns on passing, and excoriates and ulcerates the prepuce; the last drops are bloody.

Itching and sticking pains in the glans; ulcers like chancre on the prepuce.

Respiratory Organs. Coryza. Action chiefly on the larynx and trachea.

Dry cough, with dyspnœa, from tickling high in the throat; uninterrupted in the evening; provoked by speaking or stooping; it increases more and more, and then stops. Or, a violent cough, as if he should suffocate, which ends in vomiting. Sometimes, afterward, a feeling as of a hard body in the epigastrium; then comes a hæmoptysis.

(Distinguished from Belladonna by non-soreness of the larynx and no fever; from Conium by the height of the irritation; from Rumex crispus by not being affected by respiration; from Lachesis by not being excited by pressure on the trachea.)

In croup, when the cough begins to loosen, pustular eruption on the outer thorax; the axillary glands suppurate.

Cutting, drawing and aching in the lumbo-sacral region, especially in the sacro-iliac synchondroses, causing a halting gait and limping; it extends down the limb, and is not relieved by sitting, standing or lying.

Stitches in the back, and tight pain on turning. Tearing, drawing and burning pains in the extremities. Eruptions, etc.

Sleep. Disturbed by starting, by dreams, and by dyspnœa.

The pains are worse at night.

Chill at night, not followed by heat; chill in the open air (which aggravates the cough, etc.).

Sweat. Worse at night, and on the head or the back; it is clammy or sour. In the morning, when it occurs, it is sometimes general, sometimes only on the head.

Disposition. Very peevish; angry at the least trifle. Memory weak; hypochondriacal; unreasonably anxious.

General. Stitches in the joints during repose and motion. Drawing and tearing in the limbs. The hands and feet crack and ulcerate; the ulcers bleed easily, and burn and throb at night, with stitching and gnawing pain. Warts inflame and stitch. Burning, itching over the body, followed by nettle-rash. Lassitude, weakness; fainting on slight pain.

HEPAR SULPHURIS CALCAREUM.

APPLICATIONS.

Suppuration, milk crust, eczema. Ulcers, warts. Glands inflamed (high or low?). Dysentery catarrh of bladder. Prostatitis (Digitalis, Nitrum.) Croup, Bœnninghausen, 3*. Laryngeal cough, increased by slight uncovering of a limb.

---

* Bœnninghausen's powders for croup; First, Aconite[200], second, Hepar sulphuris[200], third Spongia[200]. [H. E. K. D.]

DULCAMARA.

GENERAL ANALYSIS.

VITAL POWER. *a.* Sensorium. Depressing; signs of anæmia vertigo on rising, with debility and general trembling.

b. Special senses. A partial action only; vision failing as from paralysis of the optic nerve.

c. Muscular system. Acts in such a way as to produce paralysis, or a paralyzed sensation in the tongue and in the back and extremities. These phenomena, however, succeed, except in case of the tongue and the eyelid paroxysms of sticking and tearing pains, which are indicative of a rheumatic affection of the muscles. Hence the tendency to a rheumatic diathesis may be assumed to be the leading affection of the muscular system as a result of Dulcamara. At the same time there are no indications of a rheumatic dyscrasia, except offensive sweat and urine. These affections correspond rather to the effects of simple exposure to cold and wet.

Action *upon the organic substance.* The most marked effect is shown by the action of Dulcamara upon the mucous membrane, especially of the alimentary canal and of the urinary bladder producing more or less copious discharges of mucus, altered from a normal condition, but not displaying any evidence at decomposition; and upon the lymphatic system, producing glandular enlargements (their specific nature unknown) both in the cervical and submaxillary, and in the inguinal regions. Clinical records which are rich in cases of glandular enlargements cured by Dulcamara, teach that the conditions most easily cured by Dulcamara are hæmorrhages from the nose, which occur without evidence of decomposition of the blood. A specific dyscrasia, however, is produced, as is shown by the eruptions and by the offensive sweat which allies it to rheumatic affections.

General affections. As might be inferred from the affections of the lymphatic and mucous systems, a disposition to anasarca is shown by the symptoms of Dulcamara, *e.g.*, general swelling of the limbs and puffiness of the face.

Vegetative system. Dulcamara works such an alteration as to produce copious, soapy saliva, with loose and spongy gums. Flat, soapy taste, with loss of appetite, discharge of stringy, tenacious mucus from the stomach, and yellow and green mucous diarrhœa, with griping and cutting in the abdomen before the stool. Burning in the bladder and deposit of mucus in the urine evacuated. (Vesical catarrh.)

Sphere of action. The sphere of Dulcamara is not very extensive. Its action is apparently confined to the muscular, mucous and fibrous or serofibrous tissues; and of these tissues the parts most affected are, in the muscular tissue, the voluntary muscles, especially those of the face and extremities and of the thorax; in the mucous tissue, that of the alimentary canal and urinary bladder, the air passages being scarcely affected. The cough is rather excited by stitches in the intercostal muscles and in the fibrous tissue, the substance of the meatus auditorius possibly the pericranium and the tissues about the articulations of the extremities. In addition to these tissues, the lymphatic glandular system and the special sense of vision are especial seats of the action of Dulcamara.

Sensations. For the most part, drawing and sticking pain in the substance of the tissues. The sticking, however, is not so sharp as that of Bryonia, but is as if done with a blunt instrument, and is circumscribed in location. In addition there is pain as after a blow.

Peculiarities and conditions of the pains. The pains are universally aggravated by repose; except the headache in the temporal region, which is a boring and sticking from within outward, aggravated by motion, and is probably due to a congestive condition which accompanies the Dulcamara catarrh. They are relieved or dissipated by motion and recur when the subject comes again into a state of rest. They occur or are aggravated at night, and in damp, cold weather. When the sticking pains occur in the substance of organs, their direction is universally from within outward; analogous in this to Belladonna.

Times of day. Aggravation in the evening, especially of the cutaneous symptoms.

Head. Sensorium. Vertigo. Momentary dizziness; objects appear to stand motionless; black spots float before the eyes; this occurs at noon before eating, also in the morning on rising, and is then attended by debility and general trembling, with flashes of heat in the face.

Confusion. Dull and confused feeling in the head. as if after a debauch.

Headache. The headache seems to depend in a great degree upon catarrhal or rheumatic affections of other organs. It seldom involves the whole head at once, but only a small spot is affected at a time, either by stickings or as by the pressure of a dull instrument.

The parts of the head most affected are the forehead and the occiput and nape of the neck. The temporal region, sometimes, in connection with the forehead. The pains are chiefly dull heaviness and pressing, and a pressure and a boring from within outward, and stitches and drawing pains from one part of the head to another.

To particularize :

Conditions. We have, in the forehead, heaviness, with occasional stickings, digging and boring in the substance of the brain from within outward, with a feeling as if a board were placed in front of the forehead pressing the pain back. From the left frontal eminence to the point of the nose drawing and compressive pain, aggravated by stooping.

In the *Temples.* Boring outward, with heaviness in the head, worse on motion, in connection with nasal catarrh.

Vertex. Drawing, darting from the vertex to the root of the nose.

Occiput and Nape. Tense heaviness, worse in the nape, where there is a sense of formication. Pressing outward. Feeling as if the occiput were enlarged. Pressing numbing headache from the nape upward. (Nux vomica, Spigelia, Silicea.)

The majority of the pains are aggravated on rising in the morning, and they grow worse toward evening, as the catarrh which they attend increases. The heaviness is better in the open air.

In the *Supra Orbital Region.* Perssing, tensive pain on the right side, and boring from within outward in the orbital region, contractive pain in the margin of the orbit.

(General observations on the peculiarities of pain, *e.g.*, from within outward, etc.)

Eyes. Appearance. No special changes in appearance are noticed. On the authority of Starke (upon Bitter-sweet), chemotic ophthalmia is recorded as an effect of Dulcamara; and Noack and Trinks give it the first rank among the eye-symptoms.

Sensations. Pressing pain whether reading or not, but aggravated by reading.

Sensation as if fire sparkled out from one's

eyes on walking in the sunlight; also in the chamber.

Sight. 1. *As to power.* Dimness of vision; all objects appear as if seen through a veil; beginning of amaurosis with partial paralysis of the upper eyelid. (Ptosis).

2. *Abnormal vision.* Sparks before the eyes.

Lids. Partial ptosis in the upper lid, as if it would fall. Jerking movements of the eyelids and lips (in cold air).

(General considerations, tissues, special sense affected, nerves of motion as in the ptosis; connection with other pathogenetic diseases of Dulcamara.)

Scrofulous blepharophthalmia and *adenitis;* crusty eruption on the margin of the eyelids and swelling and induration of the cervical glands. "Caspari, Archiv," 3, 3, 68.

Ears. External region. Various sensations, involving the zygoma and parotid region, viz.:

Painless pressing on the left zygoma (belongs to the face). Fine stickings in the parotid and in the external meatus. A cramping constrictive pain below the ear down toward the ramus of the lower jaw.

Pains. Meatus. Left. Pinching sticking toward the tympanum; aching, with fine stitches. Earache, with great nausea. Dreadful earache the whole night, preventing sleep; it ceases suddenly in the morning, but leaves a rushing in the ears.

Pricking and feeling as if cold air had streamed

into the ear. Tearing in the left ear, with stitches from within outward, accompanied by deafness and rustling in the ear.

Special sense. Abnormal. Clear, loud ringing. Drumming and bubbling before the ear and deafness, with tearing in the left ear and stitches from within outward. On opening the mouth a rustling in the ear, as if something were torn in two there.

General considerations; seat and tissues; concomitants, etc. Concomitants are nausea, with earache and sticking in the parotids, with the same in the meatus.)

Nose. Epistaxis. Profuse hæmorrhage; four ounces of bright red and warm blood from the left nostril, with pressure on the region of the superior longitudinal sinus.

Eruption. Pimple, with ulcerative pain in the inner left ala nasi; eruption (itching) in the angles of both alæ. (Analogous remedies, Millefolium, Ledum, Thlaspi.)

Face. Cheeks. Tearing and drawing pains in the whole cheek. Itching in the eruption. (General considerations.)

Lips. Organic. Eruption, pimples and ulcers on the inner part of the upper lip and on the anterior part of the hard palate; also externally around the mouth, with tearing pain on moving the parts.

Functional. Jerking motion of the lips and the eyelids (in the cold air).

Chin. Itching eruption.

Teeth. Numbness, as if devoid of feeling.

Mouth. Tongue. Itching, crawling in the apex of the tongue.

Functional. Paralysis of the tongue, hindering speech, occurring in damp weather. Actual paralysis of the tongue after long use of Dulcamara. (a symptom noted by three allopathic authorities).

Aspect. Rough and dry.

Saliva. Discharge of much soapy saliva. Salivation, with loose and spongy gums. (General considerations).

Neck. Drawing pain in the muscles of the right side.

Fauces. Pressure, as if the uvula were too long. Scraping in the fauces and burning in the œsophagus, with copious eructations.

Glands. Adenitis. Swollen, often very painful and sensitive; cervical and sub-maxillary lymphatic glands (with a sub-inflammatory condition), painful on every turning of the head. "Hartmann, Archiv," 8, 3, 80.

Gastric Symptoms. 1. Flat, soapy taste, with loss of appetite. Natural taste, with good appetite, yet soon satiated. 2. Appetite good, yet soon satiated. Hunger, with aversion to food. 3. While eating, repeated gulping up of soup just swallowed. Frequent pinching and distention of the abdomen. 4. After eating, immense distention of the abdomen. 5. Eructations copious, with scraping in the œsophagus and heart-burn, with constant rejection of very tenacious mucus. Empty with shivering, as if before nausea, with hiccough. Frequent during a meal, gulping up soup just swallowed. 6. Nausea and vomiting. Qualmishness and nausea. Vomiting with chilliness, or with heat and anxiety. Vomiting of tenacious mucus, with warm rising in the œsophagus in the morning. (General considerations.)

Epigastrium sensations. Distention, with empty feeling in the abdomen. Constant griping on going to sleep. Tensive pain, as from a strain. Pressive as from a blow, worse on pressure.

Hypochondria. Left: Sudden cutting. Dull sticking, increased by pressure on the exact spot. Intermitting stitches. Single pulsating stitches when sitting, relieved by rising. Right: Dull stickings which take away the breath.

Umbilical Region. Sticking. Short dull sticking. Just below the umbilicus, griping when sitting bent forward, better on rising. Griping in the morning, as if to stool. Gnawing, throbbing pain just below the umbilicus. Tearing, digging, cutting around the umbilicus. On the left side, below the umbilicus, a pressing outward, as if hernia would ensue.

Abdomen generally. Uneasiness, with frequent flatulent discharge. Dull stitches in quick succession from within outward, taking away the breath; the spot is painful on pressure, as if something would force itself out there. Pinching, sticking in the right side, not relieved by pressure. Violent griping, as if a long worm were creeping and gnawing in the intestine. Griping, as before a diarrhœa. Pain, as from a cold, such as is apt to occur in damp, cold weather.

Flatus. Rumbling in the bowels, as from a purgative, every time he stoops forward. Rumbling as before a stool, with griping and some pain in the loins. Pain as before a diarrhœa, relieved by the discharge of flatus.

Groin. Glands. Pain. Pressing pain in the glands, right and left. In the bubo, burning and sticking, worse from motion and touch. Swelling on the left side, hard and painless. Pain in the left groin, not sensitive to the touch, with sensation of coldness in the back, and rumbling in the abdomen.

Stool. Sudden and imperative desire for stool, with nausea, but a tardy discharge of hard fæces or none at all. Griping and rumbling in the abdomen, with discharge of flatus smelling of asafœtida. Desire to stool, yet no action in the rectum; great straining.

Character. Diarrhœa with flatulence several afternoons in succession. White, slimy alternately with green and yellow stools, with lassitude. Hard stools in pieces. Time, afternoon. Before stool, cutting pain and rumbling. After stool, lassitude, cutting pain.

Cures of Diarrhœa. Case of one month's duration. Cause, cold; continued during cold, damp weather, night and day, worse at night, preceded by violent cutting in the abdomen, chiefly around the navel. Then nausea, profuse cold sweat and thin liquid stools of yellowish or greenish bilious matter; sometimes, simultaneously, vomiting. In the rectum and anus, sensibility and biting, such as are caused by salt. A dose of Dulcama 3°. In one day the patient was cured and remained so. Gross, "Archiv," 1, 3, 169.

Bloody Diarrhœa. Duration, three and one-third years. The patient was a shepherd who had been in the habit of watching his flocks by night; hence, the causes were cold and damp exposure. The symptoms were violent cutting around the navel, at night chiefly. Immediately bloody diarrhœa, almost uninterrupted, and consisting almost of pure blood. On account of the pain and diarrhœa he had no sleep the whole night long. Unceasing, unquenchable thirst. The rectum protrudes; biting at the anus, as from pepper. One drop of Dulcamara, mother tincture. In four days the patient was cured and remained so. Sonnenberg, "Archiv," 4, 1, 12.

Urinary Organs. 1. Pulsation in the bladder from within outward. Painful urination; burning in the orifice of the urethra while urinating.

2. Copious discharge of urine, at first clear and tenacious, then thick and milk-white; first clear, then turbid, with gluey deposit. Turbid and offensive with offensive sweat. Slimy deposit, red or white.

Sexual Organs. Heat and itching of the sexual organs. Papular eruption on the labia majora.

Menses. First increased, then diminished.

Nasal mucous membrane. Sneezing. Mucous membrane dry. Dry coryza, with confusion of the head.

Trachea. Short, irritated cough, excited by a deep inspiration. Much coughing, with expectoration of tenacious mucus, excited by violent stickings in the right or left side of the chest. Expectoration of blood. The exciting cause is deep inspiration; stickings in the right or left side.

Thorax. External. Sternum. Painful stickings, which subsequently feel like blows, upon the sternum. Tension and drawing upon the anterior parts of the sternum on a deep inspiration. A sticking, tearing pain in the middle of the sternum, going through the whole chest to the spinal column while sitting, but ceasing on rising.

Sides. Pain as if struck by fists on both sides under the shoulders. Painful pressing as with a dull instrument when sitting bent forward, on the left side, just above the ensiform body.

Axilla. Pulsating pain in the left axilla, disappearing on motion. Same in the right axilla.

Internal. Organic. Soreness, like a digging or from a strain or injury. Pinching pain in the whole chest, increased by inspiration.

Clavicular region. Benumbing, dull stitch under the right clavicle into the chest. Deep cutting pain in the left chest, close under the clavicle, relieved by pressure.

Sternal region. Jerking and drawing under the

sternum. Pressure in paroxysms under the whole surface of the sternum. Painful sticking in the region of the sternum.

Costal region. Violent stitches, now in one side, now in the other, provoking frequent cough, with sputa of tough mucus.

Right side. Dull sticking in the region of third rib, especially on pressing thereon, when the pain withdraws to the loins, thence rises to between the shoulders; a sticking on the internal margin of the left scapula on inspiration. Digging pain, relieved by pressure. Sudden and quickly disappearing stitch between the fourth and sixth ribs.

Left side. Slow intermitting, dull stitches. Painful stitch, as from a dull knife, between the fifth and sixth ribs. Sticking pain in the region of the sixth rib. A feeling as if something were pressing out from the chest (aggravated from within outward).

(General considerations.)

Heart. Functional. Palpitation violent, externally perceptible, especially at night; one seems to feel the heart beat outside of the thorax.

Back. Sacro-lumbar region. Pain as after long stooping Dull sticking, from within outward, on every inspiration; in both loins when sitting bent together after a walk. Pain as if the body were cut in two in the lumbar region above the hips; the pain is so severe as to keep the patient in constant motion to and fro, which yet gives no relief.

Left. side. Digging, sticking pain near the sacrum. Digging over the left crista illi, relieved by pressure. Close to the lumbar vertebræ, pain as from a blow previously received there. A digging, sticking pain in the loins above the left hip, relieved by walking, but returning on sitting down. Dull stitch from within outward, on each act of inspiration.

Right side. Deep cutting pain in the loins over the right hip, ceasing on pressure, but soon returning. Darting single stickings, as if with a fork, close to the lumber vertebræ.

Dorsal region. Single, painful stitches in the middle of the vertebral column on respiration.

Left side. Intermitting, dull stitches, like sensitive throbbing, near the vertebral column. Intermitting pressure near the vertebral column, near the cervical region, when lying on the back in bed.

Scapular region. Right: Tickling stitch in the middle of the right scapula. Drawing, tearing pain on the external margin. Left: Intermitting, tearing shocks on the external side of the left scapula.

Cervical region. Painful stiffness in the cervical muscles on turning the head to either side. Stiffness. Pain in the nape, as if the head had lain awry. Contractive pain, as if the neck were getting twisted. (Torti collis.)

Extremities. Drawing, tearing in the right shoulder, above the right hip, and above and below the right knee. Upper extremities. Inability to move the arms forward and backward; the attempt produced jerkings in them. Jerkings in the muscles of the upper arm on flexing the arm and moving it backward; on extending the arm, stiffness of the fingers and inability to flex them.

Shoulders. Jerking and pulsating pains in the axillæ.

Arms. Pain in the evening in bed, and in the morning on rising. Paralyzed pain in the left arm, as from a contusion, almost only during repose; less during motion; the arm not sensitive to the touch, and having its usual power. In the whole right arm, a dull violent pain as from apoplexy, with lead heaviness, immobility and sensibility; the arm was icy cold to the touch; the muscles tense, even in repose; the arm paralyzed, could not raise it nor grasp a pen; the attempt to do so produced a sharp pain in the elbow-joint, which was also painful to the touch, as if beaten. The same icy coldness returned in twenty-four hours.

Elbows and Fore-arms. Frequent painful drawing in the left ulna. Dull drawing from the left elbow to the wrist, worse on pronation in the evening. A turning, borning pain slowly descending from the elbow-joint to the wrist; ceasing during motion, but instantly recurring on repose. A sudden jerking, griping, tearing in the middle of the left fore-arm. Left fore-arm powerless, as if paralyzed, with a similar sensation in the elbow-joint.

Wrists. Right. Sticking as with a dull point, relieved by motion.

Hands. Trembling in damp, cold weather. In the left thumb, cramping drawing; one scarcely dared move the thumb. Jerking, sticking in the first phalanx of the middle finger.

Lower Extremities. Hips. Stitches aid drawing, tearing pain in the hips. Drawing, sticking pain in the left hip joint, extending to the groin only when walking, as if at every step the hip would be dislocated; relieved by forcible extension of the thigh, the whole leaving a pain as if beaten in the parts, for fourteen days.

Thighs. Right: Sticking, tearing pain, not relieved by pressure. Drawing sensation on the anterior part of the right thigh. Drawing tearing in the posterior part of the thigh, from the middle to the knee-joint. Paralyzed sensation on the anterior part. Left: Fine sticking, posteriorly, close to the knee. Both: Constant sticking, throbbing or griping pain, ceasing on walking, but developed again when sitting. Here and there drawing in the flesh of the thighs, which is sensitive to the touch. The thighs go to sleep and are very weak.

Knees. Great weariness as after a long walk. Tearing in the knee-joint when sitting. On the internal side of the knee a rhythmic, throbbing, pressing pain.

Legs. Left: Cramp-like drawing pain down through the leg. Swelling of the leg and calf (not of the foot), with tensive pain and feeling of extreme fatigue toward evening. Gentle tearing from within outward in the shin-bone. Pain in the shin-bone, as from fatigue by walking. Pain down the posterior part of the calf. Tearing in the calf, relieved by motion of the foot. Sudden stitch in the calf, as from a needle, followed by a sensation as if blood or water flowed from the spot. Painful cramp when walking. Sensation of numbness in the calves in the afternoon and evening.

Feet. Burning in the feet. Intermitting sticking, burning in the toes.

Left. Tearing from the external malleolus forward. Pulsating, tearing pain in the great and second toes.

Right. Violent cramp in the inner ankle bone, wakes one at night; relieved by getting up and walking about. Drawing tearing about the interior malleolus. Cutting pain in the middle of the right sole, not relieved by stepping.

General Symptoms. Convulsions and spasmodic affections of the muscular system. Jerkings in the hands and feet. Convulsion, first, of the facial muscles, then of the whole body. Trembling of the limbs. Cramp pains here and there, especially in the fingers. Dull stitches here and there in the limbs and body generally, from within outward. Pains in various parts of the body, as from a cold. Great lassitude and feeling of fatigue; heaviness and fatigue in every limb, compelling to sit and lie. Great lassitude and heaviness in the limbs and debility, sometimes sudden, like syncope.

Sleep. Sleepy the whole day, with much yawning. Sleeplessness. Sleep disturbed by distracted dreams, with much sweat during sleep. Restless, interrupted, anxious sleep, with many dreams. In the evening, just on dropping asleep, starting up with fright. Sleep with loud snoring, with open mouth. After midnight, anxiety and fear for the future. Sleep restless; after four A. M. cannot sleep again; stretching and turning, with great fatigue, and feeling as if the posterior cervical muscles were paralyzed and he could not lie on them. Wakes up as if called, and sees a ghost, which constantly enlarges and then vanishes on high. Toward morning no sleep, with fatigue in the limbs, as if paralyzed. Sleep disturbed by itching on the chest, abdomen etc.; heat and stinking sweat.

Skin. Eruptions (see *Nose*). Pimples in the angles of the alæ nasi; painful.

Cheeks. Moist eruptions; itching.

Lips. Pimples and ulcers around the mouth and inside the upper lip.

Chin. Itching eruption.

Sexual Organs. Papular eruption on the labia majora; heat and itching.

Arm. Right. Burning, itching, compelling to scratch, and relieved thereby for a time; a burning vesicle appears. In the hollow of the elbow a red eruption, visible in a warm room in the morning and evening, compelling to scratch, which is followed by burning.

Hands. Covered with warts. On the back of the hand burning red eruption on going from a warm place into the air. A papular eruption.

Thighs. Burning itching, provoked by scratching.

Legs. On the outer side itching and itching stitch, relieved for a time by scratching.

General. Itching in various parts of the body; violent itching eruption of red spots with vesicles; nettle-rash; itching, sticking, and after rubbing it, burning. Fine eruption on the chest and abdomen, with moderate itching. Red spots on the body. Dryness and heat, with constipation and painful retention of urine, with the pulse soft, slow and elastic.

Swelling. Sudden swelling of the body and puffiness of the limbs, which are sometimes painful and sometimes feel numb and go to sleep.

Nettle-rash. Itching and burning after being scratched, and, before each eruption of it, needle-stickings in the whole body. Dulcamara [24] cured. Sonnenberg, "Archiv," 4, 1, 115.

Pemphigus. Child, of thirteen months, with no teeth, old-looking face, great emaciation. Great hunger, yet refuses food. Great thirst; slimy, brown, liquid stools; urine offensive, turbid when passed, and excoriating the skin which it touches. Restless, impatient. Lax, tired, cannot stand. Vesicular eruption, large as a pea, containing yellow, translucid fluid, and on a red, inflamed base, covering the whole body except the face. Sleep little and restless. Dulcamara one dose cured. Bethmann's "Archiv," 3, 2, 119.

Warts. On the hands. Dulcamara second only to Rhus toxicodendron. Stapf, "Archiv," 2, 3, 118.

Crusta lactea. Right cheek, with important symptoms of a cold. Dulcamara [30]. J. Romig, "Archiv," 15, 3, 156.

In Abdominal Typhus. Dulcamara produces good results when patients distinctly remember having taken cold; tongue is clean, no gastricismus; stools yellow, liquid, with rumbling, cutting, digging and griping pain in the umbilical region or whole abdomen. Administration followed by sweat. Bärtl, "Archiv," 20, 3, 69.

Mehlflechte. On the knee; old, obstinate, size of a dollar. Cured by Dulcamara [100], several weeks continued. Gross, "Archiv," xvii, 2, 52.

CALCAREA CARBONICA.

LIME is used in allopathic therapeutics: 1. As caustic lime in combination with caustic potash as an escharotic; it lessens the deliquescence of the potash and makes the causticity more controllable.
2. In the form of lime-water it is used externally in combination with oil as an application to burns; as a soothing application to intertrigo and eczema; also internally to correct acidity of the stomach and primæ viæ; and in combination with milk to prevent vomiting in children who are fed by the bottle. It is given, with their food, to debilitated rachitic persons and to pregnant women who are supposed to suffer from a deficiency of lime.
3. As a dry powder the carbonate is applied to inflamed surfaces, and in the form of chalk mixture is administered, along with other drugs, to control diarrhœa supposed to depend on acidity.
Ringer remarks that small doses, very small ones, e. g., one or two grains, act at least as well as large ones, because the diffusion power of lime

is very small, and but little of it is or can be absorbed into the blood.

Calcarea carbonica* or acetica was proved by Hahnemann, and regarded by him as one of the most valuable and most widely applicable of the antipsoric remedies.

We proceed at once to consider its effects in anatomical order.

Sensorium. Vertigo, especially when walking in the open air, aggravated by stooping, and most noticed in the early morning when rising or shortly after rising; accompanied by nausea and a feeling as though one would fall unconscious. The memory appears to be enfeebled.

As regards disposition, we notice first, indifference, with reticence and inertness; then depression and sadness, with anxiety about the future and disposition to weep. Finally, peevishness and much nervous excitement and irritability.

Despairing, hopeless of ever getting well. Anxiety, shuddering and awe as soon as evening comes near; with fear of death, tormenting those around him day and night.

Fear of going crazy, or that people will observe her and suppose her to be crazy.

The mind is confused, so that what is read or heard is not understood or apprehended.

Heavy aching, and pressing headaches in various

* NOTE.—In Hahnemann's provings of Calcarea carbonica and Calcarea acetica, he prepared them both from oyster-shells giving an impure Carbonate and Acetate. H. E. K. D.

parts of the head, always worse by reading and stooping. Stooping produces a bewildered sensation.

The pressing pain is from within outward, and occupies only a part of the head at a time.

A feeling of congestion alternately with a sensation of icy coldness in the head.

It is peculiar to Calcarea that the head very easily becomes cold and seems affected thereby, so that headache results and the integuments of that particular part become sensitive. A muscular strain produces headache.

The hairs fall out.

Eyes. The pupils are sometimes dilated and sometimes contracted. Hahnemann has remarked that Calcarea is peculiarly applicable to persons whose pupils are habitually dilated.

Perversions of vision are noted.

Veils, feathers, shadows or black spots appear before the eyes, making vision indistinct; it is also indistinct from straining of the body or mind, from reading, and after dinner. Also-presbyopia.

The lids itch and burn and especially the canthi. The lids are red and swollen; also the conjunctiva, with much discharge of muco-pus. The pains are aching, as if grains of sand were in the eye, worse in the evening and at night; burning and itching in the eyes; and in the lids a smarting soreness. Experience has shown the efficacy of Calcarea in scrofulous ophthalmia. (Contrast with Conium.)

Face. Eruptions of painful papules or an eczema.

Frequently a general swelling with tearing pains in the facial bones.

When emaciation occurs the face is pale or sallow.

Many perversions of hearing; noises; deafness with feeling as if something lay in front of the membrana tympani; and noise or sputtering in the ear when using a handkerchief or swallowing.

Pulsation, stitching and heat in the ear. Ear much swollen, with sudden jerking pain, causing the whole body to start. (Same in the eyelids and face.)

The sense of smell is perverted. There is an odor of bad eggs or of gunpowder (I add, of *manure*). Epistaxis frequent and profuse. Ulcers and sores in the nose and on the lips.

Nose sometimes very dry and then again plugged with yellow, offensive pus.

Neck or Throat externally. Swelling of the glands, with aching and, on chewing, stitching pains; sometimes also on swallowing. Also goitre; a most valuable remedy in scrofulous swelling.

Gums. Swollen, bleed easily, sore; aften swelling of the cheeks and ulcers on their inner surface.

The toothache is excited by currents of air (characteristic of Calcarea) or by getting wet, working in damp places (characteristic). They are tearing pains, extending up into the head, as if the roots were being torn out. Also throbbing and boring and swelling of the gums and cheeks.

Renewed by every cold drink, or by both cold and warm drinks.

Speech is difficult and clumsy.

Tongue generally white coated. Burning pain; burning vesicles, which become ulcers. Dryness, alternating with excess of saliva. (Ranula.)

Feeling of a lump in the throat; no tonsillitis.

Taste generally sour. Frequent eructations, generally sour, with burning from epigastrium upward. Frequent hiccough.

Nausea. A. M., with accumulation of water in the mouth and a vertigo; also at other times; with waterbrash. Sometimes early vomiting.

Appetite increased abnormally, alternating with loss of appetite. Increased thirst, especially for cold drinks.

Many symptoms occur after eating,—eructations with burning; nausea after drinking milk, though only half satisfied; headache, palpitation, rush of blood to the head and sleepiness.

Stomach. Aching, both when fasting and after eating, and particularly on coughing.

Right hypochondrium. Aching and swollen and hard; worse at night. This likewise throughout the whole upper abdomen during constipation, with headache and vertigo.

Contractive drawing aching in the epigastrium and across the upper abdomen, compelling to walk bent forward, and aggravated by deep inspiration.

Some sensation in the lower abdomen. Coliky pains about the umbilicus toward the uterus.

Tension in the abdomen from distention of that part of the body; large and hard abdomen, especially in children, is a characteristic of Calcarea carbonica.

Generally the abdomen pains, etc., are brought on or aggravated by inspiration.

In the groins a drawing or jerking pain and frequent swellings of the glands, which are tender and painful on motion.

Anus and Rectum. Itching, as from thread or pin-worms, and a burning, inflamed eruption around the anus.

Aching and burning, or jerking pain in the rectum.

Constant tenesmus or desire for stool is an important symptom (after dysentery, in the chronic form, very useful.) Constant desire for stool; almost no discharge.

Stool. First: Hard, thick, scanty, and evacuated with difficulty, or complete constipation.

Second: Diarrhœa of various characters, undigested, offensive, like spoiled eggs, mixed, soft and lumpy. Undigested, whitish; a stool which is first hard, then pappy, then soft. Scanty, mixed with blood. The stool does not weaken the patient. The records of diarrhœa by provers are meagre, yet Calcarea carbonica is one of our most valuable remedies in chronic diarrhœa. Hæmorrhoidal tumors appear, which pain both during motion and repose, and especially at stool, and bleed freely.

Urinary Organs. Symptoms worse at night.

Cutting and burning in the urethra during micturition. Frequent desire to urinate; varying quantity. Urine dark and offensive. Blood from the urethra. Fungoid of trigone vesicle.

Calcarea increases sexual desire and provokes emissions, but unusual weakness follows indulgence and ejaculation is tardy.

Aching of the testicles, with spasmodic retraction of the same, occurs; also, itching and burning of the genitals of both sexes.

The menses occur too early and are too copious. This is often the case in incipient phthisis. Various phenomena accompany them: Ophthalmia, headache, toothache, colic and backache.

During the interval, a milky leucorrhœa, with burning itching, worse before the menses. The least excitement brings on a return of profuse menstruation.

Calcarea, however, is sometimes indicated when the menses are scanty.

Respiratory Organs. Frequent sneezing and dry nasal catarrh, the nose being very sensitive, with headache, sometimes accompanied by hoarseness.

In the trachea a tickling irritation, as if from dust or feather-down; and cough is provoked by this as well as by eating and playing piano.

The cough is dry at night and in the evening, with shocks in the head and sometimes vomiting; in the morning it is loose, the sputa being yellow and sometimes bloody; there is often in the morning a large mucous rale an expiration in the trachea before coughing.

The chest pains are aching, and general uneasiness. If stitching pains are present, they often are not affected by respiration. Palpitation often accompanies the oppression. The oppression of breathing is sometimes distressing, and is relieved by throwing the shoulders back. Soreness of the chest, especially under the clavicles, to deep respiration, and especially to the touch. The mammæ swell; the nipples are sore when touched; the milk of nursing women fails.

Various pains in the trunk.

Painful stiffness in the back, making change of posture very difficult. Stitches very severe in various parts of the back; sudden stitches, especially between the scapulæ.

The same kind of pains in the extremities. I call attention to the cramps in the calves at night, to the sluggishness of circulation in the hands and feet, causing dead appearance, numb tingling, and excessive coldness.

Skin. Itching and various eruptions; of vesicles, papules, like urticaria (sour stomach), eczema, thin moist scabs upon the head, with swollen cervical glands; eczema behind the ears. Papules in various parts of the body; also warts, which inflame and form ulcers.

Children and sucklings becomes thick and gross, as if fat, but are pale and unhealthy.

Sleep. Considerable day-sleepiness.

CALCAREA CARBONICA.

Difficulty in getting asleep at night, and the sleep is restless. Starting in sleep, or just when going to sleep. Nightmare; cramp in the calves; much palpitation and tumult of the blood at night.

Fever. Mixed. Cold and heat partial. Great sensibility to cold at all times.

Heat attended by thirst.

Sweat copious by day during the slightest motion, also at night and early in bed, and then chiefly on the limbs. (Not as with Rhus and Silicea.)

General Action. Lassitude in the limbs; general sense of weakness after every walk, such as one feels after a fever. It even goes so far as to amount to attacks of faintness with chill; indistinct vision and nausea.

APPLICATIONS.

In every case where the nutrition is impaired with tendency to glandular engorgements.

Hahnemann says Calcarea does much good in epilepsy. Also, he says, it is seldom beneficial to repeat Calcarea upon itself.

It is indicated especially in cases of women whose menses comes too early and too copiously. It acts best after Sulphur or Nitric acid, but never well if it has been given before them.

It produces a general feeling of illness, and great sensibility to cold air; it has been observed that after washing or working in water the symptoms re-appear or are much worse.

It is useful for children who are self-willed and inclined to fatten. In itching of the scalp; children scratch the head when their sleep is disturbed or on waking. In difficult dentition of little children. (G.)

It is indicated by deafness after the abuse of quinine.

By a sour taste in the mouth or of food; sour vomiting, especially with children during dentition; also by sour diarrhœa.

By longing for eggs, particularly with children during sickness or convalescence.

When the pit of the stomach, instead of being concave is convex.

When the feet are constantly cold and damp, as if she had on wet stockings. (Calcarea phosphorica is better in uterine trouble. G.) She is very sensitive to the least cold air, which goes through her.

In fever, when there are horrid visions on closing the eyes; or headache, diminished by closing the eyes.

Hughes says Calcarea seems to be indicated not in primary but in secondary disorders of assimilation; these are scrofula, tuberculosis and rachitis. It is useful for rachitis; difficult dentition; imperfect ossification; delay of the power of walking; for scrofula; adenitis; mesenteric disease; chronic diarrhœa; eruptions, etc.

CAUSTICUM.

THIS drug is known only to the homœopathist, at least under this name. What is it?

Hahnemmann directed it to be prepared as follows:

"Take a piece of recently prepared quicklime weighing about two pounds, immerse it for a minute in a vessel full of distilled water, and then lay it in a dry cup, where it soon becomes pulverized, giving out much heat and a peculiar odor called the vapor of lime. Of this fine powder you take two ounces, place it in a mortar which had been previously warmed, and then mix it with a solution of two ounces of the bisulphate of potash in two ounces of boiling-hot water, the potash before being dissolved having been exposed to a red heat, melted, cooled again and then pulverized.

"This thickish preparation is inserted into a retort, to the open end of which the receiver—which ought to be dipped in water to half its height—is hermetically fastened. The liquid is distilled over by gradually approaching a coal fire to the report, and until the preparation is perfectly dry. The liquid in the receiver is about one ounce and a half, as clear as water, and containing the Causticum in a concentrated form. It smells like the lye obtained from potash, and has an astringent and burning taste on the back part of the tongue. Its freezing point is below that of water; it promotes the putrefaction of animal substances that are placed in it; with the salts of baryta it gives out no trace of sulphuric acid, nor any trace of lime-earth with the exalate of ammonium."

Dr. Black had several specimens analyzed, and believes Causticum to be a weak solution of potassic hydrate. Others deny any virtue to it, and reject it from the materia medica but to this proposition we oppose the physiological and the pathological tests.

The symptoms ascribed to Causticum are very many. Instead of giving a resumé of all, I will call your attention to certain groups, of which the value has been abundantly established by clinical experience.

Face. Pains in the malar bones, zygomatic arch and maxillæ; drawing pains which extend into the cheek and ear, and are most apt to occur on the right side Burning; the pains produce spasm of the muscles, a sensation of numbness on the side of the face as if asleep.

These symptoms have led to the use of Causticum in prosopalgia and in facial paralysis. In general, hemiplegia of the right side.

Wart on the nose.

Digestion. Burning and water-brash. Constipation.

Urine. Constant ineffectual desire to urinate; frequent evacuation of only a few drops, with spasms in the rectum and constipation. Evacuation of blood with the urine or instead of it; with great pain; all the sensations worse at night. (Morgan's case.)

Burning in the urethra during micturition.

Involuntary micturition when coughing sneezing or walking.

Nocturnal incontinence; not conscious of it. (Different from Kreasote and Plantago major.)

Larynx and trachea, aphonia.

Hoarseness toward evening, with dry tickling cough.

Cough, with a sensation as if the prover could not cough low enough to start the mucus, produced by tickling, accompanied by rawness.

Backache, especially in the coccyx.

Limbs. Twitchings and clonic spasms.

Rheumatic aching in the shoulder; paralysis if the deltiod; cannot raise the hand to the head; subject to pains, worse at night, causing continued motion. The same in the hips and knees; constant tearing and piercing pains, compelling constant motion, which, however, does *not* relieve (as under Rhus); always coming on at evening, and diminished in the morning. Useful in rheumatism when the fever has abated.

Convulsions.

NITRIC ACID.

HAHNEMANN says Nitrict acid is especially indicated for those disposed to diarrhœa. It is most especially effective after Kali carbonicum.

Most of the symptoms are relieved after driving in a wagon; but slight movement, especially after eating, excites heat, sweat and palpitation. It produces great tendency to take cold, and it excites pains in the back and all the limbs.

As regards the skin, the sweat-pores are black, and papules are frequent. It disposes to ulcers, and those already existing bleed readily when touched or bound up; and are the seat of sticking and burning pains, as if from nettles. Itching of the skin is a common symptoms, and, after scratching, large blotches appear. Warts itch.

Ulcers and caries, resulting from the abuse of Mercury, are relieved by Nitric acid especially if there be erethism.

A characteristic symptom is the sensation of great weakness, sometimes felt early in the morning, as lassitude in the joints and limbs; sometimes in

NITRIC ACID.

the afternoon, as weariness, even to trembling, throughout the body. As a consequence, day-sleepiness, even early, soon after getting up.

Sleep at night is disturbed; sometimes by frequent waking, sometimes by turning and tossing, sometimes by frightful dreams, and especially often by thirst and necessity to pass water. Abdominal uneasiness and nightmare.

Fever. Coldness, not only at night but also by day; coldness of the skin of the entire body, the chill chiefly at evening and on getting into bed; and mostly in the back.

Heat. Fugitive, and in frequent flashes by day; sometimes only in the hands or the cheeks, without thirst. Often a continued sensation of heat in the body without thirst; can endure but little covering. At night this heat is often intolerable, partial or general, without sweat and with thirst.

Fever mixed up.

Sometimes sweat at night, general or partial, and often only on the parts on which one lies.

Disposition peevish, ill-humored at every trifle, even at himself, especially in the morning early.

Often anxious about his own illness; constantly thinking about past troubles.

The mind is weakned; the thoughts wander, especially on weighty subjects.

Vertigo. Not only when stooping, and compelling to lie down, but also occuring in the evening after lying down, and when rising at night or early in the morning.

Head. Nothing specially characteristic about pains, or their locality. It should be noted, however, that the pains generally are aggravated by succussion, as by riding in a wagon or by stepping hard. Externally the head is sensitive, as if contused, either all over or in certain spots, as, for example, on the spots pressed when lying, or by pressure of the cap or hat (verified in practice).

Face. Tearing and cramp-like pressure in the cheeks and malar-bone, increased by touch and at night.

Eyes. General. Exterior. Dull and sunken, hard to open, A. M. Yellow and sickly hue of the surrounding skin. The conjunctiva is reddened, with an aching as though sand were in the eyes, or as if one had been looking at the sun; lachrymation, with burning and biting, much increased by reading; stitching pains, which come from the head into the eye and ear. Nebulosities of the cornea have been observed; and Nitric acid has been found very serviceable in ophthalmia from suddenly suppressed syphilitic affections.

Ears. Glandular swelling behind and below the ear, from which stitching pains extend into the ear; stitching pain in the internal ear and in the maxillary articulation.

Nose. Discharge of offensive, yellow mucus, and frequent epistaxis.

Chin. Pimples with a red areola, leaving a hard lump after suppuration. Swelling of the infra-maxillary glands.

Gums. Swollen; teeth yellow. Throbbing and sticking toothache, worse at night.

Toungue. Vesicles upon the tongue and sublingual glands; burn when touched.

Soreness of the tongue, palate and gums; and ulcerated spots on the cheeks. Great dryness of the mouth. Offensive breath, as if putrid.

Scraped sensation in the throat.

Aching when swallowing food, with sensation of swelling deep in the throat. Soreness of the uvula. Sticking in the tonsils, and deep in the swollen throat, and in the root of the tongue; worse in the evening.

Digestion is retarded and modified, as is shown by sour eructation and rising of half-digested food. Sour and bitter taste. Nausea and vomiting along with headache; most symptoms occur after eating and at night, and are attended by profuse sweat. Much flatus. Aching in the region of the liver and kidney; and at the same time a jaundiced hue. Sticking and griping in the abdomen.

Inguinal glands swollen, but often not painful.

Rectum. Soreness and chafed sensation after stool; a moist soreness at the anus and between the nates. Burning and itching. Sticking pain in the rectum, chiefly when coughing and at stool. Aching or long pressing toward the rectum and anus; stool not hard, but difficult. Hæmorrhoids protrude and at every stool bleed.

Stool. Diarrhœic; offensive and with much tenesmus. Constipation, says Hahnemann, rarer.

Tenesmus of the bladder. Urine offensive, scanty, sometimes acid, sometimes alkaline. Color dark brown; soon becomes turbid; white or clear red deposit, sometimes granular. Burning and soreness after urinating.

The sexual instinct is increased. Male urethra painful to pressure; orifice swollen and red; discharge of bloody or thick yellow mucus.

Much itching of the prepuce and glands. Swelling and drawing in the testes. Vesicles and ulcer on the inner surface of the prepuce and on the glands, as before described; also the warts.

Menses too soon, with backache and great weakness, with bearing-down pains.

Leucorrhœa of a stringy mucus of a cherry-brown color and offensive. Ulcers in the vagina.

Sneezing, dry nasal catarrh, or alternately; hoarseness, headache and cough. Throat has catarrhal inflammation. Roughness, etc.

Cough, with headache. Aching in the loins, and soreness in the thorax sputa dark, bloody. Soreness and constriction of the chest.

The back and loins ache with the least cold. Stiffness of the nape.

Aching and sticking in the extremities.

Itching, burning eruption between the fingers.

Cramp in the calves and soles of the feet at night and toward morning on stretching out the feet; painful to the touch.

CARBO VEGETABILIS.

CARBO LIGNI. VEGETABLE CHARCOAL.

CHARCOAL possesses the power of absorbing gases in large quantities in vastly greater proportions than the relation of its bulk. It condenses the gases within its pores. It does not act equally upon all gases in this way; absorbs but little hydrogen; more oxygen; large quantities of sulphuretted hydrogen, and still more of ammonia. It is used as a disinfectant and to purify water; to remove the foul smells from ulcers, etc. It is inferior as a disinfectant to volatile substances, becouse it can act only on the air which comes in contact with it. Not so good in poultice on sores as in bags, dry and granulated.

It is used in the old practice to relieve heart-burn, flatulence, ets. In does, six to ten grains.

Hahnemann says: "The disinfectant action of Carbo vegetabilis is purely chemical. The mouth rinsed with charcoal and made sweet soon becomes foul again. So do the ulcers and the excretions treated with charcoal. It is not," he continues, "until charcoal has been reduced to a state of minute subdivision by trituration, according to the rules of homœopathic pharmacy, that it produces specific effects upon the organism." The proving which Hahnemann presents us was made with the third centesimal trituration.

These symptoms may be summarized as follows:

Head. Sensorium. Indifference is the characteristic symptom. The irritability noticed seems to be a protest against disturbance of the quiet which the patient desires; and the sensibility and peevishness of disposition to be another phase of the same protest.

Memory is feeble, the course of ideas slow, with tendency to fixed ideas.

Vertigo is a marked symptom. It occurs in the bed, when sitting up after sleep; and is especially induced by quick movements of the head, stooping, walking, sitting, etc.

Headache is a marked symptom of Carbo vegetabilis. The general character is heaviness, pressure, dull ache. Thus provers complain that the head is "as heavy as lead;" that there is a weight in the occiput; or a pressure across the forehead weighing down the eyelids, etc. Even the weight of the hat seems to aggravate this symptom. A feeling of tension, as if the integuments of the head were too tight; as if a strap were drawn tightly across the forehead. Sometimes after a meal and at evening, the pain is a throbbing, with heat in the head and fullness. But generally the headache, like the vertigo, is attended with weakness and tendency to faintness. Sometimes the pains, if acute, extend to the upper maxilla.

The hair falls out.

Eyes. In the eyes we notice, first, itching and bitting, especially in the canthi, with lachrymation and soreness in them. The prominent sensation is pressure and aching in the globe of the eye. As regards vision, black spots and flames and rings and shortness of vision have been observed.

Ears. Tearing and aching from within outward. External ear swollen and hot. Parotids swollen. Ringing in the ear accompanies the vertigo. Also, there is roaring and singing. Deafness.

Nose. Epistaxis copious and frequent; black blood, generally at night. Paleness before and after it.

Face. Complexion pale or yellowish. Drawing and aching pains in the facial nerve.

Mouth. The teeth feel long, and are sore. Tearing ache. The gums are swollen and bleed, and recede from the teeth. Vesicles appear on the gums, and they bleed on suction by the tongue.

Tongue. Whitish or yellow coat. Dry mouth. Burning and biting sensation in the fauces, and scraped feeling in the throat. Aching in the throat and œsophagus as if from a swelling, which hinders deglutition, as if the throat were constricted.

Digestion. The taste in the mouth is saltish, sometimes bitter.

Appetite vanishes.

Frequent and abundant eructations, with great

accumulations of flatus in the stomach. Nausea after eating, yet no vomiting. Most of the digestive symptoms are aggravated after eating. For example, hiccough, irresistible sleepiness, with lassitude and heaviness of the legs; but especially the feeling of fullness and great distention of the abdomen.

As regards sensations, burning in the stomach, with a creeping sensation up to the throat, is very characteristic.

Also, spasmodic pain in the stomach, compelling to crouch forward, and impeding respiration. One of our best remedies in gastralgia, especially when there is much flatus and a burning ache. Similar achings and burnings in the abdomen.

In the region of the liver, stitching pain; also in the epigastrium, and thence to both sides, increased by deep inspiration.

Excessive flatulent distention, with rumbling. Flatus not always offensive. Sometimes very much so, and evacuation gives relief.

In the rectum and anus, burning, both independently of, and during, the evacuation of flatus and stool. Itching and burning, stitches and cutting pain at stool.

Stool. Ineffectual urging to stool. Stool scanty and difficult, even when not hard. Stool solid and enveloped in mucus. Before stool much pressure with, at same time, pressure on the bladder and in the back (frequent in women); at last with pains like labor-pains, and great straining; a soft stool.

CARBO VEGETABILIS. 329

Exudation of moisture from the anus; and soreness of the perinæum, with itching. (Hence used in hæmorrhoids with epistaxis.)

Urine increased; dark and red, as if mixed with blood. Pressure on the bladder. Tearing in the urethra, and the last drops are of mucus.

Sexual instinct suppressed.

Female Sexual Organs. Burning and smarting and soreness, with abundant leucorrhœa, most abundant in the early morning. Menses are too frequent, preceded by spasmodic colic, and attended by violent headache and colic.

Respiratory Organs. Catarrhal symptoms. Frequent sneezing and dry nasal catarrh; nares obstructed. Sneezing, caused by tickling and creeping in the nose, with lachrymation and biting pain in and above the nose. Sometimes an ineffectual desire to sneeze, which is very troublesome.

Hoarseness, especially toward evening. Cannot speak a loud word, or the voice becomes deep and rough, or fails. Compare Causticum, Phosphorus, Rumex, Lachesis.

A tight feeling in the chest, and constant desire to cough, from a scraped feeling and a tickling in the throat and trachea.

In cases of obstinate hoarseness, worse in the evening; in tracheitis, and asthmatic affections dependent on hydrothorax, it is very useful. Ruckert.

The cough is mostly hard and dry, and hoarse or rough-sounding; is most apt to occur after a full meal, and ends in vomiting (indication in whooping cough). It often produces pain in the chest and stitches through the head (and the pain in the chest *after* the cough is a burning as from a coal of fire). Sometimes there are tough and greenish sputa.

Chest. Aching and tearing pain and the burning after coughing. Constriction and short breath, increased at evening in bed. The breath is short, and the chest tired on waking. Cases of suspected slow tuberculosis.

Back and Loins. Aching and tearing, extending to the hips. Pain in the scapular region. Rheumatic drawing and aching from the loins to the coccyx. Burning externally about the hips and the scapulæ, and aching along the spine.

In the extremities, aching and burning pains, but especially lassitude, heaviness and even numbness; generally diminished by repose, but often in the legs a restlessness, so that one knows not where to place the limbs.

As regards the skin, fugitive itching when warm in bed. Nettle-rash, painless papules and fine itching eruptions on the hands and the salves. Ulcers are offensive; old ones break out afresh. They burn and easily bleed.

As regards sleep. Great sleepiness by day, with yawning and stretching, both in the morning and afternoon. Early sleepiness in the evening; but cannot go to sleep early after going to bed. Anxiety, restlessness; congestion of the head early

ness; external tenderness to pressure (cannot bear clothes). Abdomen full, sensitive to pressure; the feet swell; the urine is scanty.

Stool. Sensation as if diarrhœa were coming; urgency, pressure, tenesmus. Every morning, soft stool, light yellow. Diarrhœa yellow, watery, slimy, without pain, especially in the morning. Offensive diarrhœa, tenesmus, blood, also mucus. Heat and throbbing in the rectum, and feeling as if the rectum were full and stopped. Thin, yellow stools, with the greatest prostration and weakness; the stool comes with every motion of the body, as though the anus stood open.

(Verified in the case of Dr. B. Dysentery. 1870.)

Electric shocks in the rectum before disposition to stool. Rawness in the anus, with diarrhœa. Insupportable itching, with swelling, shooting, boring pains in hæmorrhoids; a bloody oozing, with swelling of the anus.

Urine. Little or none. Frequent desire; scanty and high colored. Burning in the urethra (when the urine is scanty).

Genitals. Pain in the ovarian region, as if dislocated; tender to pressure; cuttings in the left side, then in the right; drawings, shootings and bearing down. Bearing down in the uterine region, as if the menses would appear. Swelling of the labia. The menses are interrupted for a day, then re-appear again and again.

Respiration. Hoarseness. Larynx sensitive to pressure; throat rough and dry. Tickling in the throat-pit, producing evening cough; cough before midnight; after lying down and sleeping; better by expectoration. Respiration slow, difficult; the throat constricted. Worse by motion, going upstairs, and walking; soreness under the ribs, with heat, headache and drowsiness; cannot bear a hot room; chest full; must sit up. Pain in the left side near the sternum. Shootings in the left side. Pain in the region of the heart, shooting and impeding respiration. Pulse full and strong, or small and rapid.

Trunk and Externally. Stiffness of the loins. Drawing pains in the shoulders, beginnings in the shoulder and extending to the finger-ends. Numbness, especially of the left arm. Burning, shooting and stinging in the hands. Redness, heat, swelling. Itching, burnig and chapping. Drawing pain through the leg from the hip to the toes. Aching and swelling of the knee. The feet swell, are heavy, stiff, painful, swollen; and itch as if they had been swollen. They are sensitive to the least pressure.

Disposition. Irritable and restless; weak and trembling. Weakness in paroxysms, with vertigo. Fainting, with pallor, coldness and diarrhœa.

Sleep. Yawning, and great desire for sleep. Sleep restless, full of dreams. Dreams of cares and trouble. Long sleep in the morning.

Fever. Shaking chill, with urticaria after heat. Slight shiverings on the least movement while sitting in the evening; with headache, heat of the

in the night prevents sleep. (Arsenic after midnight.)

Fever. Coldness and chilliness at night, followed by heat. Great disposition to sweat, which occurs early in the morning, and is often sour.

Dr. Guernsey gives the following indications for intermittent: Chill, with a marked degree of thirst. No thirst, or but slight during the fever, but the patient wishes to be fanned constantly, as if to compensate for the lack of thirst.

Before the chill, often throbbing headache. During the chill, often much languor and apparent losing of strength.

General Characteristic are depression, not preceded by erethism or excitement.

[Carbo vegetabilis (wood charcoal) was not used in medicine until the discovery of its power to absorb gases and hold them confined in its pores, to an extent several hundred times exceeding its own volume, suggested its use, both internally and externally, in cases of decomposition, whether of food within the intestine, or of tissues and excretions of ulcerating surfaces on the intestine or the integument, evolving offensive gases. In such cases charcoal was given in large doses, or applied to the ulcerating surface. We owe our knowledge of its specific, pathogenetic and therapeutic properties to Hahnemann and his pupils, who proved it.]

CARBO ANIMALIS.

THE symptoms of Carbo animalis are, however, in the main identical with those of Carbo vegetabilis.

In those of the eye long-sightedness is noted instead of myopia.

In the face, copper-colored, dry eruption, and papules.

Swelling of the glands in the neck, axillæ, inguina, and mammæ, which are painful.

Teeth very loose; cannot chew the softest food. Vesicles in the mouth, forming ulcers.

The carbons require trituration to develop their power.

[Authorities in materia medica have been accustomed to regard substances which are nearly or quite identical in chemical composition as so likely to be substantially identical in pathogenetic or therapeutic action that they might be used interchangeably, or one substituted for another as convenience or cheapness might dictate. This notion is somewhat like that which ascribes similar or identical properties to plants of the same natural families. There is a certain basis of truth at the foundation of the dogma, but the exceptions are so numerous and so trenchant that we dare not in any single case act upon it in practice. When we come to a minute analysis of pathogenetic action, we find that even substances so nearly identical as the two carbons, the vegetable and the animal, present important differences, and may not be used with indifference the one for the other. Instances illustrating this fact are found in the Ranunculus and other families among plants, and notably in the carbonaceous group of remedies, which includes Sepia, Murex, Graphites, Carbo veg. and Carbo an. It will be interesting exercise for the student to trace the resemblances and the differences.]

APIUM VIRUS.

OPHTHALMIA; angina; erysipelas; diarrhœa; dysentery; cholera infantum; urticaria; hæmaturia; dropsy; intermittent fever; hydrocephalus; each accompanied by the characteristic absence of thirst and by drowsiness.

Disposition. Depressed.

Sensorium. Cannot collect nor direct his thoughts. Confusion of the head, especially just about the eyes.

Head. Feeling as if too full; it appears too large. Heaviness, aching-pressing, especially on rising from a sitting or lying posture; worse in a warm room, better by pressure with the hand. Pains in the head, extending to the eyes; extending over the eyes; around the eyes. During the headache, photophobia.

Eyes. Itching, burning, stinging in the eyes; lachrymation, redness; shooting, stinging pains and burning. Photophobia; lids swollen and agglutinated, and the seat of itching, stinging, burning pains.

Watery erysipelatous swelling around the eye.

Ears. Stinging and burning; sensitive to noise.

Nose. Sneezing. Swelling and stinging of the nose; dryness and swelling.

Face. Face pale; also livid; feeling of fullness; tension and swelling.

Lips. Swelling and soreness and stinging; the swelling extends to the face, etc.

Mouth. Tongue as if scalded, especially on the edges. Vesicles along the edges, especially the left, with burning, rawness and stitches. Tongue dry, fiery red, burning, sticking and swelling. Tongue coated, with diarrhœa. Mouth, fauces and throat dry. The surface is sensitive, as if scalded. The saliva is tenacious and frothy.

Throat. Pressure in the roof of the pharynx, as from a hard body.

Sticking, itching and contraction in the throat, hindering deglutition. As if raw in the throat, with tenacious saliva when hawking. Burning, smarting, sticking in the throat, especially when swallowing. Tonsils red, swollen, painful, smarting.

Stomach. Loss of appetite. Absence of thirst, with dropsy. During the heat the throat is dry. Eructations with water-brash and taste of food, worse after drinking water. Disgust, nausea with vertigo, fainting, prostration even to vomiting, with headache, swelling of the head, pain in the stomach and diarrhœa. Pressure in the stomach, prickings as with needles, and extreme sensitiveness to pressure.

Abdomen. Throbbing, boring over the left or-ileum, lessened by eructation. Rumbling, sense of nausea in the abdomen. Internal sense of raw-

face and hands. Shivering increased by warmth; followed by heat and cough.

Dr. G. gives indications for Apis in intermittent: Chill at four P. M., increased by warmth; renewed chilliness from slight movement; heat of the face and hands. No sweat. Falls into a deep sleep.

Skin. Heat and redness in the evening and at night, with excitement, headache and diarrhœa, swellings and cough.

Itching, like prickling of needles, as from insects, recurring on every motion. Burning, itching, stinging. Bright red swelling, with red streaks, along the limbs. Skin swollen, pale or red, puffed. Flat swellings, with stinging, red or pale.

Nettle-rash. Œdema. Dropsical swelling.

General. Warmth aggravates; cold relieves. Burning and stinging. Sensibility to external touch and pressure. Drowsiness. Thirstlessness.

APPLICATIONS.

See *ante*.

Diphtheria, patches gray; great debility; puffy eyelids, and swollen feet; drowsiness.

Hydrocephalus. Meningitis tuberculosis of children. "Child lies in a torpor; delirium; sudden shrill, piercing cries; squinting; grinding teeth; boring the head in the pillow; one half of the body twitching, the other paralyzed; head wet from sweating; scanty urine."

PHOSPHORUS.

SPECIAL ANALYSIS.

DISPOSITION. Phosphorus presents interesting alternations of the psychical conditions, as the following series of symptoms show:
1. Sadness, depression with forebodings of calamity; melancholy, relieved only by vehement weeping. 2. Great anxiety, uneasiness and distress, fearfulness and restlessness, paroxysms of anxiety, which feeling seems to arise from the left chest and to be attended by palpitation, 3. Great excitability, even when thinking of ill-fortune long past, a disagreeable sensation is felt in the præcordia; all the senses are too keen, especially hearing and smell; irritability, anger upon slight provocation. 4. Spasmodic laughter and weeping contrary to one's will; hilarity, very sensitive imagination. Indifference to ordinary feelings of shame or affection. Of these phenomena the proving gives no clue to the order, but we may infer from Hahnemann's observations in the preface that sadness (recurring regularly at twilight), anxiety and irritability are the characteristic modifications of disposition induced by Phosphorus.

PHOSPHORUS. 339

Sensorium. Weakness of memory, indisposition (moderate) to exertion; difficulty in collecting and concentrating thoughts; weak feeling in the head, aggravated by thinking and by loud noise, music or hard stepping; these things produce throbbing in the head, a feeling of confusion, dullness and distraction, but especially of weakness in the head. These symptoms are interesting in connection with the known waste of Phosphorus consequent on cerebral exertion, and the stimulating effects of Phosphorus in cases of exhaustion of the cerebrospinal system (as in the administration of Phosphoric acid after debauch, etc).

Vertigo. Vertigo so great as to induce falling, occurring under every variety of conditions; also vertigo when lying down, compelling to assume an upright posture.

Head. General confusion, as from too long watching, with difficulty in collecting one's ideas; heaviness, sense of exhaustion and bewilderment in the brain; aversion to mental exertion. Confusion and heaviness, more in the vertex and sinciput, along with vertigo and disposition to fall forward. These symptoms are generally better in the cool air and when the head is unconvered.

The pains in the head are of great variety, and affect equally all parts of the head. It may be remarked that they are to a great extent superficial, seeming to affect the surface of the brain, or the bones, or the scalp. They extend from the forehead into the eyes, especially the right eye, and from the vertex and temples down upon the zygoma, in the form of violent tearing. There is great external sensibility of the head. Great organs of blood affecting the head. Shocks and single stitches in the head. The pains are as follows: Tearing, affecting the frontal and temporal regions, especially on the right side, and involving the eye and zygoma.

Sticking, affecting all parts of the head.

Shocks in the occiput and parietal region.

Drawing pain generally, with exaltation of the sensorium, followed by depression.

Pressing pain, chiefly in the frontal and temporal region, as if from fullness, and yet a feeling as if it were not actual congestion; the pressure extends from the forehead into the eyes and to the root of the nose.

Throbbing in the sides of the head and in the root of the nose, extending also to the eyes and nose, recurring periodically. This throbbing is induced and increased by laughing, motion, etc., as if it arose from weakness. Burning.

Weakness. Decided sensation of weakness, so that the noise of a piano is intolerable, and the least motion, or beginning to walk, or stooping, etc., is very distressing.

Conditions. The headache generally occurs in the evening; sometimes on waking in the morning. It is aggravated by warmth and excitement, and relieved by repose, cold and the open air.

General. Fullness of the head, the ears stopped,

PHOSPHORUS. 341

with singing in them; orgasm of the blood, heat and buzzing in the head.

The scalp is tender and itches. The hair falls out; pain when the hair is pulled.

The head symptoms display the characteristics of the action of Phosphorus upon the organism. Exaltation, intermingled with and followed by depression, not merely of the vegetative system, but also and especially of the nervous energy, until finally we have in the tumultuous orgasms the quasi-congestions and yet the apparent anæmia the the cerebral mass, a complete picture of the effect of *pari passu* exhaustion; of both organic and nervous exhaustion; such, for example, as follows too free exercise of the intellectual and sexual functions, or of both combined.

Eyes. The eye symptoms corroborate, to a certain extent, the above view of the head symptoms. The eyes are dull, glassy, and as if full of sleep; the vision is impaired; it is as if a veil were before the eyes; the axis of vision trembles; black spots waver and glide before the eyes. There are sparks before the eyes in the dark, and along with these symptoms there is roaring in the head. Moreover, there are attacks of sudden blindness. The eyelids often tremble and quiver, and the eyes fill with tears and are painful when used in reading. As regards the organic affections, there is sub-acute conjunctivitis, with lachrymation, agglutination, swelling and suppuration of the lids and meibomian glands, with itching and burning pains.

The symptoms of obscure vision, better in the twilight and on shading the eye with the hand, point to cataract, in which Phosphorus has been found useful. It must also be good in day-blindness, nyctalopia.

Ears. The throbbing, roaring and buzzing in the ears, the loud resonance of all sounds, result probably from the condition of the brain to which we have referred. In addition, there is evidence of an affection of the tissues of the external and middle ears, as follows: Sticking, pressing and tearing in the external ear and in the neighboring parts of the head. Earache. Pressure. Feeling as if the meatus were stopped. Discharge of yellow fluid from the ear. Deafness, as if the ear were stopped.

Nose. Itching, tickling and soreness of the nose. When rubbed, it bleeds readily. Here we first note a characteristic peculiarity of Phosphorus; hæmorrhages are easily produced from mucous surfaces, from wounds or from ulcers, and frequently occur spontaneously. This probably suggested its use in fungus hæmatodes. It suggests its appropriateness, other symptoms corresponding, as we shall see they do, in cases of typhus; a disease in which hæmorrhages so readily occur or are provoked. The discharge from the nose is often streaked with blood; the nose is obstructed by clots.

The sense of smell is often exalted in acuteness.

Face. The face is pale, sunken, sallow; the

eyes are hollow, encircled by blue rings,—a condition corresponding to the exhaustion represented by the head, and other symptoms. Again, the orgasm of circulation is manifested in flashes of heat and redness. A definite form of prosopalgia is described as follows: Severe tearing about the lower margin of the orbit on the right side, extending under the right ear, and involving the bones of the face and the temple, as if everything were torn out and away, increasing until eight P. M. Pressure in the facial and parietal bones, and in the teeth on eating warm food, and wose in a warm room. Tearing in the maxillary bones in the evening, when lying down, relieved by moving the jaw. Violent stitch from the middle of the left lower maxilla, coming out deep through the cheeks and eye, extending to the forehead. Pressure, drawing and tearing in the lower maxilla toward the chin. The tendency of Phosphorus to affect the maxillary region, as well as its action on the lungs, is shown in the affections to which those who work in match factories, and are exposed to the vapors of Phosphorus, are subject. Necrosis of the maxillæ, beginning with toothache, passing through the stages of swelling and inflammation of the superficial tissues, and of sinuses and caries, and ending in death by pulmonary tuberculosis. (Lorniser in "Œstreicher Medikalische Jahrbucher," 1845, March.)

Teeth. The gums are sensitive and disposed to ulceration. They swell and bleed easily on the slightest touch. The teeth seem loose and decay readily. The toothache is jerking, tearing, darting, boring, generally occurring or worse in the evening or at night, after washing.

Lips. The lips itch and burn; are sensitive to touch; vesicles form on the inner edge of them. The lips and palate are dry, without thirst.

Tongue. Similar sensations upon the tongue, which is covered with a dirty white fur, has burning vesicles near its tip, and ulcers anteriorly on the surface, which bleed readily when touched.

Mouth. Insufferable itching, tickling and soreness, as if denuded of skin, in the roof of the mouth.

General dryness of the mouth, generally without, sometimes with, thirst. Much saliva of an offensive taste; bitter, sour, offensive.

Throat and Fauces. The throat affection is definite. The cervical muscles are painful on touch and motion. Stitches in the left side of the throat; also toward the ear and thence to the vertex. The fauces and tonsils are the seat of acute inflammation, which, however, is not confined to these organs, but extends into the larynx, and especially into the trachea, extending at least as far as the supra-sternal fossa, and in most cases much farther. It is characterized, therefore, not merely by soreness and difficulty in swallowing, and by a sense of constriction in the fauces, but also by rawness and roughness in the whole affected region when not swallowing; by dry, hacking cough, which is provoked not only by speech and motion of the respiratory organs, but also when the larynx and trachea are moved and impinged upon in the act of deglutition. The inflammation of the tonsils is probably confined to the mucous membrane, and is not parenchymatous. The rough, raw, scraped sensation in the throat is a very marked symptom of Phosphorus, and occurs almost always in conjunction with similar sensations in the trachea and chest. The pharynx is dry, deglutition is difficult.

Nux vomica, Hepar, Rumex crispus, Causticum, Belladonna.

COCCULUS INDICUS.

"MENISPERMUM cocculus, Cocculus indicus, Cocculus suberosus, Anamirta cocculus." The seeds or berries are the parts used in medicine.

This substance was employed by the ancients as a poison for fish, stupefying them, and rendering it easy to catch them. It is stated that the half-ripe, bruised berries, being formed into little pellets and thrown into the water, are eagerly devoured by the fish, which thereupon are soon seized with dizziness, and, after whirling around, remain motionless, and float on the surface of the water. It is stated that if the fish have eaten any considerable quantity of the Cocculus before succumbing to its influence, their flesh becomes poisonous.

The active poisonous principle of Cocculus is stated to be picrotoxin. Recent toxicological experiments have been made with this substance. It is probable, however, that this does not comprise the entire active principle of the Cocculus, any more than strychnia does that of Nux vomica or quinia of Cinchona.

In consequence of its use as a means of stupefying fish, and also as the basis of an infusion for the destruction of pediculi and other vermin, cases of poisoning with it have been recorded from time to time. It has been, and still is, extensively used in Great Britain for the purpose of adulterating malt liquors, it being supposed greatly to increase their intoxicating properties, and also to prevent the secondary fermentation.

Cocculus was first introduced into the materia medica, and used as a remedy in the treatment of diseases, by Hahnemann.

He published, in 1805, in the "Fragmenta de Viribus Medicamentorum Positivis,"—the germ of the "Materia Medica Pura,"—156 symptoms of Cocculus, together with a few observations from other authors.

He had already, in an "Essay on a new Principle for ascertaining the Curative Powers of Drugs," published in Hufeland's "Journal of Practical Medicine," in 1796, stated, on the authority of Amatus Lusitanus, some symptoms produced by Cocculus in the healthy subject, and had used this language : "Our successors will find in Cocculus a very powerful medicine when the morbid phenomena it produces shall be more accurately known."

In "Hufeland's Journal," in 1798, Hahnemann published a case of poisoning, occurring in a healthy man, from a single grain of the Cocculus seed. To this we shall recur at a later period, only stating here that Hahnemann relieved the man with Comphor.

In volume one of the "Materia Medica Pura," Hahnemann published a proving of Cocculus in 1811. Some additional symptoms were contributed by Hartlaub and Trinks, in their "Pure Materia Medica," and Hahnemann incorporated these (with three exceptions) into his own proving in the second edition of the first volume of his "Materia Medica Pura," published in 1830. This last publication we shall make the basis of our study.

In the introduction, Hahnemann says that "Cocculus will be found curative where the symptoms correspond, in certain forms of sneaking, insidious, nervous fevers in so-called abdominal cramps; and so-called spasmodic pains of other parts of the body, etc., etc.; in not a few cases of paralysis of the extremities, and in mental affections." From the publication of this proving to the present day, the records of the Homœopathic Clinique have furnished, from time to time, cases in abundance corroborating these statements; and yet, in 1848 (Canstatt's "Jahresbericht," p. 137), Tschudi announces the discovery that Cocculus "acts chiefly on those parts of the nervous system which control muscular action," and has the impudence to claim as original the suggestion to use picrotoxin "in paralysis of the extremities and of the sphincters;" and Reil, acting on this suggestion, employed a tincture of the seeds of Cocculus, with success, in chorea, in hemiplegia from cold, and in paralysis of the bladder from the same cause. ("Materia Medica der reinen Pflanzenstoffe," p. 200.)

Turning now to Hahnemann's proving of Cocculus, in volume one of the second edition of the "Materia Medica Pura," we proceed to make in conformity with a schema for the study of the materia medica published in the "American Homœopathic Review." vol. 3, the following.

SPECIAL ANALYSIS.

Head. Sensorium. Vertigo. Cocculus produces a well-marked vertigo, described as like drunkenness. It occurs when sitting up in bed, is a whirling vertigo, is always accompanied by nausea, which, together with the vertigo, comples a resumption of the recumbent position; -accompanied by a peculiar dullness in the forehead, as if there were a board in front of the head.

In the condition of circumstance this vertigo resembles that of Bryonia (it occurs when sitting up in bed, and comples a recumbent posture).

Intelligence. Dullness; distraction; difficulty in understanding what is heard or read, and in appreciating the lapse of time; the prover sits as if sunk in thought, not regarding what occurs about him.

Memory. Weakened. As a general thing the symptoms of the sensorium are aggravated by any mental effort of any kind.

Headache. Location; chiefly in the forehead and temples; somewhat in the vertex. Pains pass from over the right eye into the head; also, pressing pains extend downward in the whole head; from the temples inward.

Sensation. The chief and controlling sensations are dullness, pressure, compression, constriction; a headache is also described as compounded of the above sensations, together with digging and boring. There are also stitches in the temples, and in the right forntal region. Hahnemann gives a special prominence to the following symptom: "Headache, as if the eyes would be torn out."

Conditions. These sensations, both the dullness and the pains, and particularly the pressing pain in the head and forehead, occur in the forenoon; are very much aggravated by reading and thinking, and particularly by eating and drinking; also by walking.

The muscles of parts of the head are affected in a manner which we shall see to be characteristic of Cocculus. There is cramp-like pain in the left temporal muscle; pain as if the eyes were forcibly closed; convulsive trembling of the head.

Eyes. Lids. Pressing pain, with inability to open the eyes at night. Dryness.

Globe. Stitches from within outward; feeling as if the eyes were torn out.

Special sense. The pupils are contracted. Muscæ volitantes; a black figure seems to float before the eye, moving as the eye moves, Yet without impairing vision. Hahnemann emphasizes the symptom "obscured vision."

In the symptoms of the head we perceive no evidence of organic change. The symptoms are such as accompany gastric disturbances and the dyscratic conditions on which continued fever is supposed to depend. No organic changes seem to be produced in the eye; but the symptoms of the special sense point to commencing amaurosis, a paralytic condition of the optic nerve, similar, perhaps, to that produced by Cocculus in the muscular nerves.

Ears. Attacks of deafness, and of noise in the ears like the rushing of water, attended by deafness.

These symptoms have the same significance as those of the head.

Nose. Increased sensibility to odors.

Face. The pains are confined to the region of the malar bone and the masseter muscles, where they are pressive and benumbing and cramp-like, increased by opening the jaw. Redness of the cheeks and heat in the face, without thirst. Swelling of the sub-maxillary glands. The features are sometimes distorted.

Teeth. The teeth are long and loose.

Mouth. Dryness without thirst. The saliva is frothy.

Taste. Coppery, metallic, sour after eating and coughing; bitter taste on the base of the tongue.

Tongue. Yellow coat upon the tongue. The

tongue seems paralyzed, so that speech is difficult; pain at the base of the tongue when stretching the tongue out.

Throat. Externally. Stiffness of the cervical muscles. Paralytic drawing of the sides of the throat. The muscles seem weak and the head heavy; he must support the head; is most relieved by leaning it back.

Internally. Dryness and roughness, especially when swallowing. Dryness and high in the fauces. Burning in the palate. Sensation of swelling at the root of the tongue. A feeling of constriction in the fauces which impedes respiration. A kind of paralysis, preventing swallowing.

The above symptoms point to on organic changes, but indicate rather a kind of paralysis of isolated groups of muscles, *i.e.,* the sternocleidomastoid, the constrictors of the pharynx, the lingual.

Stomach. In the epigastrium, over the stomach and extending to the hypochondria and into the chest, a pressing, pinching, constricting, cramp-like pain, which takes away the breath; occurs and is worse after eating and drinking; also when walking; is worse from cold; is accompanied by nausea.

Appetite. Loss of appetite; disgust for food, the very smell of which is offensive; at the same time a sensation of hunger at the epigastrium; aversion to acids; bread tastes sour.

Thirst. Aversion to drinking, and yet great thirst.

Nausea. Great nausea is a characteristic symptom of Cocculus. It is provoked by eating, drinking, by motion, by becoming cold, especially by driving in a wagon; by sudden change of posture. It occurs in connection with the headache and the pains in the intestines.

Eructations. Bitter, putrid, causing sore pain in the epigastrium and chest. Incomplete eructation, hiccough and spasmodic yawning.

The attacks of nausea sometimes produce fainting.

Abdomen. Pressure; sticking and cutting pains in various parts of the abdomen, chiefly around the navel. Feeling of emptiness in the abdomen.

Flatus. Rumbling in the abdomen; great distention; incarceration of flatus; severe flatulent colic at night.

Hypogastrium. Constricting pain, with pressure toward the genitals, and qualmishness in the epigastrium. Disposition to inguinal hernia, with pain and soreness. Rupture-pain worse on the right side; fullness in the groin with a sensation as if all would give way there. (Singular and characteristic symptoms.)

Stool. Constipation. Stool followed by violent tenesmus in the rectum, producing faintness, also diarrhœa; small frequent stools, each accompanied by flatus.

Rectum. Disposition to stool, but the peristaltic motion in the upper intestines is wanting.

Anus. Itching.

Urinary Organs. Frequent discharge of watery urine.

Genital Organs. Sore and sticking pains in the testes. Itching of the scrotum. Alternate excitement and depression, the former being probably the primary action. Menses suppressed. Menstruation difficult, attended with violent spasmodic pain in the abdomen and loins, increased by motion cold and contact.

Respiratory Organs. Dyspnœa, as if from constriction of the larynx. Sneezing, coryza disposition to cough, from an irritation high up in the larynx; from constriction of the chest. The cough is increased by indulging the disposition to cough, as is the case with the cough of Ignatia. Fine stitches in various parts of the chest; feeling of emptiness in the chest; palpitation and anxiety.

In the above symptoms no local organic affection is evident. They may all be ascribed to an affection of the spinal marrow or nerves (functional or organic).

Back. Spasmodic constriction through the whole length of the spine, especially on motion.

Sacrum. Paralytic pain extending over the hips, interfering with walking, along with an anxious, apprehensive disposition.

Loins. Paralytic pressure, tearing, drawing as if broken, as if stiff. All these pains are increased by motion and by cold.

Upper Extremities. Paralysis of the hand when writing. Pains in the bones, as if bruised; in the arms, felt on lifting the arms. The arms go to sleep. Hot swelling of the hands.

Lower Extremities. Paralytic immobility, extending from the sacrum. Sore pain of the thigh. Inflammation and swelling of the knee(?). Burning in the fet.

Sleep. Coma. Coma vigil. Absence of sleep from anxiety and bodily restlessness. Anxious dreams.

Fever. No definite typical fever. Constant chilliness, while yet the skin is hot In the evening chills run down the back. Exhausting sweat during motion.

Disposition. Mild, indolent, despondent in the face of difficulties, excessive anxiety, fearfulness; intolerance of noise or any disturbing influence.

GENERAL ANALYSIS.

Vital Power. Cocculus exercises what may be called a purely depressing action upon the vital power. This action is called pure because it is not, so far as we know, dependent upon any change in the organic substance. Thus the sensorium is benumbed, as the marked vertigo and confusion show. Of the special senses, that of vision is so distinctly impaired as to remind one of incipient amaurosis; but the most marked action of this character is exhibited in the voluntary muscular system, paralysis more or less complete being produced in the eyelids and in the muscles of the face, the tongue, the pharynx, and of the extremities, particularly of the lower extremities of this nature, perhaps, are the symptoms of the inguina, resembling hernia.

Organic Substance. While the action upon the vital power is, as has been seen, very marked and definite, that upon the organic substance is scarcely perceptible. The circulation is but little affected. The evacuation is scarcely altered, though, as might be expected from the depression produced in the general vital power, the secretion from the surface of the intestine is diminished. Eruptions are mentioned in the proving, but in so indefinite and isolated a way that we can hardly attach to them any physiological significance.

Sphere of Action. Pre-eminently the system of animal life. The vegetative system is hardly affected at all. The voluntary muscular system first, and then the sensorium, are the primary seats of action. In addition to the above, and not evidently connected with it, must be mentioned the action of Cocculus upon the stomach and digestion. Nausea, extending to the point of vomiting, and accompanied by faintness and by severe vertigo when lifting the head, is a characteristic symptom. The nausea is felt from the epigastrium to the throat. It is accompanied by a sensation of constriction around the waist, is aggravated by eating, drinking, by motion, by mental exertion, and in the open air. The taste is bitter and metallic.

The appetite is completely wanting.

Sensations. A general sensation of lassitude, which makes the least exertion, even standing, very irksome. Syncope often follows any bodily exertion. In the extremities, drawing and digging pains in the bones, but more frequently a weakness as if paralyzed. Sometimes this sensation is accompanied by twitchings of isolated groups of muscles.

Periodicity. Not at all marked in Cocculus.

Peculiarities. The symptoms of Cocculus in general, and particularly those of the head, are aggravated by eating, drinking, any bodily or mental exertion, by tobacco smoke, and by cold air. They are accompanied by a great intolerance of fresh air; in fact, all the functions of animal life seem to be more or less torpid, and intolerant of any stimulus. There is a constant disposition to sleep, and yet the sleep is restless, interrupted by frequent wakings and startings, so that in the morning one is still sleepy. As regards the disposition, the prover seems sunk in deep thought of an unpleasant and rather sad character. Nevertheless he is easily roused to anger.

In many respects Cocculus reminds one of Pulsasilla, which also depresses the vital power, but the symptoms of Pulsatilla are ameliorated by cold and by motion, and the disposition of Pulsatilla is gentle and yielding. In its action upon the digestive organs, Cocculus resembles Nux vomica; the characteristics, particularly the conditions of aggravation, distinguish them. Moreover, Nux vomica affects the vegetative system quite as much as the animal. Cocculus resembles Ignatia somewhat in the almost simultaneous appearance of seemingly incongruous symptoms. It is probable that we shall find a closer analogy to Cocculus in Tobacco than in any other remedy.

APPLICATIONS.

Hahnemann recommends Cocculus in certain kinds of insidious, nervous fevers. In this Hartmann agrees with him, and says: "Particularly in cases which have been produced by frequent fits of anger, or are accompanied by great disposition to anger." Hahnemann recommends it also in several kinds of spasm, as, for example, in menstrual colic, resulting from sudden suppression, or hindered coming on of the menses; in spasmodic flatulent colic. Its chief application, perhaps, is in the treatment of paralysis of the extremities, particularly in hemiplegia. Cocculus has proved a very valuable remedy in sea-sickness; and has cured many persons of a tendency to nausea and faintness from riding in a wagon. Dr. Curie has found Cocculus a valuable remedy, along with Nux vomica and Antimonium crudum, in the various forms of dyspepsia from over eating and drinking, which are common among a certain class of the English people.

The following remarks by Dr. Wurmb ("Clinische Studien," 1, Typhus, p. 124) give a clear picture of that kind of slow nervous fever to which Cocculus is adapted :

After dividing typhus into several groups, in all of which the systems of vegetable and animal life are affected to an equal extent, he says that other cases occur which may be divided into two groups. "In the one, the system of vegetable life is profoundly involved, while the animal life is scarcely at all affected. For this group Veratrum is the chief remedy. In the other, the animal life is pre-eminently involved; vegetation is hardly affected. For this group Cocculus is appropriate." He says : "The patients complain at first of lassitude, prostration after the slightest exertion, difficulty in thinking, loss of memory, loss of appetite, and invincible disposition to sleep. They soon feel so weak that they must keep the bed, and they fall into an apathetic condition, which ends in actual coma. If awakened out of this, they complain of vertigo, of a feeling as if a heavy load were pressing upon the head, of weakness, and a paralyzed feeling in the limbs, but especially in the eyelids, which they can hardly keep open. Sometimes, instead of the paralyzed feeling, there is a sensation of twitching and jerking. The patients think correctly by slowly. They soon fall back into the comatose condition; the expression of countenance is devoid of all signs of mental activity. This condition is not uninterrupted; for there occur sometimes intervals of moderate excitement, during which the patients, awakened from their stupor, look eagerly around, move themselves quickly, and, by the hastiness of their replies, seem to seek to hide their lack of force; sometimes there is mild, uneasy delirium.

"In this torpid condition of the nervous functions the rest of the organism participates but little. The pulse is weaker, it is true, but seldom sinks below the average frequency, often even rises above it. The temperature remains normal or changes but little; the skin is pale but lax; the tongue moderately coated sometimes even clean; the bowels generally constipated, diarrhœa rarely present; the respiratory mucous membrane almost never involved.

"Symptoms of a blood dyscrasia, such as exanthemata, decubitus, hæmorrhages, are never observed. The spleen is always swollen."

Among the applications of Cocculus must not be forgotten its use in inguinal and femoral hernia, of which several cases are recorded as cured by Cocculus; among them one in which four herniæ existed simultaneously. Precisely what cases are curable by Cocculus it is not easily to say *a priori*. Other remedies, as, for example, Nux vomica, Aurum and Nux moschata, have also cured hernia. Until the functional pathology of hernia shall be better understood, it will be impossible to divide the affection into groups corresponding to the different modes of treatment, or different remedies which experience has shown to be useful. While

COCCULUS INDICUS.

the affection is, by most practitioners, regarded as exclusively a mechanical accident, to be met by surgical methods, the history of many cases and experience in their cure, shows them to be amenable to dynamic agencies.

In all of these applications, as in others which may be made of Cocculus to the treatment of diseased conditions, the similarity of the symptoms must be our only sufficient guide.

CONIUM MACULATUM.

SPOTTED HEMLOCK.

UMBELLIFERÆ. It is a native of Europe, but is naturalized in the United States.

The active principle is conia, a yellowish oily-looking transparent fluid, lighter than water, of an acrid, nauseous, tobacco-like taste. In smells like tobacco and mice. It is very volatile, slightly soluble in water,—less so in warm water than in cold water,—readily soluble in alcohol, ether and oils. It is alkaline. Its combinations with acids do not easily crystallize, and are very soluble and poisonous.

It was known in ancient times, but has not until recently been used as an internal medicine. It was a means of killing political offenders. Socrates drank it, and his death is thus described:

"After swallowing the poisoned cup he walked about for a short time, as directed by his executioner; when he felt a heaviness in this limbs he lay down on his back; his legs and feet first lost their sensibility and became stiff and cold; and this state gradually extended upward to the heart, when he died convulsed." This is the brief account given by Paul of Ægeria. Xenophon relates that he continued to talk with his friends and disciples both while he walked and after he lay down. This gives us evidence that his mind retained its normal condition after the limbs had refused to fulfill their functions.

Conium that grows in southern latitudes is thought to be more powerful than that which grows in northern climates. It should not be subjected to heat, because the active principle is volatile; hence the extract is often inert. The most active preparation is the juice, succus conii; and this is almost identical with the homœopathic tincture.

Conium was recommended by the ancients as an anodyne for pains, and as useful in erysipelas and in phagedenic ulcers. Dioscorides recommended the bruised plant to be applied upon the genitals to remedy nocturnal pollutions, and upon the breasts of girls to prevent their development. Pliny and Avicenna recommended poultices of Conium and corn-plaster to remove tumors of the breasts and testes, and to repress the secretion of milk.

In modern times it has been applied for the same purposes; and at one time it gained a high though undeserved reputation for the cure of cancer.

It is remarkable that while this substance, or its active principle, is one of the most active and rapid poisons, yet some animals, as the goat, sheep and horse, eat the plant with impunity.

The following case of poisoning from eating a Conium salad illustrates its action in large doses: "In this man was first noticed weakness of the legs, so that his gait was staggering. As the weakness increased, he tottered as if drunk; and his arms began to be similarly affected. Loss of all voluntary motion followed, and he was unable to swallow. Lastly, the muscles of respiration were affected slowly by paralysis, and he died of asphyxia. Up to the time of death his intelligence was unimpaired, but his sight was destroyed though his hearing remained. There was no recided spasmodic affection of the muscles."

Gradual paralysis, then, of the voluntary muscles seems to be effect of Conium; first the lower, then the upper extremities, then the muscles of the trunk, and finally those of respiration. Let us inquire, How is this paralysis produced? It may be by affections of the muscles themselves, or of the brain and cord, the centres of action, or of the nerves, the conveyors of stimulus to act. Is it due to changes produced in the muscles by Conium? Probably not, because muscles taken from an animal completely paralyzed by Conium act energetically under a galvanic current, and do not act when the current is passed through the nerves supplying the muscles; but only when the current is passed through the muscular substance itself.

It cannot be that the spinal cord is affected, because if the artery and vein of one limb be ligatured, and the animal then paralyzed by Conium, the limb thus protected is moved energetically, as in health. Neither can its action be on the brain, because in this case the poisoned blood passed as freely to the brain as to the cord ; nor was intelligence impaired. It must, then, affect the motor and the periphery sooner than they trunk of the never.

The sensory nerves do not appear to be affected.

Dr. John Harley, of London, has recently published a work containing proving upon the healthy subject, of Conium and some other drugs. He says :

"The first effect of Conium is a depression of the mother function; and its last is the complete obliteration of all muscular motion derived from the cerebro-spinal-motor tract.

"After taking 3iij of the succus conii, I set out walking, and three-quarters of an hour after the does I felt a heavy, clogging sensation in my heels, a distinct impairment of the motor power. I felt that the go was taken out of me Vision was good for fixed objects, but accommodation was sluggish. Continued exertion removed these symptoms. the mind was not affected."

Dr. Harley sums up the action of Conium as follows: "It exerts its power chiefly, if not exclusively, upon the motor centres within the cranium; and of these the corpora striata are the parts chiefly affected. The sensory part of the nervous system is not affected." From this view of the physiological action of Conium Dr. Harley concludes that "in selecting Conium as a remedy for nervous diseases we must be guided by that simple view of its physiological action which is stated above, and we must ask 'is there irritation direct or reflex of the motor centres?' If so, we hope for good from Conium."

Harley, therefore, recommends Conium in convulsions, chorea and muscular tremor, in pertussis, and spasm of the œsophagus and stomach, in spasm of the glottis; in paraplegia and concussion of the spine; in exhaustion of the sexual organs; also in ophthalmia, especially the strumous variety, which he ascribes to spasm of the orbicularis and corrugator supercilii. He regards it as a palliative in cancer, in that it allays muscular spasm, and thus mitigates pain.

CINA.

THE Wormseed or Tartarian Southernwood, of which the unexpanded flower-heads are used in medicine, is found in Asia Minor, the Levant, Africa and Persia. The flowers have a strong order, and a bitter, camphoraceous taste.

Sensorium. Head. Vertigo, with blackness before the eyes, faintness and staggering, immediately relieved by lying down; occurring on rising from the bed.

Confusion, as a result of headache, as if the whole head were screwed together.

Headache. General. Violent headache, with feeling of general illness; headache the whole day, a tearing pressure which extends also to the zygoma; pressing headache all day; in the evening it occupies the forehead also; headache as if the whole head were screwed together, with confusion; immediately after a meal, dull drawing internal headache, increased by reading and by mental labor; headache alternating with pressing pain in the abdomen.

Special. Forehead. External pain, a pressing

from above downward, as if a weight were gradually sinking down there; benumbing internal headache, especially of the sinciput, but also of the occiput. Externally, a pressing, benumbing pain in the forehead and temples, which finally involves the whole head; pressure upon the frontal bone, and at the same time, internally, an undulation as of waves dashing; pain above, as if the frontal bone were violently compressed from both sides.

Left Forehead. Confusing drawing from the left frontal eminence to the root of the nose. In the left frontal eminence a paralytic tearing, with benumbed sensation in the head, and, immediately afterward the same in the right side.

Temporal Region. Pinching tearing, increased by pressure. Left side: Drawing pressure, like fine tearing, relieved by moving the head. Right side: In the forehead, above the temple, powerful dull stitches, deep in the head, which threaten to benumb one.

Vertical Region. Right side: Numbness in a small spot. Left side: Dull stitches in the brain.

Conditions. The headache is increased by reading and reflection, but relieved by stooping.

Review. The sensorium is indirectly affected by Cina; the vertigo resulting evidently from changes induced in the vegetative system. The vertigo appears to be connected with an anæmic condition, occurring with faintness on rising from the bed, and immediately relieved on lying down. The headache corresponds to the vertigo in its anæmic character, as is seen by the relief which results from stooping, notwithstanding the aggravation from mental exertion and the character of the pains, which would lead one to suspect congestion. Hence Cina corresponds well to that anæmic condition of the brain—the result of depletion, and which is yet so often mistaken for congestion—described by Marshall Hall. The pains in the head are located chiefly in the frontal and temporal regions, as much externally as internally, and point strongly to affection of the cutaneous nerves of sensation distributed to these parts. The pains are pressing, screwed-together pressure from above downward and tearing. Similar pains in the roots of the nose, the eyelids and eye, and in the zygoma and face, point to the efficacy of this remedy in neuralgia.

General. Dull headache, with affection of the eyes.

Orbit. Convulsive motions of the corrugator supercilii.

Eyes. General. Dull headache, with affection of the eyes; dull pain in the eyes on reading and mental labor.

Aspect. A sick appearance around the eyes and in the face.

Lids. Weakness of the upper lids, so that the eyes can scarcely be opened (Dulcamara). Burning and itching in the canthi and margins of the lids, compelling to rub them, with a scanty secretion in the inner canthus in the morning.

Globe. Pressing pain internally in the eyes, generally with dilatation; dryness of the lids and pressing, as if sand were in the eye; pressing pain on reading a little.

Vision. In the evening, when reading by a candle, everything appears as if seen through a veil; relieved for a short time by wiping the eye. On reading, dullness of vision, relieved for a short time by violent rubbing of the eye.

Review. Blue margins around the eye, indicative of abdominal disease. The nerves of the lids, as well as that of the special sense, are evidently involved, weaknss of vision resulting from the latter. A moderate degree of conjunctivitis and blepharitis is also induced, aggravated by using the eye and compelling to rub it frequently. Rubbing removes the dimness for a short time.

Ears. Spasmodic jerkings in the external ear, like earache. Below the mastoid process dull sticking, like a pinching pressure, aggravated by external pressure, as from a blow or shock.

Nose. Boring in the nose blood comes.

Face. Infra orbital region. Dull pressure, excited or aggravated by external pleasure.

Zygomatic Region. Pain, as if both zygomata were seized with a pair of tongs and compressed; aggravated by external pressure. Cramp-like jerkings in the zygoma, a pain which even when gone may be re-induced by external pressure, by which, however, it is induced as continuous pricking or paralytic pain. Periodic twisting, tearing pain in zygoma, wandering from one part to another.

Inferior Maxillary Region. Right side. Dull sticking pain in the ramus, increased by pressure. Left side. Fine stickings as with needles in maxilla, increased by pressure with the hand. Jerking pain in maxilla.

Inferior Maxillary Glands. Pressing pain.

Expression and Aspect. Pale, and livid around the mouth; puffed and bluish face. The child leans its head on one side.

Cervical Region. Paralytic feeling in the nape of the neck. Boring stitches in the right cervical muscles, synchronous with the pulse; relieved by motion of the neck.

Review. A variety of prosopalgia is distinctly represented by Cina. The supra and infra orbital nerves and that portion of the facial nerve which is distributed over the zygoma, are involved in this affection; and it occasionally extends to the inframaxillary region. It differs from that of Graphites in not involving the malar region. The pain is a compression and pressure more or less acute, sometimes as with tongs, and is always increased and frequently re-induced by external pressure.

Toothache, as from soreness. Inhaled air and cold drinks penetrate painfully the teeth.

Mouth. Dryness and roughness of the mouth, and especially of the palate, with qualmishness.

Deglutition. Inability to swallow; drink rolls around audibly in the mouth a long time.

Worms. Lumbricoides are passed from the mouth of a child.

Appetite. Great hunger shortly after a meal. Thirst.

Gastric Symptoms. Eructations. In the morning, before eating, empty eructations. After a meal, eructations tasting of the ingesta, and gulping up of a bitter-sour fluid.

Epigastric Region. Qualmishness, with chill. Nausea; with empty feeling in the head. Frequent hiccough.

After a meal, straight across the epigastric zone, a pinching or cramp-like pressure. A pain which embarrasses respiration. A digging, crowding pain, as if beaten.

Left Side. Dull sticking, increased by external pressure, and diminished by deep inspiration. Pressing pain in the navel.

Umbilical Region. Above the umbilicus, boring pain, relieved by external pressure.

Left Side. Intermitting, fine stitches, like griping, while sitting. Sudden, deep, sharp stitches, especially when inspiring, and at the same time stitches in the inner side of scapula; P. M. Violent pain as if navel were forcibly pressed inward, or had been struck; increased by respiration. Twisting pain increased by pressure. Odious feeling of warmth in abdomen, which became cutting pain.

Abdomen. Hypogastrium. Just over the pubis an internal pulsation.

Flatus. Constant noiseless motion of flatus.

Rectum. On discharge of flatus, violent stitches in rectum.

Urine. Frequent desire to urinate, with copious discharge. Urine is turbid as soon as discharged.

Uterus. Metrorrhagia of a girl ten years old during the use of Cina.

Review A depraved state of the digestive organs is set forth by the few symptoms we have touching the intestinal tract. Dryness of the mouth; affection of the apparatus of deglutition; canine hunger shortly after a meal; qualmish distress at the epigastrium, and winding and sticking pains around the umbilicus, with peculiar sickish pressure in the epigastric zone. These symptoms correspond remarkably to those of helminthiasis, as do also the sickly, pale and livid expression of countenance and the constant disposition to bore in the nostrils.

Nasal Membrane. Left nostril. Burning deep within, as if hæmorrhage would ensue or as if produced by brandy. On the septum, a burning pain as if a scab had been torn away. Worse when touched. Violent sneezing, with bursting sensation in the head and temples, which continues for some time. The same, with bursting feeling in chest, which continues, especially on the right side.

Coryza. Constant pressure of movable tenacious mucus in the nose; discharge of purulent matter; coryza in the forenoon, obstruction in the evening.

Review. No clearly defined inflammatory coryza; but a disposition to ulceration corresponding to that of helminthiasis, and a tendency to hypersecretion of mucus and to formation of pus.

Larynx and Trachea. Sensations: Tickling irritation, rather deep in the trachea, disposing to cough, which is followed by white mucus sputa. The same in trachea under the manubrium of the sternum, with a similar discharge.

Secretion. Dryness. Feeling of dryness posteriorly in the throat; a catarrhal sensation; increase of mucus in the larynx, ejected by voluntary coughing and hawking; mucus hangs in the larynx in the morning on rising, compelling to frequent hawkings, and soon re-appearing again. In the morning, constant production of mucus, compelling to hem and hawk, etc.

Respiration. Difficult, loud respiration; short, rattling (in the throat) respiration.

On walking in the open air, short, rattling respiration, as if much mucus were upon the chest, yet no disposition to cough; very short respirations, with occasional interruptions; child, very short-breathed with loud rattling in the chest.

A kind of constriction of the chest; the sternum seems to lie too close, and respiration is embarrassed; dyspnœa, with anxiety and much sweat.

Sounds of Chest. Rattling in throat and chest; a loud whistling puring, heard only during inspiration.

Cough. Exciting Cause. Deep inspiration; tickling deep in the trachea, and just under the manubrium of the sternum; feeling as of down in the trachea on inspiration.

Character. Violent paroxysms from time to time. Hoarse cough (with disposition to vomit), the paroxysm consisting of but few coughs, and recurring after a considerable pause in the evening. The same in the morning, provoked again by inspiration. In the morning after rising, violent hollow cough toward the upper part of the trachea, by which mucus is slowly loosened. Morning cough, so violent as to bring tears into the eyes. Before coughing, the child suddenly rises up in bed and looks wildly around; the whole body becomes somewhat rigid; she is unconscious, as if an epileptic spasm were coming on, and then cough ensues. After coughing, the child cries out "au! au!" and gurgling downward is heard; she is anxious, bites at the air for breath, and is very pale in the face; the paroxysm lasts two minutes. When coughing, pain in the upper part of the chest under the sternum, and when after a time mucus has been loosened and discharged, sore and burning pain in this part as if something had been torn away.

Chest. Sternal Region. Pain under the sternum, a cramping pain when running; a spasmodic digging, as if the chest would burst.

Painful digging superiorly under the sternum.

Left Side. Sudden, spasmodic, constrictive pain; an outward pressing pain, now in the left chest, now in the loins; the latter as if from much stooping, worse on expiration; pinching pain, increased by every inspiration.

Between the second and third ribs, pinching pain; pinching, sticking pain; pricking, burning, intermitting, fine stitches in the side on one of the true ribs; dull stitches near the sternum, upon the costal cartilage, increased by pressure and by expiration; diminished by inspiration; sudden jerking stickings between fifth and sixth ribs.

Clavicular Region. Near the sternum, under the clavicle, on deep inspiration, two dull, piercing stitches in quick succession; on expiration, nothing is felt; on pressure, very painful.

Right Side. Between the sixth and eighth ribs, jerking sticking pains, not affected by respiration or pressure; in the middle of the right side, under the ribs, a boring, sticking pain, relieved by pressure.

Heart. Palpitation; great anxiety in the præcordia, as if he had suffered some evil in the heart; when walking in the open air.

Review. The symptoms of the respiratory organs indicate a catarrhal affection of a light grade, with nervous excitement, quite disproportioned in its great severity to the former; and not merely local, but involving also the whole cerebrospinal system. Indicative of the catarrhal state, we have accumulation of mucus in the pharynx, larynx and head of the trachea, with loud rattling in the upper part of the trachea and rattling respiration, the catarrh being confined to these organs and the primary bronchi; while the excessive nervous irritability is exhibited in the undue violence of the exertion made to remove this mucus; the cough so violent as to bring tears into the eyes, as to produce pain under the sternum and soreness, and also in the susceptibility to cough on unusually deep respiration, a state of things analogous to that irritability of the cutaneous tissues which induces pain when pressed upon. Hence, probably, the dyspnœa, which is one of the symptoms of Cina, and the feeling of constriction of the chest. The participation of the general nervous system in this over-excitement is shown in the spasmodic affection which precedes a paroxysm of coughing, and which simulates so closely a paroxysm of whooping-cough. This preponderance of the nervous over the local affection indicates the role which Cina plays in whooping-cough and in spasmodic asthma.

The external chest is affected by varieties of dull and fine stitches, generally increased by pressure and by inspiration. So far as defined they resemble intercostal neuralgia.

Back. Lumbar Region. Pain as if beaten, not increased by motion. Paralytic pain. After a meal, sensation as if the loins just above the hips were constricted by a tight band. A sensation of fatigue as from long standing, felt also in the whole spine on bending sidewise or backward.

Spinal Column Generally. Pains and sensations. Tearing, jerking pain; sticking pain, relieved by motion but returning on repose. Even in bed, when lying on the back or side, pain as if broken.

Scapulæ. Right. Tearing, sticking in the upper part of the spine toward right scapula. Pain in scapulæ when they are moved. Sticking pain on external margin.

Extremities. Upper. Drawing, digging, tearing pain in all parts of the extremity, from the top of the shoulder to the hand, not affected by pressure or motion, or if relieved by pressure returning again when the pressure is removed. Paralyzed feeling in the whole arm and hand, it sinks by one's side. Paralyzed feeling, as if the arm, hand and fingers were asleep. Paralyzed feeling through the middle of the arm, one can hardly venture to move the arm; soreness on pressing the affected spot. Contracted sensation like cramp in the forearm and hand, relieved by motion. Little jerking stitches in the hands. Spasmodic contraction of the flexors of the fingers and thumbs.

Extremities. Lower. Hips. Iliac Region. A boring, from within outward, below the glutæi, while sitting, relieved by pressure and motion, but returning again (characteristic in the muscular affections of Cina). Glutæi pain when sitting, as if fatigued thereby. When walking, pain in great trochanter, as from a fall. Spasmodic cramp and drawing tearing in the right thigh, relieved by violent motion. Paralytic pain near the knee.

Stitches near the knee and upon the patella.

Hot flashes, not unpleasant, as from a hot coal near the knee.

Sticking and cutting pain in the toes, as if they were loosed, and in the leg, not relieved by motion. Spasmodic motion of the foot in a child. Clonic spasm of the left limb, followed by paralytic extension of it.

Review. The pains in limbs and back appear to be of a neuralgic nature; and when more pronounced this affection shows itself under the form of paralysis or convulsions, thus corresponding with the spasmodic affection of the larynx and respiratory muscles, and indicating the appropriateness of this remedy in certain forms of chorea. The pains are in general not affected by motion or pressure, or if relieved by pressure return again.

Skin. Burning, fine stitches in various parts of the body, relieved by scratching. Pricking, itching, crawling sensation in various parts of the body, relieved by scratching. Violent itching at night; eruption of red, itching pimples, which quickly disappear. Transparent, miliary eruption.

General Symptoms, involving several parts of the body. Dull stitches here and there, now in limbs, arms, feet and toes; now in the side or back; now in the bones of the nose, but especially on the posterior part of the crest of the ilium (on the hip); dull stitches, sometimes like pinching, pressing or shocks or itching; the spots feel sore and as if beaten when pressed upon.

Spasmodic stitches and tearings in various parts of the muscular system, often only instantaneous, involving also the head and chin.

Convulsions. Convulsive movements of the limbs; paralytic jerkings in various parts of the body, especially in the limbs.

Epileptic convulsions, with consciousness (eclampsia). In the afternoon, an attack of spasmodic extension of the body; then trembling of the whole body, with blue lips and whining complaints of pain in the chest, throat and all the limbs; paralytic pain in arms and legs.

Characteristics. The child is very feeble, lax and ailing; painful sensibility in the limbs of the whole body on motion and touch. The attacks are worse early in the morning and in the evening, and the symptoms are most violent always after eating.

Review. The disposition to that amount of nervous erethism of the nerves, which expresses itself in neuralgic pain, is exhibited in the pains felt in various parts of the body. It is characteristic of these pains that they pass quickly from one part of the body to another, are much aggravated and re-provoked by pressure. The convulsions correspond also to the crethism of the nerves of motion already remarked. In the convulsions thus produced, it is to be remarked that the sensorium does not at all participate, even the epileptic (so-called) convulsions being unattended by unconsciousness.

Sleep. Frequent yawning, as if one had not

slept enough. While sitting, great sleepiness; he must lie down; sleepiness the whole day long; invincible; sleepiness; restlessness at night, frequent tossing and discomfort in every position; sleeplessness; tossing during sleep, with pitiful outcry and complaint of bellyache; awaking with cries, groaning and hiccough, with restless motions; dreams; anxious, tiresome, unpleasant, busy dreams.

Febrile Symptoms. General groups: Fever, vomiting of food, then chilliness over the whole body, followed by heat with great thirst; daily fever at the same hour; chill, followed by heat with great thirst; daily fever at the same hour; chill, followed by heat without thirst; daily fever at the same hour with very short respiration; fever daily, afternoon; several attacks of chill, with thirst and coldness of the hands and feet; followed by heat of the face, which however, is pale, but especially heat of the hands and feet, with cutting pain in the abdomen.

Special Parts of the Paroxysm. Chill. General. Yawning, trembling of the body, with a shuddering sensation; shivering over the upper part of the body toward the head, with horripilation, even by the warm stove; shiverings run over the body, so that one trembles even by the warm stove.

Partial. Coldness of the face with warm hands; cold cheeks; pale, cold face, cold sweat of the forehead; of the forehead and hands; of forehead, nose and hands.

Heat. General. Chill over the whole body, with hot cheeks without thirst; strong fever, with vomiting and diarrhœa; heat in the evening, and during the night.

Partial. Heat, mostly of the head, with yellow complexion and blue rings around the eyes; feeling of heat, and heat with redness of the face; burning heat over the whole face, with red cheeks and thirst for cold drinks; palpitation.

Review. The intermittent of Cina is evidently not of a type to which violent paroxysms belong. The paroxysm is often preceded or attended by vomiting of food or pain in the abdomen. It recurs at the same hour daily. The chill is not very severe, is sometimes partial, and if so, confined to the upper part of the body, and is not relieved by external warmth. It is sometimes attended by thirst, but the relation of thirst to the members of a Cina paroxysm is not well defined. It is sometimes attended by short respiration. The chill is often accompanied by warm hands and by hot, though pale, cheeks (calor mordax?), and by cold sweat of the forehead and nose and hands, either or all. The chill presents more characteristic features than the heat.

Heat. The heat may be general or partial. If general, it is attended by red cheeks and desire for cold drinks, and occurs at night. It is often partial, confined generally to the head; the face being at the same time yellow, with blue rings around the eyes.

Sweat. Beside the cold sweat of the forehead, nose and hands, which accompany the chill, no mention is made of sweat.

We thus see the type of intermittent in the paroxysms is which reaction is very imperfectly established. This accords well with the disposition of Cina to produce a cachexy, the stress of which falls upon the abdominal organs—a cachexy closely resembling probably that of helminthiasis.

Disposition. The child is very whining and peevish and complaining; weeps piteously if one go to handle or lead him. Great earnestness and sensibility; cannot take a joke. Indifference to all impressions. Restlessness. Greediness. Cannot be composed by things at other times agreeable, or by caresses.

GENERAL OBSERVATIONS.

Action on the Vital Power. Cina does not exercise any very strongly marked action on the general vitality. The sensorium is in no special manner directly affected. It is involved secondarily in the anæmic cachexy which Cina produces. Of the special senses that of vision alone is affected, the power of the visual organ being simply reduced in degree. A similar action is exerted upon the voluntary muscular system, paralytic sensations and partial temporary paralysis occuring in the extremities; but this paralysis is not pure and simple, but is complicated with convulsive muscular contractions, the co-ordinating power appearing to be in abeyance, a state of things which at once calls to mind the disease, chorea.

Action on Organic Substances. Of this we know little. That Cina, however, does strikingly impair the nutrition is shown by the yellowish, livid complexion, the paleness about the month, and the blue margins about the orbits; and the locations of these phenomena point to the abdomen and the digestive canal as the primary seat of the organic alterations, whatever these may be. They suggest those which result in the cachexy of helminthiasis.

The sphere of action of Cina is not very extensive. The nerves of sensation, especially about the face and extremities, are affected, as the neuralgias show; those of motion, as the convulsions exhibit; those of special function, in connection with those of sensation and motion, as the convulsive action of the laryngeal and respiratory organs show, together with the hyperæsthesia of the laryngeal mucous membrane. The distress in the epigastric region, the frequent vomiting of food in other affections, pains in the abdomen, and the peculiarities of the intermittent fever paroxysms, chill, with vomiting of food and imperfect reaction, show the influence of Cina upon the abdominal organs.

Peculiarities of Pain. The abnormal sensitiveness of individual nervous filaments is aggravated by external pressure, and the pain generally is so aggravated or reproduced.

Aggravations. The symptoms of Cina are all worse after a meal, at night and early morning.

Periodicity. Marked in the febrile symptoms. The paroxysms of intermittent recur at the same hour every day.

THE ART AND MODE OF PRESCRIBING.

THE spirit of homœopathic practice requiring the administration of a single remedy at a time, there is no room for the compounding of drugs in prescriptions. When it is required to order a dose of any quantity of a remedy from a pharmaceutist, it suffices to inscribe the name of the drug and to add in plain English the form in which it is desired, with the potency and the quantity.

Nevertheless, the venerable antiquity of the art of rightly marshaling drugs in the serried ranks of a complex prescription, demands a passing notice at our hands.

The writing of a prescription involves two things:

1. That we know what drugs we desire to associate together, and in what relative quantities.

2. That we know how to express our desires in the terms of the art.

The first demands scientific knowledge of a high order, embracing a full acquaintance with the chemical and physiological actions and reactions of drugs.

The second requires an acquaintance with the language in which prescriptions are written (generally, but not necessarily, the Latin), and with the symbols of the apothecary.

It is not a matter of indifference what drugs are mixed in a prescription.

Drugs of which the united or joint action might seem desirable, may yet be chemically incompatible in such way that through their mutual action a third and altogether different substance may be formed. This third substance may be simply inelegant and inert, or it may be noxious and poisonous. Of the former we have an example in the following prescription:

℞ Tinct. Ferri chloridi f ℥ss.
Quiniæ sulphatis gr. xx.
Syrupi rosae Gallicae f ℥ijss.
Misce. Signa. Sumat æger cochleae magnum quaque hora in apyrexiam.

By the action of the iron upon the tannic acid of the roses ink is formed and a precipitate occurs. The object of adding the syrup of roses, viz., to give a fine color, is completely frustrated by the addition of the iron. But this is not noxious, though inelegant.

Again, the incompatibility many spring from the tendency of the ingredients of form a noxious product, as in the following effervescent draught, which has twice, in New-York, caused instant death :

℞ Sodæ Bicarbonatis gr. xx.
  Potassii Cyanidi gr. iv.
  Aquæ destillatae f ʒijss.
  Solve.
  Deinde adde—
    Succi limonis recentis f ʒj.
  Misce. et bibat æger, misturâ effervescentre.

In this case the citric acid decomposes the cyanide of potassium, and hydrocyanic acid is formed as the draught is taken. It proves fatal. Again, the incompatibility may come from the ingredients being physiological antidotes, *e.g.*, morphine and strychnine.

℞ Morphiæ acetatis gr. viij.
  Strychniæ sulphatis, gr. ij.
  Panis q. s.
  Fiant pillulæ minimæ quadriginta.

It is probable that these pills might be taken freely without the physiological effect of either of these powerful alkaloids being experienced, because they antidote each other.

It is requisite, therefore, for success, in writing prescriptions, that one know the chemical and physiological properties and relations of drugs.

Again, it has been found by experience that certain combinations of drugs possess properties not known to be possessed by any of the ingredients. The Dover's powder, or pulvis ipecacuanhæ composita is an example of this. Such

knowledge is hit upon by chance, and is a matter of memory. Presupposing the possession of knowledge to select the drugs suitable to be associated in a prescription, the form of composition of the prescription is merely technical. It may be done as well in English as in Latin. The following is an instance of a correct and quite harmless prescription:
Carminative for an infant.

    ℞ Cretæ præparatæ.
        Sacchari albi aa ʒj.
        Acaciæ pulveris ʒij.
        Aquæ cinnamoni f ℥iv.
Misce. Signa. Sumat cochlear parvum bis vel ter die, pro re nata.

As an example, at one and the some time, of the mode of writing prescriptions, and of the padantic and nonsensically stilted language and manner in which simple and familiar beverages are sometimes ordered, let the following serve :
Agreeable refrigerant.

    ℞ Succi limonis recentis f ℥ij.
        Corticis limonis recentis magnopera tenuis ʒss.
        Sacchari albi ℥iv.
        Aquæ Crotonis glacialis O iij.
Misce. Cola. Divide in amicis. Sumat quisque quantum libet.

Or the following:
Haustus stimulans calorifaciens et roborifaciens.

390   THE ART AND MODE OF PRESCRIBING.

    ℞ Spiritus frumenti Borbonica f ℥iv.
     Aquæ bullientis O ij.
     Succi limonis recentis f ℥iss.
     Corticis limonis recentis magnopera tenuis ʒss.
     Sacchari albi ℥iv.
     Infusi theæ sinensis ℥ij.
 Misce. Teneatur mistura calleda.
  Divide in poculis octo. Sumat quisque amicus unum is animum oblectandum.

The whole art of prescribing consists first in knowing exactly what you want to give the patient, and in what doses; and then in writing your directions so clearly and intelligibly that the apothecary may fully understand you.

HOMŒOPATHIC PHARMACY AND POSOLOGY.

The preparation of drugs in the homœopathic pharmacy is simple. We have: 1. Triturations. 2. Tinctures. From each of these forms preparation are made, called, indifferently, *dilutions, attenuations* or *potencies*.

Metals, chemical salts and some dry vegetable substances are prepared by trituration with an inert substance, such as milk sugar, which is especially suitable from the hardness and sharpness of its crystals, and from its non-hygrometric properties.

Vegetable substances that are prepared in the form of *tinctures* may be divided, according, to their mode of preparation, into three classes.

  1. Roots, barks and leaves that are dry. These

THE ART AND MODE OF PRESCRIBING.

are coarsely powdered, and a tincture is prepared by the process of percolation.

2. Plants which contain a large quantity of juice. These are bruised, mixed with an equal weight of alcohol, the mixture kept in a cool, dark place for a day or two, and then subjected to pressure and filtered.

3. Plants which contain but a small quantity of juice are bruised, mixed with double their weight of alcohol, and then treated as class No. 1.

The alcohol and milk sugar used must be carefully purified.

The attenuations, dilutions or potencies (as they are variously called) are prepared by triturating the preparation obtained as above with milk sugar, or by mixing them with alcohol, according to one of two different scales, known as the decimal and centesimal, respectively. Thus, if one grain of metallic gold be triturated with one hundred grains of milk sugar, this forms the first centesimal trituration. A grain of this first trituration, triturated again with one hundred grains of milk sugar, forms the second centesimal trituration; and so on. If with ten grains instead of one hundred, they are the first and second decimal triturations. With alcohol instead of milk sugar they are dilutions or attenuations; all are called potencies.

These attenuations or potencies have been carried to very high numbers. In the way I have described, I know them to have been carried to the two hundredth; of higher, prepared positively in this way, I have no personal knowledge.

PATHOGNOMONIC SYMPTOMS AND CHARACTERISTIC SYMPTOMS.

DR. VEIT MEYER, of Leipsic, in 1850, told me an anecdote of Hahnemann, which, so far as I know, has never appeared in print. It was related to him by Dr. Franz Hartmann, then recently deceased, who in his early days had been a pupil of Hahnemann, and was present at his consultations with patients.

Hartmann relates* that one day a patient came to consult Hahnemann. The malady was condylomata (figwarts). Hahnemann examined them and then questioned the patient for a half-hour, noting symptoms in his record book. He then closed his book, consulted the "Materia Medica" for a few moments, went into the next room, brought out three powders, and said: "Take a powder every three days; come again the fourteenth day, and pay now four dollars." The man paid and retired.

* In this paper (written for delivery before the Onondaga County Homœopathic Medical Society, October 18, 1864), the disease here designated as "condylomata" (figwarts) was spoken of as hæmorrhoidal tumors, and the patient as a female. Its present version is taken from a note-book written by Dr. Dunham, at Leipsic, dated 1856.—[H. E. K. D.]

"What then did you give, Herr Hofrath?" "What!" replied Hahnemann, "have yau listened to the examination and do you not know? You must study the 'Materi Medica'!' So Hartmann said no more, for Hahnemann never told his pupils what remedy he gave, fearing to encourage routine practice. The fourteenth day the patient came again, the warts were but one-third their previous size. Hahnemann gave him two more powders, to be taken every fifth day. "Come again the fifteenth day; this time you pay nothing." Hartmann, surprised at the rapid diminution of the warts, said again, "But, Herr Hofrath, what did you give?" "Do you not yet know? study then 'Materia Medica.'"

The fifteenth day the man returned; no trace of the warts was to be found. Hartmann could not contain himself. He came to Hahnemann's study at an earlier hour than usual and opened his record book to learn the remedy given. It was Chamomilla[30]; three powders. The two on the second day were sugar of milk alone.

More astounded than ever, Hartmann could not contain himself, and when Hahnemann came in; "Herr Hofrath," said he, "I have committed a great crime. The desire to know with what remedy you cured the figwarts so burned within me that I opened your book and ascertained it, and now I pray you, on what grounds did you give Chamomilla?" "Ah, have you done that?" said Hahnemann; "then take the book and read further, read the 'Symptomen-codex' and see if it were possible to give any other remedy than Chamomilla, when such symptoms were present," And so it was. Even Hartmann was satisfied that Chamomilla was the only suitable drug.

And yet the prescription was made without any regard being had to the chief objective symptom, to the very feature which, from a pathological point of view, was the central, pivotal fact of the case. To make such a prescription might seem "like playing 'Hamlet' with the part of Hamlet left out."

A great many most brilliant cures have been made by prescriptions precisely similar to this one of Hahnemann's. Nay, an entire class of case, and, by no means a small one, must be cured in this way, if they are cured at all.

What are generally called organic diseases, well-defined and tolerably far advanced structural modifications of the nobler organs, we can never expect to see produced in any proving. Much less can we look for provings that shall exhibit analogues of the various forms of chronic organic disease, benign or malignant. Occasional accidental provings, in the way of cases of poisoning which come to our knowledge in a medico-legal way, may chance to throw light on these spheres of action of drugs; but these sources of information are infrequent, and always very imperfect and impure.

The science of therapeutics would be forever most imperfect, were we compelled to rely on the knowledge we can gather from such data.

For example, a proving can hardly be expected to be carried so far as to exhibit unequivocal signs of pneumonia. And although some cases of accidental provings in the shape of poisonings have shown us that certain drugs which we know to be curative agents in treating pneumonia do actually produce the organic phenomena of pneumonia, yet this knowledge, while it may confirm our faith in these drugs as proper remedies in cases of pneumonia, to which they correspond, would nevertheless lead us astray and ensnare us if we should allow them to withdraw our attention from other drugs which have not as yet been known to produce the organic signs of pneumonia. If, for example, because it is known that Tartar emetic, Phosphorus, Aconite and Bryonia have produced actual pneumonia, we should allow ourselves to look upon these as the sole remedies for this disease, we should be in danger of neglecting other remedies, such as Lycopodium, Sulphur, Chelidonium, Cepa, and a number of others which, though never known to produce the organic symptoms of pneumonia, have yet shown in practice a power to cure that disease speedily and completely when their general symptoms corresponded to those of the particular case in which they were given.

If this be true of a disease which is, pathologically considered, so simple as pneumonia, how much more likely is it to be the case with regard to affections which depend upon more complex and elaborate changes in the processes of assimilation and nutrition; such as tubercle, cancer, lupus, and many others; or (not to go so far) as the benign affections of the skin and glands, or even as the exanthematous fevers. It is manifest, that while symptoms resembling the general, constitutional symptoms that accompany all of these complaints, may be produced in provings of drugs, yet the organic phenomena which are pathognomonic of the malady, and in the absence of which the disease could not be diagnosticated, cannot be looked for in the pathogenesis of remedies.

But these organic phenomena, these pathognomonic symptoms, for such they are in most cases, are the very ones on which the diagnosis depends. If, therefore, the diagnosis and the prescription are to be worked out by the same method, and are to be made on the basis of the same symptoms or series of symptoms, then an accurate homœopathic prescription would be a rare thing, and in the majority of grave and serious affections, it would be an impossible thing; yet so many successful prescriptions have been made in such cases as to show that it is not impossible, nor indeed always very difficult.

But a prescription is always based upon a correspondence of the symptoms of the drugs with the characteristic symptoms of the case in hand. It follows, therefore, that those symptoms which the prescriber regards as characteristic symptoms, are not at all the same which the diagnostician regards as pathognomonic symptoms; they are not the phenomena from which the malady gets its name, those which depend upon, and indeed constitute, its pathological anatomy.

In the case related by Hartmann, the symptom pathognomonic of the case was the tumor. This was the "pathological anatomy" of the case. By this symptom the case was classified. From this, it takes its name, and this was the symptom of chief importance to the diagnostician.

But the proving of Chamomilla did not contain this symptom. Consequently had Hahnemann regarded this symptom as a characteristic symtom from the point of view of the prescriber, he would not have been able to select Chamomilla as the remedy. He did not so regard it.

The symptoms which he regarded as characteristic of the case, and for which he sought and found in Chamomilla corresponding symptoms, were the general constitutional, for the most part subjective, symptoms,—the symptoms of mind and disposition, and the conditions of time and circumstance, such as aggravation, amelioration, etc.

Cases still further illustrating these facts are to be found in the clinical records. It happens sometimes that cases of disease are cured by drugs that had not, at the time they were so used, been known to produce the pathognomonic symptom of the malady they seem to have cured, whereas subsequent more extensive provings, or accidental observations in cases of poisoning, have shown that these drugs are capable of producing and do produce these organic changes, these pathognomonic objective symptoms.

A considerable number of cases of albuminuria, some of them, no doubt, cases of Bright's disease, have been recorded as cured by various remedies.

Some of these remedies are not yet known to have produced albuminuria in the healthy subject. Others are known to have done so.

One of them, Arsenic, has cured a number of cases. It has almost always been selected because of the correspondence of its general constitutional symptoms with those of the cases in hand. And indeed the correspondence, in this respect, with the general symptoms of Bright's disease, is very striking. I myself once cured with four doses of Arsenic^{200}, a most severe case of post-scarlatinal dropsy, which had already lasted ten days before I was called to it, growing steadily worse until death seemed imminent, and in which the urine in the test-tube became nearly solid on applying heat, the entire quantity of urine passed in twenty-four hours being less than two gills. In this case, of course, the pathognomonic symptom for the diagnostician would have been the albumen, the blood discs, and the casts in the urine (they were all there).

The symptoms which guided my choice in the selection of the remedy were the general symptoms, the character of the pains, their aggravations and ameliorations, the prostration, thirst, temperature, posture, etc., etc., all of which were so characteristic of Arsenic that I could not hesitate a moment. I did not know at that time that although Hahnemann's proving does not contain this pathognomonic symptom, albuminuria, yet this symptom has been produced by Arsenic, together with all other objective signs of Bright's disease, in healthy cats in numerous instances, by Dr. Quazlio of Munich; and again it was observed, with equal minuteness, in two remarkable cases of arsenical poisoning recorded by Dr. Maclayan in 1852. (Editor "Medical and Surgical Journal.")

Phosphorus has been found to produce Bright's disease; Mercury has produced albuminuria. Cantharides have produced objective symptoms corresponding to, at least, the first stage of one form of Bright's disease.

Now if we had a case of. Bright's disease to treat, how should we select a remedy? The fact of the drug having produced albuminuria in the healthy subject is common to these four drugs, and is perhaps true of several others. How should we choose among these drugs? Why, by the general subjective symptoms. But these symptoms alone, without the objective symptom, albuminuria, have already, in a great number of cases, been sufficiently good guides, to enable us to select not merely this group, but the exactly appropriate drug in the group.

Thus it appears that these general constitutional symptoms are not only a sufficient, but they are a more accurate guide, than the objective pathognomonic symptom.

They are also a more comprehensive guide. They enable us to employ, and direct our attention to, remedies that we should not be led to employ if we confined our attention to the pathological anatomy of the disease under treatment.

For example : Apis has cured many cases of albuminuria. The general symptoms of Apis correspond well to some cases of this disease. Yet we find no record of albuminuria in the proving of Apis. Nor is it likely that we shall ever have toxicological data to complete our proving in this respect, because Apis is not a substance likely to be employed as a posion.

It is possible that as Arsenic and Phosphorus and Mercury have accidentally been found to be capable of producing pathologico-anatomical conditions corresponding to those which they have cured, so Chamomilla may have been, or may some day be, found capable of producing hæmorrhoidal tumors. If so, the fact will be interesting; but it will not make it one iota easier to prescribe Chamomilla for hæmorrhoids. For the prescription, if we would have it an exact one, must be based on the correspondence of the general and subjective symptoms, and on the times and conditions of their occurrence and aggravations.

Upon these slightly desultory remarks three propositions might be based.

1. The point of view from which the pathol-

ogist and diagnostician regard a case of disease, and that from which the therapeutist or prescriber regards it, are radically different. And inasmuch as therapeutics, as a science, have hardly received any systematic cultivation, while great and successful attention has been paid to pathology and diagnosis, it has happened that the manner in which disease has been studied, discussed and described by medical authors,—contemplating it rather as a natural phenomenon to. be studied and classified, than as a condition of the individual patient, for which an individual specific is to be found,—has been unfavorable to the purposes of the prescriber, obscuring rather than elucidating those points which are to be his chief guides, and exalting into a position of prominence features which are to him only of subordinate value.

2. The arrangement of materia medica on the basis of a pathologico-anatomical schema, as is desired by some, would be, first, impossible, second, useless, third sure to mislead.

3. It is probable that while to the diagnostician, the pathological anatomy of a case is the fact of prime value; to the prescriber the diathesis, general and special, is that to which he is chiefly to look for his indications.

VALEDICTORY ADDRESS

To the Graduating Class of the New-York Homœopathic Medical College, by Professor CARROLL DUNHAM, M. D., Dean of the Faculty. February 29th, 1872.

Gentlemen of the Graduating Class:

THE immediate object of your patient endeavors is attained. You have completed one stage in that curriculum of medical study which must end only with your lives. The officers of the college formally attest this evening that you have mastered the rudiments of medical knowledge. The faculty, who have directed your labors, and who have witnessed with no ordinary pleasure your faithful industry, now bid you a kindly farewell as pupils, and at the same time extend to you a hearty welcome and fraternal greeting as members of the medical profession.

You are eager to enter upon the life for which you have become fitted by the years of training which close to night; and to-morrow's sun will see you speeding in various directions toward the scenes of your respective future labors. The career upon which you are about to enter is so peculiar in its nature and in the demands which its honorable and successful prosecution will make upon you, that you will bear with me, I am sure, if I ask you to tarry a moment and survey it with me, as lies before you glowing in the morning radiance wherewith the hopefulness of youth ever gilds the future.

Hitherto, you have been encouraged and stimulated in your work by the companionship of fellow-students, and aided and directed by the counsels of preceptors. In your essay in practice, you have felt that older and wiser men were beside you to guard you from error and to supply your deficiencies. But from the present movement, you must depend upon yourselves. You must trust to your own knowledge and resources to meet whatever emergencies may present themselves, with rarely a friend at hand to counsel and encourage, with none to share your responsibilities, however great, unless you resort to a formal consultation, which a young physician sometimes hesitation to do, since it is often, *though wrongly,* regarded by the public as a confession of incapacity.

This isolation in responsibility is peculiarly oppressive. because a physician cannot select his case according to his own estimate of his knowledge and ability. He settles in a neighborhood, offers his services to the inhabitants, and he must take the cases as they come, however trivial or however serious they may chance to be, and do his best. It is not with us as with our cousins of the legal profession, a neophyte in which may decline to grapple with a capital case until he has proved his weapons upon smaller game. And the newly fledged priestling would scarcely aspire to a metropolitan charge, preferring to warble his first tremulous notes, over the brink of a rural pulpit.

But no liberty of choice is available for *you*. Your very first case may be the most difficult you will ever encounter, and, if you be placed in charge, you must meet the difficulties, calling what aid may be within reach; but, aided or not, never flinching from the responsibility so long as the patient demands your services. For the cases which are intrusted to us brook no delay. If the lawyer be not ready for trial, an accommodating judge may grant a postponement. But if you be not ready in a case of cholera or of hæmorrhage with the right expedients, at the right time, the laws of nature move on in their destructive course,— the case is closed against you, and from this judgment there is no appeal.

While your inevitable isolation involves difficulties, it brings also dangerous temptations peculiar to our profession. The advocate conducts his case in open court, subject to the wisdom of the judge and the criticisms of the bar. By them are tested the faithfulness of his work, the thoroughness of his researches, and the soundness of his conclusions. The preacher has always in his flock at least a dozen critics, keen to detect a heresy, prompt to denounce a backsliding, and swift to lay charges before the presbytery or the bishop.

But *you* will be seldom observed by any save the anxious relatives, who believe in your skill but have no means of testing it; who hang in confidence upon your words, but rarely comprehend them; asking only that you bring the loved one back to health, and ready to give you all the credit of the restoration. Or if they be distrustful, they are still almost helpless in their position toward you, inasmuch as they have little or no knowledge to direct them in seeking out or weighing evidence in medical matters. For, although every one in the community knows a little law, and all of us are so instructed in theology that the minutest arrangements and relations of this world and the next are as familiar to us as the affairs of last week, yet the laws of life and health, and the simplest principles of medical science, are as a sealed book to almost the whole non-medical community.

Who, then, shall know it if you err in diagnosis, if you fail to detect disease at the time when it is curable.—if you let the decisive movement glide away without the remedy which it requires? No watchful expert will stand beside you as you sit idly at the bedside while life ebbs away, though *you* might stay the tide; none tarries to note that *you* were at fault when you left your patient for your slumbers, and Death came while you slept. The desolate hearth and the motherless children may be witnesses against you before the judgment-seat of the All-Seeing, calling you to answer for neglected opportunity, for love of ease, for slothfulness of judgment and tardiness of action. But in most instances, if your conscience accuse you not, you go in peace.

Realize, then, how tremendous are the responsibilities involved in your isolation. Cherish the tenderness of your conscience; never allow yourself to disregard its warnings. The more you are withdrawn from observation and criticism, the more you become a law into yourselves. Act always then as under the immediate eye of the Omniscient.

Wherever you live, you will have professional neighbors, who will be, of necessity, your rivals or competitors, and who yet ought, for every reason, to be your friends. For they are those upon whose aid and counsel you would rely in cases of great difficulty or danger, and you should not lightly do any thing to alienate their regard.

As homœopathic practitioners, members of a branch of the medical profession which is still a decided minority, you will find in your neighborhood practitioners outnumbering you as six to one whose relation to you will be, at the best, one of armed neutrality,—or, if the past be any criterion of the future, one of uncompromising hostility; men who will deny you the ordinary courtesies of professional intercourse, who will not heistate to injure you as a practitioner at every turn, and who hold themselves absolved, as toward you, from every obligation of medical ethics,—acting apparently upon the principle that a homœopath has no right which a "regular" is bound to respect.

Demeanor of this kind from members of your own profession, whose interests and aims are one with your own, and from whom your only ground of difference is that you have perceived the advantage of a better way of curing than theirs, will be hard to bear. Remember, however, the provocations they receive. Your medical faith and practice are a direct contradiction of theirs. Whereas they bind upon the people burdens grievous to be borne, your expedients are positively pleasurable to the sick. You parry as with airy nothings the dread reaper's scythe, which their ponderous battle-axe so often fails to beat aside. Every patient who recovers under your gentle ministrations is a public protest against their harsh and damaging procedures.

As regards the conduct of physician toward their colleagues in the various contingencies of professional life, medical associations in this country have framed and adopted codes of medical ethics which define the duty of practitioners toward each other, toward their patients and the public. I commend these codes to your careful study. But I know of no general rule more likely to guide you aright in your dealings both with members of your own school and equally with those of the opposing school, then that which is taken as the basis of the code of ethics adopted by the National and all the State and Country Homœopathic Societies in the United States, and which is no other than that which is the basis of the great Christian code of ethics: "As you would that men should do to you, do ye even so to them." If you add to this golden rule the aphorism also expressed in our code of ethics: "The paramount object of the physician in all that he does should be the greatest good to the patient;" and if you plan your professional life intelligently upon these great principles, you will not often go astray.

Consistently with these principles, you will find our code of ethics somewhat more liberal than those of other schools. Whereas the latter forbid consultations or associations with physicians who adhere to a certain or to any system or "dogma" of medical practice (as though the man who has no coherent system, no faith in any principle, could be a safer practitioner than he who has a system and a reason for his faith), *our* code enjoins upon us to consult with any honorable practitioner of good reputation as a man, no matter to what school he may belong; and this because the patient has the right to enjoy the benefit of whatever knowledge or skill may exist within his reach, and we have no warrant for circumscribing this right by declining the consultation.

Our code forbids the adoption of special creeds, as tests of orthodoxy in medicine, on the ground that our present knowledge is as nothing compared with what remains to be found out, and that creeds as tests of orthodoxy are barriers to progress in knowledge, and are allowable only when we have learned all that is to be known and when progress is merged in possession. These very precepts must make you tolerant of your "old-school" neighbor, though he be intolerant of you. Govern your demeanor toward him by the strictest observance of the golden rule. Never let a word of aspersion, detraction, or unbrotherly reproach escape your lips. Give him full credit for his professional knowledge, and for his achievements. You can afford to wait the verdict of the court of final appeal, the common sense of the people.

Gentlemen, you will encounter sundry little unpleasantnesses at the outset of your career as physicians. Some patient will object to you on the score of your youth,—most unreasonably as it may appear to you, conscious, as you are, that the wisdom of gray hairs reposes underneath your waving locks. But a patient intrust to a physician the present facts of his case and their possible sequences, and he may be pardoned if he feels some hesitation at confiding these to the inexperienced hand of youth. This objection is, however, often urged with unseemly persistence, for it is obvious that the patient need not employ you if he do not choose. A professional friend of mine once lost his temperature when a patient for the twentieth time objected to his youth, and retorted: "Sir, you must have lived your long life to little purpose if you have not learned that there may be *old* fools in the world as well as *young* ones."

You will be apt to find great difficulty in collecting your bills, in proportion to your youth. This seems peculiarly unjust, for the young doctor is usually straitened in means, and has greater need of prompt returns than his seniors. In this, as in many other concerns, you will realize how true is that scriptural axiom which seems to be a statement of what *is* rather than of what *ought* to be: "Unto him that hath, shall be given." When you shall have acquired so large a practice as to have no longer any great pecuniary anxiety, you will find those prompt to pay their bills who, in the early days of your poverty, were very neglectful.

Then, again, in your first years of practice, you will be sorely tried by a want of confidence in your professional skill. In a case of no great real gravity, friends will become alarmed, require a consultation, and ascribe to your older colleague the credit of a cure which you were abundantly competent to effect unaided. Or, what is still more trying, when you have carried a patient safely through a dangerous illness and he is just on the verge of convalescence, a panic may arise in the house, counsel may be demanded, or the case withdrawn from your charge and placed in other hands. You will have the chagrin of feeling that your honest and good work has been unappreciated and your reputation for skill has been damaged.

These trials certainly are difficult to bear, and there may be a deal of injustice involved in them; scarcely so much, however, as you would at first suppose. Remember the golden rule, which is to be your guiding principle, and in imagination put yourself in the place of the public, and then ask whether you would not act much as they do. It is not the way of the world, nor is it a good way, to pay a bill unless vouchers are presented, nor to yield to authority unsupported by credentials. What do you ask of the public when you offer them your professional services? You invite them to confide to your skill the health, comfort,—it may be, the lives,—of themselves and their families; to admit you to their houses on terms more intimate and confidential than those on which any other human being enters; to suffer you to observe their most secret ways, their holiest joys, their hidden sorrows, their carking cares. Can you expect them to do this easily, willingly or unreservedly, until anxious observation of your character and conduct shall have satisfied them that you deserve this confidence?

Win the confidence of the community in which you live, and the little unpleasantnesses which mark your early career will cease to vex you. For if one should object to your youth, a dozen zealous clients will reply, "It is an old head on young shoulders;" and will tell of the great men of history who have reached the acme of their fame before their heads were gray. If your bills are called exorbitant, another will remark, "Capacity and devotion are cheap at any price." Of, if a patient's friends speak of a consultation, or of placing the case in other hands, they will hear, "I would sooner trust one good head than a half dozen divided minds;" or the more homely aphorism, "It is not wise to swap horses while crossing a stream." Your first business, then, must be to win the confidence of the community in which you seek your practice.

But you will say to me, is not this unfair? for have you not just said, the public are not competent to judge of professional skill, and often through ignorance discharge a physician who is on the verge of a great success? This is so; and if there were no other means of winning confidence than by the methods of strictly medical and surgical procedure, you might well despair of being rightly estimated. But, though the public are not competent judges of your prescriptions, they are in the main very good judges of your qualities and acquirements in certain other matters which are almost as important to your success in the care of the sick.

To these, I wish to call your attention in the few moments which remain to me. I assume that you will be unceasing in your labors to master your profession, to keep fully acquainted with all that is achieved by its many workers in various lands, and to add something yourselves to the common store of knowledge. Your clients can witness your industry, though they cannot measure the results. They will closely watch your doings to note whether you faithfully devote yourself to those who seek your aid. Among your first patients will surely be many poor persons, who seek the new doctor, hoping, perhaps, to be treated at less cost. There will be many chronic cases who, having despaired of help at the hands of the old doctors, catch at the straw of a new man's coming. It is not so pleasant to take care of the poor as of the rich. Their houses are cold and untidy, the atmosphere is unsavory and the patients are uncouth. Now, if you undertake these cases at all, you are bound to bestow upon them the same unwearied attention and faithful study and tender care that you would give your wealthiest patient. Their health and lives are as precious to them as ours to us. You have no right to set a lower value upon them. If you assure the responsibility of the cases, you must fulfill the obligation. This is your duty; and I dislike to adduce any other and less elevated consideration. It is, however, a fact that nothing will more surely introduce you to the most desirable and lucrative practice than a faithful, honest and successful treatment of the poor. For every pauper knocks and takes alms at the gate of a dozen of the benevolent rich; and the greatful commendations of the penniless widow whom you have freed from pain, will reach the heart of those whose good word is a passport to success. As you advance in years and in knowledge of the world, few things will surprise you more than the intimate relations which exist among all classes of society. No act of yours, praiseworthy or blamable, can remain hidden. Even in this world, your good or evil deeds will find you out. From the very beginning, then, let every case be treated with your utmost skill and with untiring fidelity.

You will further win the confidence of your patients and of the community by showing that you understand not only how to treat the diseases and injuries of the sick, but that you understand the nature of that which is the subject of your ministrations, the body and mind of man. Recollect that, while you are studying your patient, you are yourself the object of study, and frequently by persons accustomed to observe keenly and weigh the characters of men; and demean yourselves accordingly.

You will succeed in this just in proportion as you possess and cultivate what is called *tact,* which may be defined as the power of adapting your speech and behavior to the mind and circumstances of those with whom you are dealing. It is an every-day affair to you to be called to a patient; but to each patient the calling a doctor is a mementous matter, and the sickness which requires it is a thing of prime consideration. Act, then, as though the case were equally important in your mind, and give it your undivided attention. Let neither word nor action show that your thoughts wander from the patient in whose behalf you you are called. Give ample time for a full understanding of the case, bearing with your patient's prolixity of statement if it amount even to garrulity, and withdrawing as soon as your directions are given and clearly understood. For, however welcome you are as the bringer of relief, when that has been accomplished, your presence can be only a restraint. Even if friends, or attendants, or the patient himself would fain beguile you into general conversation, break it up as soon as you can courteously do so. You impair your usefulness as a physician by establishing any other relations with the patient, at least during his illness.

Do not regale your clients with the incidents and experience of your European tour, or the sufferings of your cousin who was in the war; with the performances of your new microscope, or the wonderful acquirements of your children. However polite may be your patient, she will surely give a sigh of relief as you go, and will dread the next visit. Never introduce into conversation with your patient, or in his presence, subjects connected with politics or theology, nor allow yourself to be drawn into such discussions in the sick-room. On these subjects people differ widely and feel deeply. Your professional duties will bring you into contact with patients of all parties and sects, and you should be equally acceptable to all. Do not misunderstand me. As no man is more contemptible than he who, to gain business, is non-commital in matters of principle, if your opinions be squarely asked for, state them without passion, but so explicitly that there can be no mistake. If, when led to the subject, you can, by an effective word, kindle in your patient's soul the love of country, of liberty, of justice, you will have done your duty as a citizen, and not exceeded your privileges as a physician. And it may be your good fortune to sustain, by a word of encouragement in the hour of extremity, the Christian's hope and faith; but if you have seen many of differing creeds meet death, you will hardly venture to obtrude the halting dogmas of theology between the flitting soul and its expectant Maker.

Never talk about your patients to anybody, least of all to other patients. Even when narrating a case to a professional brother, conceal the name and identity of the patient. No fault is so inexcusable and so offensive as neglect of this duty of silence. There is sometimes a great temptation to cite to a patient the case of another, as an illustration or a warning, to enforce our precepts, or perhaps to give proof of our skill and penetration in diagnosis or treatment. But see what comes of it. No sooner have you left the house than our patient says, "What a shocking case is that of Mrs. B! How badly would she feel if she knew that we know it! But if Dr. S. talks so freely of her case, what, think you, will he say of me and my case? I think, my dear, I cannot have Dr. S. any more. Let us send for Dr. Blank." So you are dropped from this family, and wonder that they can have failed to appreciate your skill; when in truth they think very highly of your skill, but deplore your carelessness of speech, which is the only reason of their ceasing to employ you.

You who are fresh from your studies of anatomy know that the outer ear of ordinary men is a blind tube, through which the waves of sound flow in and impinge upon the tympanum; but the ear of the doctor should always have an extra tube, leading from the tympanum to a bottomless pit of forgetfullness.

If you would do for your patient the best that could be done, you must study his nature, the effect of his occupation upon mind and body, his particular relations public and private. The diversions, often more valuable than medicine, which you recommend to the student worn with plodding among his books, must be very different from those which you advise for the statesman or the merchant, weary of the concourse of men and the rush of affairs. In every case, you must appreciate the immediate circumstances of the patient. Whereas, at a time of case and quiet in business circles, you would keep your patient at home in bed; if there is a panic abroad, it might be the highest wisdom to take the risk of encouraging him to go to business, for to remain at home hourly expecting tidings of his failure might drive him mad. Your greatest skill will often be displayed in a judicious balancing of risks.

Again, it will tax your insight into human nature to come at the remote causes of the disease which you are called to treat. You may wonder why a mother has not long ago been cured of an ailment apparently so amenable to treatment. You will understand it when you learn how heavy a heart she bears for the wildness of her eldest son. The pallid face and drooping form of the maiden is due, of course, to impoverished blood. You may wonder that the iron she has taken has not brought back the roses to her cheek. They will bloom again with a glory that will gladden your heart if, perceiving the remote cause of her disease, you can induce her parents to withdraw their opposition to the suitor who has won her heart.

You may suppose that you have done with the dry bones now that you have left the dissecting room. But, gentlemen, the proverb teaches us that "there is a skeleton in every house," and the skeletons in your patients' houses will often intrude themselves between you and your cure, and must be the subject of your anxious study if you would do all the good you may in your profession; for whatever in the occupations, relations or circumstances of your patients may in any way affect their health or perpetuate their maladies, becomes a legitimate object of your investigations.

And if, comprehending these things, you, in perfect honour and respect for your patients, with "saving common sense," advise them wisely, you will command their confidence and fasten them to you as "with hooks of steel."

Such are some of the difficulties, duties and obligations of the profession which you have chosen.

Need I tell you of its glories and its pleasures?

The subject of your life-long study will be,—not fabrics, nor wares, nor stocks, the works or machinations of men, but the noblest of God's creation,—that which he made in His own image,—the body and mind of man.

And your labors will consist not in strife of wits with your fellows, wherein he who is worsted gets hurt; nor in bargainings, wherein, too often, the gain of one is the other's loss; but in the endeavour so to comprehend and put in operation the forces of nature that, under your guidance, the higher may be set in conservative opposition to the lower and destructive forces.

It is not possible to conceive of a purer and keener pleasure than attends success in this endeavor.

May you enjoy it in full measure!

And at the close of long and busy careers, may you have the pleasant consciousness, not only that you have made some permanent additions to the common stock of knowledge for the common good, but also that many men and women have been the happier for your lives.

INDEX.

	Page.	Vol.
ACONITUM	66	I.
ALLIUM CEPA	105	II.
ALOES	366	I.
ANAMNESIS, THE	49	II.
APIS	333	II.
ARSENICUM	178	II.
ART AND MODE OF PRESCRIBING, THE	386	II.
BELLADONNA	213	I.
BRYONIA	89	I.
CALCAREA CARBONICA	307	II.
CARBO ANIMALIS	332	II.
CARBO VEGETABILIS	325	II.
CAUSTICUM	317	II.
CHAMOMILLA	108	II.
CINA	367	II.
COCCULUS	346	II.
COLCHICUM	157	I.
COLOCYNTH	231	II.
CONIUM	362	II.
CYCLAMEN	80	II.
DULCAMARA	287	II.
EUPATORIUM	115	I.

	Page.	Vol.
EUPHRASIA	98	II.
GRAPHITES	393	I.
HELLEBORUS	311	I.
HEPAR	280	II.
HYDRARGYRUM	208	II.
HYOSCYMUS	278	I.
IGNATIA	122	II.
KALMIA	187	I.
KREASOTUM	164	II.
LACHESIS	401	I.
LACHESIS	243	II.
LEDUM	173	I.
LYCOPODIUM	256	II.
MATERIA MEDICA AND THERAPEUTICS .	1	I.
MEMOIR OF THE AUTHOR	vii	I.
MILLEFOLIUM	177	II.
MUREX	158	II.
NATRUM MURIATICUM	266	II.
NITRIC ACID	320	II.
NUX VOMICA	349	I.
OPIUM	301	I.
PATHOGNOMONIC SYMPTOMPS AND CHARACTERISTIC SYMPTOMS. .	392	II.
PHOSPHORUS	338	II.
PLATINA	129	II.
PODOPHYLLUM	239	II.
PREFACE	v	I.
PRELIMINARY OBSERVATIONS . . .	61	I.
PRINCIPLES OF HOMŒOPATHY . . .	1	II.
PULSATILLA	57	II.

	Page.	Vol
Rhododendron	182	I.
Rhus	121	I.
Sabina	175	II.
Secale	169	II.
Sepia	138	II.
Silicea	316	I.
Spigelia	196	I.
Stramonium	288	I.
Study of Materia Medica	19	I.
Sulphur	381	I.
Symptoms, their Study; or How to Take the Case.	25	II.
Therapeutic Law, The	39	I.
Valedictory Address	402	II.
Veratrum	272	II.

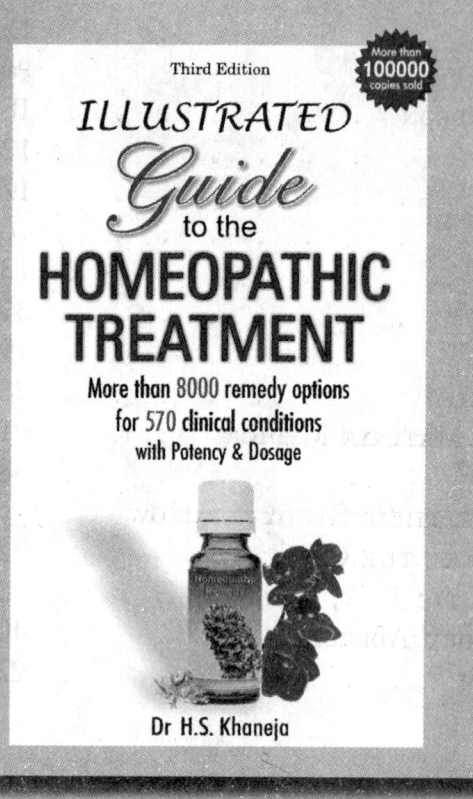

Illustrated Guide to the Homeopathic Treatment

Dr HS Khaneja

- Includes author's commentary as well as views of stalwarts like J. T. Kent and H. A. Roberts to give a wider perspective of each topic
- An Intern's tool on the subject
- Contains knowledge about medicines, diseases, their causes and their prevention
- Methods of surgery and comparisons of the conventional treatment with the homoeopathic treatment are given
- New chapters on Adultery, Adrenalitis, Athelete's foot, Autism, Chlorosis, Pelvic Floor Prolapse and Vulvodynia have been added

ISBN: 978-81-319-0164-9 | 776pp | PB